T0138296

HEALING POWERS

MORALITY AND SOCIETY

A Series Edited by Alan Wolfe

Fred M. Frohock

HEALING
POWERS

Alternative Medicine,
Spiritual Communities,
and the State

THE UNIVERSITY OF CHICAGO PRESS
Chicago & London

Fred M. Frohock, professor of Political Science at Syracuse University, is the author of *Special Care: Medical Decisions at the Beginning of Life*, also published by the University of Chicago Press.

The University of Chicago Press, Chicago 60637
The University of Chicago Press, Ltd., London
© 1992 by The University of Chicago
All rights reserved. Published 1992
Printed in the United States of America
01 00 99 98 97 96 95 94 93 92   5 4 3 2 1

ISBN (cloth): 0-226-26584-6

Library of Congress Cataloging-in-Publication Data

Frohock, Fred M.
    Healing powers : alternative medicine, spiritual communities, and
the state / Fred M. Frohock.
        p.   cm. — (Morality and society)
    Includes bibliographical references and index.
    ISBN 0-226-26584-6 (cloth : alk. paper)
    1. Alternative medicine.   2. Alternative medicine—Social aspects.
3. Medicine, State.   I. Title.   II. Series.
    [DNLM: 1. Alternative Medicine.   2. Holistic Health.   3. Mental
Healing.   4. Religion and medicine.   5. Sociology, Medical.   WB 885
F928h]
R733.F79   1992
362.1'042—dc20
DNLM/DLC
for Library of Congress   91-36941
                                                                     CIP

♾ The paper used in this publication meets the minimum requirements of the American National Standard for Information Sciences—Permanence of Paper for Printed Library Materials, ANSI Z39.48-1984.

CONTENTS

Healing Powers is a book about a single issue: whether unorthodox beliefs on health and healing ought to be shielded from state regulation when (a) life is at stake and (b) the competence of individuals to select therapies cannot be demonstrated successfully. The negotiation of this issue takes the author (and readers) on an expedition of sorts, a narrative journey that explores a variety of claims for extraordinary healings along the way and also examines the lives of those who engage in healing practices. The aim is to reconstruct, to *enter* the spiritual life that is at the center of so many unorthodox healing beliefs, and in particular to examine two claims found in all spiritual communities: that humans have access to alternative realities and that these realities have healing powers. At the end the book returns to the problems of regulation and political power that occur when different beliefs about reality compete in a liberal political society.

The methodology of the work is drawn from a variety of disciplines and orientations. The least controversial, meaning the most conventional, is the examination of material in the standard prose sections. These sections include overviews of the history of medicine and selected religious traditions, medical practices and norms, mind-body problems, rationality across radically different beliefs, spiritual and secular discourses, and the vocabularies of governance that help define liberalism. A second set of methods, still within conventional boundaries, produces the biographical studies of individuals engaged in healing practices. These sections are reconstructions of material obtained in taped ethnographic interviews. Selections from the tapes are introduced at various points in the work to emphasize some idea or story, or to shift the flow of the work in a different direction.

The unconventional research methods, those that make one wonder whether the writer is a fit intellectual companion, are the use of fictional techniques and a guiding fictional voice ("Luke"). The fictional techniques reproduce narratives related by the subjects in the interviews; they do not create fiction as such (as in novels, poetry). My aim in using these techniques is to provide access to interior or subjective levels of experience that linear texts cannot. The Luke voice is wholly imaginative, not anchored in the research data gathered for this study. But even here the text is used to present views on human identity, not simply to tell stories, and includes references to the appropriate philosophical literatures. Igor Stravinsky once said that music is too important to be just beautiful. The conviction driving these latter texts is that literature is too important to be just fine writing. It must be, and is here, at the service of philosophy and social inquiry.

I hope I am not giving away too much when I say that the book is also designed to be self-reflecting. It comments on itself at various points, an exercise made possible by the use of different methods in producing rival texts. The competition among texts intensifies in the final chapter as objective and subjective, secular and spiritual, are brought into sharper contrast. The use of narratives is also exploited more fully at this stage by introducing a variety of stories at different levels, with Plato's allegory of the cave competing with set pieces and street narratives. The fragmentary deployment of texts in this last chapter heightens in particular the competition between narrative and linear approaches in the study.

The goals of this study are easy to state, although they become more complex as they are pursued with different methods in the work. At the simplest level, the book is a study of liberal dilemmas that occur when incompatible ontologies enter public space. But this immediately leads to a second goal: understanding the beliefs that produce the dilemmas. So the work is also an exercise in "extended sympathy," an effort to present beliefs in the way that those who hold the beliefs understand them. This second goal is complicated by the logic of spiritual beliefs, which often rely on nonlinear modes of exposition. The goal of extended sympathy then even more strongly requires techniques that can introduce subjective perspectives that may not fit objective frames comfortably. These techniques include both biography and fiction.

A third goal is normative. One part of this goal is to suggest practical solutions to the legal and political dilemmas addressed in the work. These solutions follow closely the presentation of different beliefs about reality. They are influenced by the need to forge rationalities that cut across at least partially incommensurate beliefs. The other part of the goal is to point out the failure of liberal principles to negotiate the problems of incommensurability successfully. Liberalism, at least in its classical incarnations, is not a suitable political philosophy to resolve or even manage disagreements over the meaning of human experience at the levels sometimes found in spiritual-secular disputes. Finally, the work aims to display a set of methods not typically employed simultaneously, and to invite discussion of their logics and effectiveness in studies of human experiences.

I am indebted to a number of places and individuals in completing this work. Three cities I love deeply figured strongly in the project. I wrote the first words in the book when the Luke voice started talking to me in London during the summer of 1988. I know there are people who will scoff at that sentence and the possibility that a voice can talk inside the head of a writer, providing him with words and sentences that he records on paper. But I am not interested in pursuing an argument along these lines. It simply happens, as many writers will tell you in trusting moments. I also wrote the final revisions on the book in London during the summer of 1991, received word while still in the city from Doug Mitchell, my editor, that the book had been accepted by Chicago for publication, and signed the contract there before returning to Syracuse.

The second city is Madrid. I returned there (after being away far too long) to teach in the Syracuse program during the spring semester of 1990. My younger daughter, Christina, then a philosophy major at the University of North Carolina at Chapel Hill, joined me in the city for that memorable spring. Since even at that time she was moving with frightening speed beyond my abilities in things philosophical, having her around in class and living with me provided fine opportunities to discuss the material with her. (She is used to this. My daughters' bedtimes stories as children included Theseus's ship, the Cretan paradox, and Lewis Carroll's puzzles. Why use ordinary childhood tales when philosophy is so much more dramatic?) But Christina's nocturnal social life was even more decisive. Madrid comes alive after midnight, and Christina and her friends were often out late, sometimes until dawn. I never have been able to sleep when my daughters are out. A good deal of the book was written on those nights while I waited up. *Now* I am grateful.

The third is New York City. My older daughter Renée was in law school at Fordham during the research and writing stages of this work. I will always remember those conversations she and I would have after I had spent a long day in the city doing research on psychic healing. Over dinner I would describe the literatures and interviews (without breaking confidentiality rules), and she would listen quietly before destroying the more extravagant claims with her lovely critical and skeptical intellect. Renée, more than anyone else, helped me to reenter my own worlds after I had immersed myself in spiritual communities.

Among the many individuals who assisted me in the research, three were unusually helpful. Catherine Bodnar searched medical literatures and routinely found the right pieces early on for me to read. Greg Reef's assistance was crucial in the middle and final stages of this project, especially when I was trying to continue the work while in Madrid during the spring of 1990 (an effort that gives fresh meaning to the old phrase "action at a distance"). My main research debt is to Robert Daly, a friend and colleague who has taught me more about medical ethics than I sometimes recognize. He read several versions of the manuscript on various occasions and made many helpful comments on both style and substance. Pat Miller read a very early draft of the work and, in addition to comments, directed me to relevant literatures for chapter 5. I am also grateful to the many undergraduate students in the two classes I taught on bioethics when I was working through these ideas and using some of the draft material as required reading. There is nothing like teaching undergraduates to force clarity of thinking. I hope some of this clarity has found its way into the book. I am also pleased to record my debt to the graduate students in my fall 1990 seminar on rationality. The course provided a forum for discussions of reasoning in various discourse communities and translation across radically different systems of belief. Unfortunately, these areas remain as complex and intractable as ever, which is why they are appropriate topics for graduate seminars.

I offer a general and profound thanks to the individuals interviewed for this book. The stories and points of view they shared with me in these sessions were vital in helping me to understand the depth of the moral and legal dilemmas sometimes occasioned by competing beliefs on healing. I also extend my thanks and apologies to the staff in the political science department at Syracuse University, whom I drove crazy on a few occasions while pushing myself and everyone around me to get the material out in tangible form. The staff in our London center were helpful at a crucial time in producing the final version of the manuscript. I also acknowledge Random House's permission to reprint the section from Gabriel García Márquez's novel, *Love in the Time of Cholera*, found on page 61. Finally, my gratitude to my wife, Val, who continues to live with me and love me even when the writing dominates the very center of my life. Only someone who has tried living with a writer could appreciate what that means, to her and to me.

London, June 1991

INTRODUCTION

The healing arts are both ancient and modern. They are found in some form in all human societies, and only humans practice them. Many animals seek and eat substances with curative powers, but human animals consciously medicate themselves with an understanding of illness and the possibility of cure.

Illness can be simple or complex. Everyone is familiar with sickness that can overwhelm the self, seeming to inhabit both body and mind. But sometimes illness requires a separation between self and symptoms, self and condition of the self. One can have certain experiences—fainting, say, or visual disturbances—that can indicate an illness one may come to know only by inference from the symptomatic experiences. Hobbes reminds us that our reflective powers force us to entertain the terrifying prospect of death and the end of consciousness. No less disturbing must be the knowledge that one can be ill, gravely ill, and not know this directly. How welcome is the possibility of cure for creatures who can both feel and know, and sometimes only suspect, their own illnesses. One does not know whether to envy or pity the other animals who do not share in such vivid thoughts.

Healing occurs originally in religious practices. Among the more impressive powers claimed by priests past and present is the ability to cure illnesses and restore health. More recent traditions separate religion and medical therapy. Citizens of most industrial societies seek help for illness in a hospital or a doctor's office rather than a church or a synagogue. Secular practitioners have even appropriated the health of the mind. Psychotherapy of one type or another is currently the dominant approach to mental problems in the Western world. It is a robust industry. A study conducted by the National Institute of Mental Health in the early 1980s found that 16 to 25

1

percent of all adult visits to a doctor in the United States were for treatment of mental disorders. Some of the most popular television shows and newspaper columns offer standard medical advice for securing and holding onto mental health.

Yet the separation between religion and the healing arts is not complete. The spiritual flourishes in the popular imagination as a source for healing. Beliefs in spiritual possibilities are widespread. A recent Gallup poll revealed that 50 percent of the American population believes in angels, 46 percent believes in ESP, and 37 percent believes in devils. The poll reports that college graduates believe in clairvoyance in greater numbers than those who do not go to college at all (27 to 15 percent). Horoscopes remain important features of newspapers and magazines. Astrologers continue to draw distinguished clientele. Many of these beliefs and services accept the reality of spiritual effects on health. The resulting practices are often institutionalized in healing ministries found within numerous religions and cults, including both traditional religions and evangelical faith healers following roughly in even longer traditions of folk miracles divinely inspired. Even the materialistic celebration of mental health as a condition for physical fitness inspires an attention to the spiritual dimensions of life.

The Catholic practice of combining spiritual renewal with physical and mental healing is typical of orthodox Christian traditions of religious healing. The beginnings of Christianity are filled with talk of miracle cures that sometimes include resurrection from the dead. Almost one-fifth of the Gospel texts describe the healings of Christ and discussions of these events. These healings often began with the Jewish tradition of anointing individuals (and objects) with oil to consecrate them. Then the individual was cleansed of a disease and/or evil spirit through prayer. After the ninth century, these practices were codified into a sacrament for the dying instead of a healing ritual ("Extreme Unction"). From the Council of Trent in the sixteenth century until the Second Vatican Council in the 1960s, the practice slowly returned to its original aim of restoring health. The more recent formal expression of the Church, passed in the Second Vatican Council, renamed the sacrament "Anointing of the Sick" and redefined the practice as an effort to comfort and heal those who are ill. In addition, the Catholic Church tolerates and even encourages healing ministries whose purpose is to continue the early traditions of faith healing through prayer and the laying on of hands.

One characteristic shared by all mainstream Christian traditions of healing is the acceptance of modern medical treatment as a complement to faith. This acceptance is not found in some of the evangelical movements.

The Pentecostal and charismatic movements, which emphasize the Holy Spirit and the supernatural in general, conduct healing sessions where prayer and divine intervention are deemed sufficient to cure a wide variety of illnesses. Standard medical therapy is sometimes not seriously entertained and on occasion is viewed as hostile to the spiritual renewal that is seen as vital to health. Often the petitioners who seek cures have exhausted standard medical remedies, or just prefer to experience what they believe is a supernatural intervention, a personal and often highly emotional contact with the healing powers of Jesus. Both Pentecostalism, a movement that began in the early part of the twentieth century, and the charismatic renewal that duplicates and extends Pentecostal practices to standard Protestant and Roman Catholic churches, yield moderate variations that tolerate modern medical practices. But both of these evangelical movements often claim that faith is a more powerful instrument of cure than medical technology.

Unions of healing and religion invariably rely on a holistic understanding of the individual that urges therapy for both soul and body, and promotes a linkage of physical well-being with spiritual salvation. Sometimes health is defined in such a way that medical therapy is regarded as useless. Christian Scientists believe that illness is an illusion and, as a consequence, efforts at healing are not needed. The founder of Christian Science, Mary Baker Eddy, had a legendary confrontation with injury and debilitation. She discovered that the powers of the mind could dissolve what is commonly taken to be illness. Put simply, she was injured in a fall and faced a prolonged and perhaps permanent condition of invalidism. She transformed her attitudes toward her physical condition and discovered that the mental transformation alone was decisive in eliminating her physical problems. In a language that Christian Scientists do not always find comfortable (there being no such thing as illness and therefore technically no "cures"), we would say that she was healed by changing her mental state. The guiding belief in Christian Science is that God is both good and in all things. Therefore, anything that is real is good. Sickness is an illusion created by a false belief that is not founded in principle. Dispel the belief with a belief based on principle—that the real is good—and illness vanishes.

Many forms of spiritual healing are secular, however, and not even loosely aligned with any formal religion. Psychic healing is a variant on spiritual therapy that is usually conducted without the imprimatur of religion, and without the resistance to conventional medicine found in Christian Science and some evangelical movements. Healers in psychic traditions maintain that various meditative efforts can provide access to an alternative reality that has healing powers. These powers can be directed at specific wounds or illnesses by a healer who acts as a conduit, or generalized by means of meditation to the whole person. Those who practice such healing generally agree that the techniques can be taught, though the role of personal attributes in contributing to the success of particular healers is not fully understood. There are also a variety of secular healing methods drawn from homeopathic and other traditions that amend and sometimes reject conventional medical therapies. These unorthodox therapies usually rely on explanations—of illness and cure—dismissed by medical science.

Medical professionals respond to unorthodox healing techniques and philosophies with mixed feelings ranging from resistance to qualified support. There is little doubt that most physicians regard any deviation from the set of best therapies in conventional medicine as an unwelcome alternative. But a number of holistic methods have found their way into medical practice. Therapeutic touch, for example, is now taught in some nursing schools, and meditation is used successfully by patients in a number of clinics and hospitals. Even radically unorthodox techniques are sometimes brought into medical practice, therapeutic touch and meditation joining hypnotism, biofeedback, and acupuncture (all outside the pale of conventional medicine at some point in the past). Physicians also occasionally accept creative variations on medical treatment. Moderate versions of macrobiotic diets are grudgingly accepted and sometimes endorsed by physicians (though as preventive medicine, not cure). Some obstetricians supervise home births, and doctors have even been known to encourage prayer as a complement to medical therapy. Medicine can be a complex package of common and uncommon techniques, even though many of the explanations for the healing effects of unorthodox techniques—in particular contact with an alternative reality—are not generally accepted by health-care specialists.

On occasion, however, disagreements over therapy lead to conflicts that are divisive and deeply troubling to all participants. It is an axiom of medical practice that competent individuals can select or refuse medical care. Christian Scientists, for example, can ignore illness and seek health by means of their religious resources if they are competent adults. Unfortunately, tests of competence cannot always be generalized across conventional and holistic medical communities. Sometimes a view impeccable in a spiritual community—for example, a refusal of medical treatment on the grounds that God has promised a cure—can be taken as an indication of mental incompetence in a medical setting. Then there are the moral and legal problems of children, who are not deemed competent because of age. Should the state respect the traditional authority of parents to choose medical therapy (or not) for their children when the choices are based on idiosyncratic understandings of reality? Or should parents be legally required to act in the best interests of their children as fixed by conventional medical beliefs and theories?

There are no easy answers for these questions. They indicate breakdowns in political and moral discourses that revise our understandings of a liberal state. One of the enduring mysteries in liberalism is how the state can resolve disputes among communities that have different and often mutually exclusive visions of the good life. The mystery centers on one of the primary tenets of liberalism: that justice cannot depend on any particular view of human life and, as a consequence, the state must be neutral in adjudicating among the ends that individuals and communities pursue. Unfortunately, political procedures that resolve disputes are often absorbed in moral perspectives, a fact of life that can be observed in many moral conflicts requiring a political settlement (for example, slavery in the nineteenth century, abortion in the current political system). Protecting the state from partisan morality is exceedingly difficult in such circumstances.

Spiritual and medical communities enter this difficult public space when disputes over treatment follow competing beliefs about reality. Many profound disagreements over therapy are located at the margins of a reality shared by patient and doctor, and are resolvable through mutual adjustment of expectations and needs. But some disputes can be mapped back to different views on the structure of the natural world and the meaning of human experience. Differences of this magnitude are bound to control understandings of consent, liberty, competence, and even nonliberal vocabularies of beneficence and community well-being. It is not clear how a liberal state can maintain neutral procedures to resolve, or even define, disputes when the competing communities have appropriated all relevant political vocabularies. Also, since the issues in these disputes are often the primary goods of health and life, the traditional conflicts between individual liberty and state authority quickly assume new levels of difficulty. The invitation is plain. An exploration of the healing arts leads us toward an examination of fundamental problems in political discourse, including the ancient and modern boundaries of the religious and the secular, of church and state, and the rules for accommodating these contrasting beliefs in a single political order.

The examination is informed by the peculiar nature of medical practice itself. Medicine seems to occupy a position somewhere between science and those spiritual and sometimes mystical discourses from which modern medicine historically derives. An increasing reliance on clinical theory and data makes medicine more like science than folk healing; for medical practice today is influenced strongly by the Cartesian separation between mind and body, and the dazzling technological advances of modern scientific inquiry. Spiritual reasoning, by contrast, views humans in a holistic perspective that includes spirit as well as body and often accepts realities not accessible to scientific inquiry. But many practitioners of conventional medicine tell tales of truly mysterious diagnoses and healings that cannot be reduced in some obvious way to scientific explanations. These narratives enlighten the conflicts between contemporary medicine and spiritual or holistic healing and complicate deeply held and contrary beliefs about the nature of the human person, the relationships that humans have with each other in political societies, and the realities that humans experience.

The depth and range of these topics require the variety of research methods on display in this book. But there is also a core premise in this work: that narratives can serve as a source of enlightenment. We are storytellers, all of us, and the languages we use to tell stories are sometimes as important as the stories themselves. The individuals who have roles and places in the medical and spiritual discourses examined here relate stories that are drawn from the intellectual contexts in which they live. When we listen to these stories, we can hear and see realities while examining the narrative materials used by the teller. In this way, stories are both the instruments used to express or represent truths as well as the materials critical reflection addresses.

With the exception of the Luke sections, the narratives introduced here are renditions of occurrences in both spiritual and secular communities that were related in the interviews. They are not literal renditions in all respects, however. The author obviously cannot enter the heads of individuals and report with accuracy on their thoughts, especially when they are dying. Some imaginative reconstruction must be permitted. Also, a few minor facts have been altered in some of the narratives, and two of the narratives are composites. These modifications are needed to protect the identities of individuals. The most extensive (and least important) shift from the literal is represented by the use of fictitious names. Only five surnames are real: Loverro, Dubansky, LeShan, Randi (for a single quote), and Twitchell. These five individuals are known publicly either because of their works or the court cases in which they were involved, and it is important that their actual names be used so that the ideas and events connected with them can be introduced. No such gain figures in the use of the other names; the research material is just as good with shields protecting these individuals' identities. But it is helpful to remember that the people are real even though their names are not. Even the slightly modified narratives and the two composites describe events as reconstructed from interview material and other evidence.

The "truths" expressed by the individuals who populate this study are often fantastic. Some of the stories told by those interviewed can be accepted as true only by suspending all belief in ordinary reality. I am not concerned here with the truth of these tales, usually spun by those who sincerely believe in extraordinary happenings and possibilities. That individuals have such beliefs, and that they offer narratives to explain them, are my main considerations in this study. I offer a map of these beliefs, not a truth table to falsify or maintain them. The map is to be used as a guide to cross and recross a set of practices in standard and unorthodox healing.

A final comment on method amounts to a cautionary tale. It is a mistake to think that ethnographic material falls into the hands and heads of social investigators. Research efforts must be at least moderately aggressive in getting at the beliefs of practitioners. Sometimes these efforts include interviews that are as intense and prolonged as therapy sessions, leading the practitioner to levels of self-discovery that might remain fugitive to more passive explorations. Of course the investigator is then part of the social event. How could it be otherwise? Social reality consists at minimum of theoretical explanations, explicit commonsense beliefs, tacit ideas, and (unavoidably) the intellectual frameworks provided by the student of society that guide and influence the material reproduced in a work like this one. We are all both Heisenberg's atoms and the light that moves them.

It helps to recognize this condition (restriction, opportunity) in identifying the range of interpretive devices created and discovered through research activity. All that follows is such interpretation distributed through various modes of expression, crafted at every turn to provide entry into certain practices and beliefs.

The importance of the entry is itself beyond dispute. In this exercise we will encounter a variety of spiritual, scientific, and moral discourses that negotiate some of the more profound areas of human experience. These discourses are especially helpful in framing, and sometimes answering, the questions, "What is real?" "What does human life mean?" And perhaps the deepest puzzle of all, "Who are we?"

L U K E

I have distinct memories of two events in the years just before the illness. One is a moment standing in the street a bit down from my house. It was getting dark, though everyone was still out and playing. My sisters were rocking in a swing on a porch right in front of where I was standing. A dog kept running to the end of the block and then turning and running back. Twice, I remember this, he ran by me. The air seemed flattened and brisk when he went by. Then, on the third run, he just jumped up at me and knocked me down. Later, one of my sisters, I can't remember which one, told my mother that he went for my throat and just missed. He bit down hard on my collarbone. I was four years old.

The other event I remember is a fight. A boy about my age, I think I was almost five then, hit me in the face. I hit him back twice and he went off crying. I remember sitting on a stool in our kitchen afterwards. My mother had given me an apple and I was just eating it and trying not to cry. The juice, the skin, the taste of the apple, and me just not about to cry. And my mother looking at me from her ironing.

Then, when I became sick, I remember my mother crying at night and my father's voice slower and deeper as he calmed her. He was always unhurried, his rhythm just a step or two behind my mother's pace. Her crying would stop and they would talk in low voices, my mother's more intense and rapid, as if demanding something from my father. Then she would cry some more. At some point they would stop and the night would be so still that nothing seemed to move, not even insects. Usually then I would drift off to sleep. On some nights they would turn to each other and I would hear the bed moving against the wall slowly and then faster, my mother's voice now issuing instructions on pace. All of this was very comforting since I knew it was about me, the worry and sadness, even the lovemaking at the end of the talking.

I remember the place my parents rented on Watson Street in Key West. It is the first memory I have of my existence. My crib was in a room down a hall. If I stood up and looked through the bars I could see the yellow walls leading to the living room where my mother would sit using the telephone. One night I was in a state of terror over dying, though I have no recollection of what brought it on. I called my mother back to my crib again and again that evening, asking her if when you died that was all there was, you were nothing. Finally, as much to calm me as anything, she provided the right assurances. No, she said kissing me, you live on after you die, no one dies finally. Later, when I was an adult, I used the doctrine of dualism to reassure my older daughter after a teenage boy had drowned one Sunday afternoon in the apartment pool. The body dies, I told her as she sought meaning and comfort from me, the soul lives on afterwards.

It would be comforting now to know where the soul and body are distinct, and even who I am in my current state. I do know, or think I know, that I had no existence before March 1, 1948, the day I was born. The world existed, or I believe it did, for many years before that day, but I, as this human subject, was not a part of it. This thought is one of many I cannot fully get my mind around. In a way it is easier to describe that world without having to include myself in it. I am not there as some irreducible subject experiencing the world—tasting it, feeling pleasure and pain. But the descriptions all begin and end with someone doing the describing, seeing the world within the familiar vocabularies of human experience. The events seem to require a subjective frame in order to *be*, to occur. And I am not there to provide the frame, the lens through which I know and have experiences.

Then I am present in the world at 3:35 A.M. on March 1, 1948, fourteen months after my parents married each other. Existence with no awareness of the self or the world. No self there as a reflective creature. Just a recipient of my parents' affection and love, my brain recalled now in memory as only a dormant instrument. But from that point in human time I have a location, an opening that no story of the world can close. I am conscious. All complete descriptions of the world must include me, but I cannot be described merely as an object in the world. My subjectivity resists closure. It is also the source and condition of all accounts I make of human experience.

These thoughts are deeply troubling to me. I am not even sure I am having them, or who is having them.

When I was six years old our family doctor told my parents that I had a form of cancer, a condition that was later verified by a specialist in Miami. The treatment was chemotherapy administered over a period of several years. The effects at first were devastating. My hair fell out. I felt hollow, my body grieving at the abusive therapy. We would drive to Miami for the treatment, and on the return trip I would be vomiting almost constantly in a container my mother held for me. I remember colors. The flat grey of the highway as we sped over it. The blue of the waters on the Florida Keys. White rags that my mother dampened to rub over my forehead.

I cannot remember the pain of the treatment or of the cancer. These experiences seem distant, as if experienced by someone else. I see myself, as another, on a table in a room dominated by metal. A nurse injects a needle into my spine, taking something out and putting something in. Sometimes I just take medicine in a blue or an orange cup. Then, in later visits, more pills, followed sometimes by the soft clicks and movements of a white and grey X-ray machine positioned over me by a technician who leaves the room. After each visit I am a small boy throwing up in a basket, myself as other in distress. Now I see my mother holding this boy as he walks down a corridor outside to the white daylight of a Miami sun. This is the objective picture that my memory now serves up for critical inspection.

Later, when the cancer was in remission, my parents began the other journey on treatment. It started by accident. A black woman who worked in the place where my mother got her hair done happened to be a faith healer. One thing led to another, and my mother visited the church where Faith (that was her name) prayed and ministered to the sick. My mother witnessed the afflicted being healed, or so she thought. We began making regular visits. I remember the hands of Faith on me, hot and black against my skin, her eyes closed as she prayed aloud with her head tilted back. The congregation seemed to be agitated, dancing to the words, the lights in the church like small fires along the top of the walls.

If health is an equilibrium of the body, a balance at which the organism flourishes to its own rhythm, then who is to say that Faith did not have the power to restore this balance? She claimed the power to tune the human instrument, to reclaim the self from a misery stretching endlessly away from the natural fulcrum of health. Only the stretch was not endless. At some point later in the paths marked off by medical therapy I lost another balance. Something changed in my state of being. That other equilibrium, the chemical arrangement at which I and no other existed, that precise point in the physical world at which the self that is me emerged as a subject, was altered irretrievably. I diminished, contracted, and then expanded like air in a balloon. I became an agent within an object. My soul was cut loose from its physical center.

1

RATIONAL DISPUTES

Caleb

Caleb Loverro was three and one-half years old when his parents acciden-
tally broke one of his legs while trying to fit him into the back seat of their
car. The fracture puzzled and alarmed the Loverros. The car seat had collapsed on Caleb's leg, but not with a pressure they thought sufficient to fracture the bone. They took him to the emergency room at Lourdes Hospital in
Binghamton, New York, for treatment. A routine blood test revealed a low
platelet count. The attending physician, a pediatrician, recommended that
they transfer him to University Hospital in Syracuse for further evaluation
and treatment. The Loverros rode with their son in the ambulance that took
them the seventy-three miles to Syracuse.

The Loverros had noticed earlier that their son was "not quite right."
Caleb was born on October 19, 1983. He was seemingly healthy until
March of 1987, when he began complaining of leg pains. By April he had
stopped running and playing and began to crawl to get from one place to
another. The Loverros had taken Caleb in for an examination in April.
X rays and a blood test revealed nothing extraordinary. The doctor said that
Caleb was slightly anemic. The Loverros assumed that the boy had some
metabolic disorder and began treating him with dietary supplements, especially minerals. Both Joseph and Gillian Loverro are vegetarians and believe
that macrobiotic diets can cure many diseases. In mid-May, Caleb's father, a
licensed chiropractor, noticed that his son's liver and spleen were enlarged.
The Loverros had planned to consult a physician again after a brief vacation
with their son. It was while returning home from that trip, on May 31, that
Caleb's leg was fractured.

More sophisticated tests conducted at University Hospital revealed that Caleb was suffering from acute lymphocytic leukemia, pre B type. One test showed that Caleb's bone marrow was contaminated with more than 90 percent leukemic cells. A spinal tap revealed no sign of leukemia in the central nervous system. This was considered evidence that Caleb's leukemia was still in the early stages and increased his chances for a full recovery. The standard treatment for this type of cancer is chemotherapy.

The chemotherapy protocol for leukemia developed over years of research and clinical use consists of four phases. The first, remission induction, is designed to saturate the body with toxic chemicals for about four weeks to reduce the number of cancer cells from about one trillion to one billion. The next two phases of therapy, prophylaxis and consolidation, continue the chemotherapy at lower doses. Even though clinical tests are unable to detect cancer at the one billion cell level, experience has shown that the cancer is almost always still present. Discontinuing therapy at this stage usually results in a relapse that is considerably more difficult to treat and has more severe side effects when therapy is resumed, including impaired mental functioning. The final phase is maintenance. Here drugs are continued for extended periods of time to ensure that all of the cancer cells have been destroyed. The most common drugs used in chemotherapy are vincristine, methotrexate, L-asparaginase, prednisone, ara-c, and 6-mercaptopurine. Each has side effects that are especially severe in the first phase of treatment. Some patients suffer considerably from these drugs for at least a few hours and sometimes longer.

Stephen Dubansky, a specialist in pediatric hematology and oncology, was the physician overseeing Caleb's case. He recommended to the Loverros that they enter their son on a three-year chemotherapy protocol named ALINC 14. These protocols treat a group of children with the best therapy available for leukemia and maintain data on the results. These data are then used to improve treatment for future patients. ALINC 14 was designed on the basis of data gathered from the previous treatment group, ALINC 13, which involved over eight hundred children nationwide. Since the survival rate for ALINC 13 was 53 percent, doctors were reasonably certain that the modification in therapy represented by ALINC 14 would result in a survival rate at least as high and probably higher than that of ALINC 13. The protocol was not experimental as that term is usually understood. The purpose of the study was only to learn how to use the standard drugs better. Accepting the protocol was voluntary and withdrawal was to be allowed without prejudice. The alternative was a chemotherapy program designed for the particular patient.

The Loverros immediately consented to both the initial efforts to stabilize Caleb's condition and the induction phase of the chemotherapy. But
they expressed reservations about the duration of the therapy program and
declined at first to enter Caleb in ALINC 14. Five days later, however, after
extensive conversations with each other and with Dr. Dubansky, they signed
the consent forms for the protocol. The inductive phase of the treatment was
immediately beneficial to Caleb. The pain and fever abated, and he re-
gained some of his old energy. By June 9, 1987, one week after treatment
began, he left the hospital.

In early July, tests indicated that Caleb's cancer was in full remission.
The bone marrow test established that the tumors in his body had been reduced to one billion or fewer leukemic cells. But the side effects of the therapy were terrible. Like all chemotherapy patients, Caleb suffered from
nausea, vomiting, headaches, irritability, and temporary reduction in white
blood cells. His parents began questioning the need for long-term therapy in
discussions with Dubansky. In late July, Caleb was hospitalized for the second phase of the protocol, requiring injections of methotrexate. Blood tests
taken at that time were normal, with no leukemic cells in evidence and a
normal white blood cell and platelet count. But leukemic cells were still assumed to be in the bone marrow and in other parts of his body.

The dialogue that the Loverros and Dubansky entered during those
summer months was aided in the beginning by shared perspectives. Dubansky is a vegetarian and, like Gillian Loverro, writes poetry. They exchanged poems, literatures on holistic medicine and the efficacy of
chemotherapy, and views on the history and logic of medicine. They explored compromise proposals, including treatment with both macrobiotic
diets and chemotherapy. But they could not reach an agreement on continuing Caleb in therapy for the three-year duration of the protocol.

The disagreement became a dispute in August. The Loverros called
Dubansky and said they would not be bringing Caleb in for his August 11
appointment. This appointment was to begin the consolidation phase of the
therapy. The Loverros explained that they were going to Chicago for a consultation with a Dr. Keith Block to explore alternative forms of treatment.
They asked that copies of Caleb's medical records be forwarded to Block.
Dubansky, deeply concerned for his patient by this time, agreed to do so. But
he also urged that Caleb continue in the chemotherapy program. The
Loverros promised to bring Caleb in for treatment on August 20. They did
not. Instead they called to say that they were going to Boston to take a macrobiotic cooking course given by Michio Kushi, founder of the East West
Foundation in Boston and leading guru of nutritional therapy for cancer.

Dubansky asked that they postpone the trip. They refused. On September 1, after returning from Boston, Gillian Loverro called and advised Dubansky that they were withdrawing Caleb from the protocol and would treat his cancer with a macrobiotic diet.

It was too much for Dubansky. The prospect of a severe relapse in his patient was unbearable. He called county officials. They responded in ways that he did not fully anticipate. State police and social workers descended on the Loverro home and charged Caleb's parents with felony first-degree reckless endangerment. The County Department of Social Services obtained legal custody of Caleb. They allowed him to remain at home only as long as his parents kept him in the chemotherapy program. A local church raised money for the Loverros' legal fees, and they began a legal battle to regain custody of their son and acquire the legal authority to determine appropriate medical treatment for his leukemia. Dubansky was dismayed. He did not want the Loverros arrested and hoped to avoid a legal dispute over treatment. But he was convinced that Caleb's only chance to live was to continue the chemotherapy.

On May 4, 1988, a court of law ruled against Mr. and Mrs. Loverro. Family Court Judge Patrick Mathews said that the couple was not qualified to make medical decisions and so could not determine Caleb's therapy. He described the Loverros as intelligent and loving parents. But he also noted that their decision to take Caleb out of chemotherapy was not supported by a single licensed physician. He ruled that Caleb's best interests were served by continuing the chemotherapy, and so ordered it. Dubansky expressed hope that the decision would set a precedent for avoiding such disputes between parents and physicians over therapy. Caleb was dutifully taken to University Hospital at the prescribed times to complete the chemotherapy program.

The Loverros

Joseph Loverro studied biochemistry as an undergraduate at the State University of New York at Binghamton. He was interested in nutrition and immunology, and took some graduate courses in these fields while he was at SUNY Binghamton. He had no desire to go to medical school in spite of these interests. His goal was to attend graduate school and earn an advanced degree in a science field.

Somewhere along the way Loverro met a chiropractor who explained the practice and philosophy to him. He immediately felt a deep sense of appropriateness, an accord between the practice and what he now views as his innate ideas about the human body and its environment. He applied to chiropractic colleges instead of graduate schools. He also began taking all the courses he could find in alternative therapies, including acupuncture, homeopathy, and herbal medicine. The Canadian Memorial Chiropractic College accepted him, and he began his studies in the fall of 1980. In 1984 he graduated and started practicing in Owego, New York.

One of the main principles in chiropractic medicine is that the body heals itself. The primary function of the health provider is to remove interference, internal or external, that is impeding the self-healing powers of the body. One cause of interference that chiropractors stress is in the nervous system, which can be inhibited by misaligned segments of the spine or extremities. When that interference is removed through manipulation of the bony structure, the energy flow resumes and a healthy state is restored. Structure, in chiropractic theory, is directly related to function. Setting the bodily structure in order permits natural functions to operate successfully.

Loverro recognizes limits in this theory. An organic condition that has altered the body's structure beyond its ability to repair itself will not yield to chiropractic manipulation. He is puzzled at the frequency of what he considers documented stories about remarkable chiropractic restoration thirty to forty years ago and the relative paucity of these accounts today. He feels that there are more complications in the environment today. Bad food and carcinogens in the air and soil so compromise living areas that removing structural impediments in the human body may no longer be enough. But these are limits set by the environment. Loverro also recognizes the need to introduce other, more conventional medical support for some human illnesses. Malignancies of any sort fall into this category. Chiropractors in New York can now order a full range of laboratory tests, from simple blood tests to CAT scans. If Loverro discovers a cancer in any of his patients, for both legal and medical reasons he will refer the individual to an oncologist. He does not believe that manipulation of the bodily structure will cure cancer in and of itself.

Loverro does not subscribe fully to conventional medical therapy either. He believes that health is best restored through an amalgam of techniques. One set of approaches ensures a harmony between the individual and the environment, in particular, the use of foods and herbs to calm the body and release its energies for self-healing. Another set is bodily manipulation, as in chiropractic and a variety of techniques found in traditional Chinese medicine (including acupuncture). Healing and health for Loverro are holistic states that can be secured through an understanding and use of organic energies and environmental influences. He rejects certain therapies in conventional medicine as both useless and dangerous. One is chemotherapy. Loverro regards this protocol as an invasive destruction of the body and its capacity to cope with disease.

When the Loverros signed Caleb into the chemotherapy protocol at University Hospital, they were concerned to do whatever had to be done then and there. Immediately after this decision, Joseph Loverro began calling everyone he knew who was knowledgeable about leukemia and its treatment. He called his professors at chiropractic school; people in the Midwest, in Texas, and in California whom he had heard about; local colleagues. He also began reading everything he could find in the upstate New York area and elsewhere on chemotherapy. He and his wife came to one quick conclusion. They would accept and use whatever methods were necessary to save Caleb's life, both in conventional and holistic medicine. In those first days of the chemotherapy, they wanted "to arrest the situation, get things under control" until they could settle on the best medical treatment for Caleb.

The Loverros began to accumulate a lot of information from all over the country. In sifting through it, they decided to do two things: one was to develop a nutritional program to support the chemotherapy regimen; the other was to find a way to wean Caleb off chemotherapy. They had signed him onto a three-year program even though they knew from the beginning that they did not want Caleb receiving chemotherapy for that extended period of time. Both of the Loverros appreciated the remission rates that the physicians cited to them: a 53 percent recovery rate based on the particular diagnosis of Caleb's condition. But they also found claims for a 70 to 80 percent success rate with nutritional methods, though with less precise experimental controls and no scientific papers supporting these claims. Joseph Loverro still felt more comfortable with the nutritional approach, given his own background affinities for holistic medicine.

The main objection the Loverros had to chemotherapy was that every child in the protocol received basically the same program of treatment. Joseph Loverro believes that one of the most attractive features of holistic medicine is that treatment is individualized. Every patient is tested for particular medical needs and therapy is tailored accordingly. Loverro found the standardized form of chemotherapy protocol hostile to his deepest instincts. He can accept standard therapy in the acute phase of a disease, though even here he has reservations, but he finds it incomprehensible that all of the children in the protocol continued to receive the same treatment with no variation sensitive to their progress. He began exploring alternative treatments that would address Caleb's specific problems, a program sensitive to his particular strengths and weaknesses.

The effects of the chemotherapy reinforced the Loverros' convictions that some alternative treatment had to be found. Caleb suffered from the expected nausea, vomiting, and lethargy. But he also had neurological reactions where he would shake uncontrollably. These spasms did no good for the Loverros' state of mind. During one phase of the treatment, intraspinal chemotherapy, Caleb was listless, almost paralyzed. He was especially affected in the early stages of this treatment, which consisted of spinal taps and regular injections of chemicals into his spine. This phase of the protocol lasts two and one-half years. After one of the first sessions in this therapy, Caleb was virtually paralyzed for four days, lying in his bed moaning, awake constantly, unable to move his arms and legs. What Joseph Loverro found galling is that the cancer was never found in Caleb's spinal fluid. The drugs were injected as a precaution. The Loverros eventually figured out which homeopathic preparations are supposed to counter trauma to the spine. When they gave these to Caleb, he began handling the injections better, to the point where he would walk, jump, and play on the same day he was treated.

During the summer the Loverros began taking Caleb to medical facilities in Philadelphia, Chicago, and Boston looking for cancer programs that used holistic medicine. They intended to transfer their son to one of these programs once the induction phase was completed and he was in a consolidation phase. Their goal was either a reduced chemotherapy program combined with diet therapy, or perhaps a complete nutritional program with no chemotherapy. They finally settled on Keith Block, a doctor in Chicago who had agreed to supervise Caleb's treatment. They visited Block the week before the Labor Day holiday and arranged for Caleb to have blood tests at their local hospital so the Chicago physician could begin a review of his condition. All summer they had been discussing this alternative with Dubansky. He was adamantly opposed to the change. After returning from Chicago, the Loverros called University Hospital in Syracuse and informed Dubansky that they were switching Caleb's medical care to Dr. Block in Chicago.

Events proceeded swiftly from that point. Dubansky lodged a complaint with the child abuse hotline stating that what the Loverros were doing was "homicidal." The next day, Wednesday, the Loverros were visited by a plainclothes New York state trooper (an investigator) and a social service worker who asked where Caleb was. Here at home, the Loverros reported. The social service worker said that the county had a report that Caleb was not receiving medical care. Joseph Loverro informed the woman (and trooper) that he was receiving care, had in fact just been to the hospital for blood tests, and that they had made arrangements with another doctor to take care of him. The Loverros thought that the incident was over when the trooper and social worker left the house.

The next day, Thursday, the same two individuals visited Joseph Loverro at his chiropractic office. They wanted to know where Mrs. Loverro and Caleb were. Out running an errand, Joseph Loverro responded. The social worker asked him if he would sign an order placing Caleb in their custody so that they could take him to the hospital for tests. He refused. The social worker then produced a court order to take custody of Caleb. Loverro found out later that another state trooper was at that time staking out his home waiting for Mrs. Loverro to return. When she did, the trooper turned on his lights and pulled her over to the side of the road. He asked her to move into her driveway. At that point he explained the court order to Gillian Loverro and said that he was going to have to take Caleb away. Gillian Loverro explained that Caleb had special needs that no one would be able to meet, that no one could care for him like she had. The social worker eventually joined the policeman and announced that they were taking Caleb to University Hospital in Syracuse. Mrs. Loverro insisted, pleaded that she be allowed to come along. With some irritation (reports Joseph Loverro) the social worker agreed, observing that such procedures were highly irregular.

Both Joseph and Gillian Loverro went up to Syracuse that day and stayed with Caleb while doctors examined him and continued chemotherapy over the weekend. Before leaving Owego Joseph Loverro had arranged for a hearing on the custody order. Since the Labor Day weekend was almost upon them, the earliest open date was the following Tuesday. One physician in the hospital quietly advised the Loverros to pick their child up and simply leave with him. Instead of fleeing, which the Loverros later felt may in fact have been the best action to take, they hired a lawyer to represent them.

At a court hearing on Tuesday another surprise was waiting. The Loverros were arrested and charged with a felony, reckless endangerment of the welfare of a minor. They were fingerprinted and mug shots were taken. These charges followed Dubansky's description of the Loverros to the district attorney as extremely dangerous. (Two months later the charges were dropped.) The Loverros wanted to minimize trauma for their son. They agreed at the Family Court hearing to allow the county to have custody of Caleb. In turn, the boy would remain at home as long as they continued him in the chemotherapy program. The county also agreed to pay Caleb's medical bills (since they were insisting on treatment). In the meantime, the Loverros waited for the court hearing. The hearing in May of 1987 led to the ruling that Caleb had to complete the chemotherapy program.

The physician in Chicago dropped out of the picture when Caleb's case became a legal issue. The Loverros had no realistic option but to continue therapy. In the later stages of the protocol a public health nurse would come to their house every day with a pill for Caleb and would not leave until she was satisfied that the boy had taken the medicine. One practical consequence of this requirement was that the Loverros could not go on any trips, even weekend excursions, without getting permission from the University Hospital medical staff. The Loverros had to make Caleb available for the scheduled treatments and medicine.

Joseph Loverro reports that his son is "doing great." The chemotherapy program is over. Caleb seems to be clear of cancer. He is socially well adjusted and apparently healthy. During the chemotherapy he would sometimes get sick and the medicine would weaken him even more. But the medical staff was always reluctant to suspend the treatment. They would think that the Loverros were trying to stop it altogether. Caleb has survived both the legal and medical wars. His parents still believe that the medical staff and the state were wrong in what they did. They also remain apprehensive about future court orders if Caleb suffers from any additional health problems. Joseph Loverro's thoughts on Stephen Dubansky are extremely negative. He does not trust him. He does not respect him. He still cannot understand why he acted as he did.

The Loverros had a second child in November 1989. The baby is a boy who appears to be healthy in all respects.

Dubansky

Stephen Dubansky graduated from the University of Maryland medical school in 1970. He regards himself as a product of the 1960s and the protest movements of that decade. He was arrested three times for demonstrating against the Vietnam War. He mentions this to point out that as a youthful member of the counterculture, he carries no a priori bias against alternative medicine. He is antagonistic to pseudomedicine, however.

Dubansky did graduate work at the Albert Einstein Institute in New York City for a year, then returned to the University of Maryland where he completed his residency in pediatrics. In his final year he was named the chief resident in pediatrics. He did a two-year fellowship at Denver Children's Hospital in Colorado and went into general pediatrics back in Maryland. After practicing pediatrics for seven years in various ways—alternative medicine, HMO, private practice in a medical group—he still was not satisfied intellectually. So he went back to the University of Maryland to specialize in a field that seemed to him to offer more of a medical challenge than general pediatrics. He came to University Hospital in Syracuse in 1984 as a pediatric hematologist oncologist. Dubansky is on the teaching faculty at the hospital. His primary responsibilities include taking care of children with blood disease and cancer. The hospital has over four hundred active patients in this category. Dubansky also teaches fellows, residents, and interns in the department of pediatrics, and does clinical research in his specialties.

Caleb Loverro, Dubansky recalls, "presented to our hospital in early June of 1987 with a several month history of fatigue and primarily bone pain that began in one of his knees." The pain had increased to the point where Caleb had been unable to walk from about six weeks prior to admission. Dubansky remembers that Caleb's father was treating the child with multivitamins, calcium supplements in particular, given the relationship between calcium levels and bone integrity. But Caleb's symptoms got progressively worse. The day prior to his first visit to University Hospital his leg twisted in his car seat and, because of the underlying disease, the bone just cracked. The first time Dubansky saw Caleb the child had a pathological fracture of the tibia, and he was suffering from excruciating pain elsewhere in his legs.

A simple blood smear told Dubansky that Caleb had leukemic cells in his body. The bone marrow test conducted the next day confirmed the diagnosis of acute lymphocytic leukemia with over 90 percent of the bone marrow replaced by leukemic cells. Dubansky reviewed the blood work that Caleb's father had ordered six weeks earlier. He concedes that to many medical personnel it would look normal. But to him and to his staff at University Hospital, it was clearly abnormal because at the time the child did not have enough nutrifil (a type of white blood cell) in his blood, indicating even then some kind of process affecting the bone marrow. Caleb's fractured leg was immediately treated and placed in a cast. Dubansky also noted the swelling of Caleb's liver and spleen, which he feels Joseph Loverro did not fully appreciate as a sign of serious trouble.

The family history taken at that time indicated no previous experience with, or interest in, organized health care. The parents, it became clear, had a general distrust of organized medicine. Dubansky was both curious and sympathetic at first. He has his own serious reservations about how medical care is organized in the United States, especially the "egomaniacal, holier-than-thou, brighter-than-thou, medical god standpoint" that he finds and loathes in modern medicine. But in conversations with the Loverros, he could not get anything out of them, no reasons that might explain their mistrust. Caleb had been born at home. Dubansky understood this. He had attended a number of home births when he was in private practice. The child had also never seen a doctor before the first signs of the illness. Dubansky had some qualms with this, but he had encountered such resistance before. The problem he had was with the Loverros' responses. They provided no general rationale to account for their distance from standard medical care.

It became clear to everyone very quickly that the Loverros were going to be a difficult family. Usually the nurses take care of these patients and their families because the hospital unit has a large volume of patients, and the doctors are trying both to supervise treatment and do research. But Dubansky volunteered. He wanted to show the Loverros some real sympathy. He knew that most medical doctors tend to be very critical of this type of patient relationship. They do not like to be questioned, and they do not enjoy having conditions placed on their therapy recommendations. But Dubansky thought it would be an interesting challenge for him and "something that I would like to do." He wanted the Loverros to discover that there are doctors they could trust and perhaps even like.

Dubansky explained to the Loverros the treatment that he recommended. It consisted of two and one-half to three years of chemotherapy. The initial six weeks of remission induction is standard everywhere in the United States. Then, depending on your location, there are either two years or two and one-half years of additional therapy. The experimental portion of the protocol was in the consolidation period. Dubansky's medical unit is a member of a national consortium of children's cancer centers called the Pediatric Oncology Group. The consortium is trying to increase survival rates for childhood leukemia to 100 percent—the ultimate goal. There is general satisfaction with the six-week induction phase because 98 percent of the children go into remission right away. But there is some speculation that more aggressive treatment in the consolidation stage might improve the cure rate. So the research design of the protocol called for random assignment of the participating children to one of four different consolidation treatments during this eighteen-week middle period. Then all of the children would get the same maintenance therapy for (in this case) two and one-half years. No experimental drugs were to be used. "It was not rat medicine," Dubansky stresses. "These were standard medicines purchasable with prescription." The only experimental part of the protocol was the use of four different combinations of drugs in consolidation to see which combination would be most effective. (It turned out that none of the four combinations was appreciably better than any other. The data indicated that the effects on the cure rate did not differ significantly.)

The Loverros hesitated. They gave verbal permission to start the therapy on a provisional basis. But they would not sign the consent form for the protocol at first. Then, after a few days ("without any cajoling," Dubansky reports), they agreed to the therapy. Dubansky thinks that the reason was Caleb's condition. The child was obviously very sick, with extreme pain in his legs, swollen organs, abnormal blood counts.

Dubansky was pleased to observe that Caleb "went into a perfect, easy, simple, uncomplicated remission without difficulty." His parents had by this time returned with him to their home. They would bring him up on a regular basis, weekly at first, for his treatments. Towards the end of July, after Caleb had been in remission for a few weeks, Dubansky told the Loverros that the tests showed a normal bone marrow and now Caleb needed to enter the consolidation phase. At that point Dubansky began sensing a reluctance in the Loverros. They wouldn't come for appointments. They began giving him reasons for not being able to make the trip from Tioga at a certain time. Dubansky tried to be flexible. He set Caleb's appointments to meet the Loverros' schedule. The Loverros also began making unusual demands. Caleb needed a special diet. Fine, Dubansky said. He arranged for Gillian Loverro to cook special food in the hospital kitchen when Caleb was readmitted for the start of consolidation in late July. Mrs. Loverro also did not want Caleb to have sugar in his IV (IV fluid is D5W with water or D5 and saline). No problem. Dubansky went to the pharmacist and made special solutions for Caleb. He believes that he acceded to every one of their demands during this period.

When Caleb was six weeks into the consolidation phase, the Loverros called to cancel a scheduled admission to the hospital. They had to attend a macrobiotic cooking course in Boston. Dubansky asked, "Couldn't you go some other time?" No, it was the only time it was to be given in the east, and for financial reasons they had to go to Boston because the only other course of this nature was scheduled for Los Angeles. Dubansky said, "Okay, fine, go," but extracted a promise from them to bring Caleb in the following week. He was still trying to show the Loverros that there are no hard and fast rules, that the medical establishment is not some evil monolith. The Loverros went to the cooking class.

When they returned, Gillian Loverro called. Dubansky could tell from the conversation that they were heavily into macrobiotic alternatives now. But the key message was "We won't be coming next week."

Dubansky replied, "I thought you were."

"No. We have decided to seek another opinion."

"Who is that?"

"Dr. Keith Block in Chicago."

"What kind of doctor is he?"

"He is a doctor. A real doctor."

"Fine. Is Caleb going with you?"

"Yes. Dr. Block is just going to see him and tell us about his diet. How to treat him with a diet."

Dubansky paused. He recalls that he was smoldering. "Listen," he replied. "Here is my limit. I'll see you next week, yes? When you come back. Any more delay will be dangerous for Caleb because we are early on in his treatment. That is it." This call represented a delay for the second week in treatment.

The Loverros returned from Chicago and Gillian Loverro called. "We are not coming in anymore."

"Pardon me?"

"Well, Dr. Block has told us that this cancer can be cured by macrobiotic diet alone, and we have decided not to bring Caleb in for any more treatments."

Dubansky entered his final plea. "Please come up and talk to me. You went all the way to Chicago. Give me a chance to explain to you simply, nicely, why this treatment is important. Give me the same courtesy you gave to Dr. Block way out in Chicago. Let me talk to you."

Pause. "Let me ask my husband." Pause again. "No, we are not coming."

Dubansky replied, "Threatening is not my thing. But I must tell you I have a higher moral obligation than to let you leave this boy on his own. If you were my patient, and you as an adult wanted to do this thing, fine. But you can't do this to Caleb because it is a homicidal act."

The use of the word "homicidal" was influential in galvanizing the social service staff and was scrutinized intensely at the later trial. Dubansky used it in the conversation and then in his letter to the county. He is unapologetic. He did not say, or mean to imply, that the Loverros were homicidal maniacs. But he was convinced that Caleb's chances of a cure would go from 53 percent or more to zero. In that sense he viewed the Loverros' attempt to withdraw the boy from therapy as no different from someone who drinks a bottle of whiskey and then gets in the car to drive—or worse, because Caleb had almost no chance to survive the adventure. Dubansky's last words to the Loverros on the phone were: "I will not stop with this. I will pursue this and we will treat this boy come hell or high water. We are going to treat him. One, because I love him. Two, because that is my job. I can't stand by and see him die unnecessarily."

Gillian Loverro replied, "We are not coming."

The next time Dubansky saw either of the Loverros was two days later when Gillian and Caleb appeared in a police car with a social worker. Dubansky reports that he spent at least an hour with this mother explaining that he felt very badly that he had hurt her, that the last thing he wanted was to have Caleb removed from their home, and that he would not allow that to happen unless Caleb did not come in for therapy. Caleb was admitted to the hospital and therapy resumed.

Two weeks later the district attorney called. His office wanted to prosecute the Loverros and remove Caleb from their home. The DA asked Dubansky to testify for the county in the trial. He replied that he absolutely would not. The DA was nonplussed. Dubansky had called to report neglect that could have resulted in the death of a child. Now he would not testify, would not back the DA up in court? (By this time the events were in all the newspapers.) The DA, the social worker supervising the case, and the head of child protection all drove up to Syracuse to see Dubansky. He told them that they could not prosecute people for what they think, that "this is not Nazi Germany." (He remembers using these exact words.) The DA subsequently dropped the charges of felony reckless endangerment and child neglect.

Dubansky read everything he could find on macrobiotic diets during the uneasy summer months leading up to the break with the Loverros. He asked the Loverros for material, and they brought him a lot of literature. He still believes that the macrobiotic diet in its moderate forms is healthy for adults. But he holds to a crucial distinction between maintaining health and curing disease. He points out that if you don't smoke, you don't normally get lung cancer. But after getting lung cancer, stopping cigarettes is not going to cure the disease. He also confesses that he has trouble when advocates of holistic therapy start talking about yang and yin tumors, and how yang foods should be eaten for yin tumors and yin foods for yang tumors. He gets lost at this point and tries very hard not to laugh at these proposals.

In preparation for the trial he conducted his own survey. He sent a letter and questionnaire to every board-certified pediatric hematologist oncologist in the United States, asking if they had ever had a child treated with unorthodox therapy, and if so, to provide a report on the outcome. He collected some thirty responses, including descriptions of vitamin C, peach pit, and macrobiotic therapies. Every patient on these therapies died. A typical response was the following: "Diagnosis: Stage IV neuroblastoma; refused all therapy in favor of a macrobiotic diet; outcome: painful, wasting, horrible slow death." Dubansky could not find anywhere in his surveys and in the medical literature one single proven case of cancer cured through macrobiotic diet.

Dubansky was obviously relieved at the Family Court ruling, though he knows the judge's decision was not based on the merits of the case but on the absence of testimony by a New York State-licensed physician on behalf of the Loverros. But he believes the main goal was secured. Caleb Loverro completed the therapy protocol. The maintenance phase of the therapy was conducted at Caleb's house at his parents' request. They did not want to come up to the hospital. So Dubansky arranged for a public health nurse to drive twenty miles each way every day to the Loverros' home to give Caleb a pill. He would not allow the Loverros to give Caleb the medicine because he says he knew it would go into the toilet. Caleb also received an injection from the nurse in his home once a week. The final result of this complete chemotherapy program was successful. Caleb's prognosis remains excellent. Dubansky can't imagine that he will not beat this disease now. In Dubansky's words, "He has done very, very well." Dubansky still feels pleased with what he did and has no regrets. He reports that he can sleep well at night and look at himself in a mirror "because I know that I did everything that I could possibly do in as gentlemanly a way as possible, while yet keeping this boy's interests at heart." A colleague at another hospital, when Dubansky had called for advice, responded, "What, are you crazy? It is a loser. Don't do this—let them do what they want. If they want to kill themselves, fine." Dubansky believes that the enormous commitment of time and emotion was worth it. "I feel as proud of this as anything I have done."

Ancient and Modern Medicines

At one level, the dispute between the Loverros and Stephen Dubansky is ethical and can be negotiated by exploring the responsibilities of the physician to his patient weighed against the authority of parents to decide on therapy for their children. But at another level, one more basic than ethics, the dispute is over cause and effect, and closely follows different understandings of evidence and inference. These more substantial disagreements create the Rashomon effects so strongly displayed in the accounts of the disputes provided by each party.

The Loverros accept causal relations between diet and healing that Dubansky does not, and rely on forms of healing (such as homeopathy and chiropractic) that are not grounded in conventional realities on which current medical practices are based. Dubansky endorses the causal effects found in a chemotherapy program that the Loverros think is destructive. He also uses traditions of medical science that have empirically mapped the human body on evidence accumulated for centuries. The Loverros rely on other traditions that exceed these scientific constructions with more holistic projections of mind, body, and environment. One way to describe these differences is to say that the Loverros define as natural what Dubansky regards as metaphysical or spiritual, and that from the Loverros' perspective Dubansky has a restricted view of nature that finally limits his therapeutic practices. Dubansky, in turn, sees the Loverros as dwelling within a reality that is largely conjectural, with no anchor in empirical science.

A rational perspective on such disputes is not readily available. It is too simple to say that the Loverros are wrong and perhaps even crazy, and that Dubansky is right and comfortably sane. The most painful feature of the Caleb Loverro episode is that the parents and doctors are both sincere and loving caretakers, concerned to do what is best for Caleb, and each is rational and competent in terms of the discourse community to which they subscribe. Almost equally unbearable is the fact that Caleb was less than four years old at the time of the dispute and thus incapable of deciding which program of treatment met his best interests. It is also necessary to observe that the lives of individuals can be at stake in these disputes, as Caleb's was, and neither love nor reason may effectively guide the principals to a decision regarded as right by both sets of parties.

Only one path to enlightenment may be open to us in this kind of disagreement and resulting dispute. It is the path that takes us directly through the reasoning employed by individuals who define healing in unorthodox terms, and by the physicians who are the practicing descendants of modern science in medicine. If the rules of inference and evidence, and the senses of reality, found in these patterns of reasoning can be put on display like landscapes arranged on a canvas, then we will be in a better position to explain how the Loverros and Dubansky could end up polarized over medical care even though they shared the same good motives.

One striking feature of the dispute over Caleb's medical care is its familiarity. In listening to the participants one feels strongly that the story has occurred before, many times. Of course it has. The dispute over Caleb's therapy echoes long traditions of differences over health and healing, and what is real, what false, in human experience.

The story of medicine begins with ideas much like those endorsed by the Loverros. The opening thought in all medical care is that there is both hostility and symbiosis between human beings and nature. Humans become ill as part of the natural order of things. Early medical treatment used nature, primarily plants, as balms to soothe and sometimes cure these illnesses. This equilibrium between human life and nature is inevitably favorable to the species or the human race would not have survived. But for individuals the desire for cure, especially when the illness is fatal, is not likely to be deterred by considering favorable prospects for the species. Medicine begins from the natural preference for health rather than illness within the balance of evolutionary adaptation.

Mystical discourse controlled medical practices for most of human history. Serious illness was not regarded as natural but as caused by spiritual effects that could be reversed by spiritual means. The doctor and shaman were one, and the use of exorcism to free the patient from possession or the use of talismans to ward off evil spirits were variants on medical treatment. Early medicine was relentlessly holistic, treating both body and soul, and even refusing to distinguish them in diagnosis and therapy.

From antiquity to the present, physicians seem to be interested in the natural mechanisms of the body. But the concept of the body as a natural entity is not clear in early history. The body itself was often shielded from inspection by religious codes. Chinese, Greek, and early Roman physicians gained anatomical information from animal cadavers since religious beliefs prohibited cutting into dead human bodies. Often the bodily organs were used in divination. The reliance on livers from sacrificed animals to predict the outcome of illness in Babylonian medicine is typical of such practices.

The basic functions of the body were framed in metaphysical or spiritual vocabularies in early medicine. Hindu culture viewed the body in terms of three elementary representatives of divine universal forces that were later taken into Greek medicine: spirit, phlegm, and bile. Traditional Chinese medicine was developed on the dualistic principles of yin and yang. Yin is the female principle represented by the earth. It is passive and dark. Yang is the male principle. It is active and light, and represented by the heavens. These principles must be in balance in the body for health to be achieved.

Diseases are classified under these two principles as well. Basic physiological processes are specified as proportionate relations fixed by yin and yang. One of the main beliefs today in nutritional treatment of cancer is that tumors can be classified as either yin or yang. Breast cancer, for example, is a yin cancer, while colon cancer is in the yang category. Since yin and yang complement one another, therapy requires "attacking" a tumor with its opposite type of food. Yang foods like root vegetables are supposed to be antagonistic to the yin breast cancer, yin foods like leafy green vegetables are thought to destroy the yang colon tumor. Both of the Loverros are sympathetic to such nutritional therapy.

It is remarkable from a modern perspective that any effective understanding of the human body could be gained from inquiries in which material and spiritual variables are so completely fused. The most profound contributions of early physicians, however, may be in the holistic perspectives that controlled medical practice in antiquity. Historians generally mark the start of the slow and uneven abandonment of magic in medicine to the beginnings of classical Greek philosophy. By the time of Hippocrates (fifth century B.C.) the material causes of disease were beginning to replace supernatural explanations in medicine. But the materialism enlisted by Hippocrates was robust by any standards. He viewed humans in a social and physical context that itself could facilitate or compromise health. He stressed natural cures based on sensible diets, congenial living conditions, and temperate climates. One could say that Hippocrates maintained the cosmic perspectives of ancient medicine in materialistic terms, without the earlier dominance of spiritual causes; and that body and mind were still being treated together, but in more nearly secular terms.

The modern dominance of material explanations in medicine evolved slowly, with abrupt accelerations from scientific discoveries. By the beginning of the nineteenth century, the science of physiology was well established and the human body (with the exception of the brain) had been mapped completely in its gross anatomical form. Medicine was by that time more science than magic, chemistry rather than alchemy. Body had begun to dominate mind in diagnosis and treatment. The most influential philosophy in medicine was the Cartesian separation of mind and body, and a gradual conception of medicine as a practice that addressed those physical mechanisms that seemed governed by natural laws rather than spiritual forces. Even the mind itself was addressed in more or less scientific terms with Freud's development of psychoanalysis in the late nineteenth and early twentieth century, a medical specialty that both supporters and detractors viewed as an effort to study the mind independent of both the body and those supernatural influences assumed in religious discourses.

The synoptic perspectives of antiquity were found in public health movements in the eighteenth century, when the effects of the environment on health and disease began to be appreciated. The sense of community that had infused early Greek life was reintroduced in modern form with the thought that communal efforts are needed to prevent disease and prolong life. But the efforts were not invocations of gods or spirits from an external reality. They were designed to clear the environment of *physical* causes of disease. The commonplace attention to personal hygiene in many religions had unwittingly reduced disease. The modern efforts to cleanse the body and its environment were grounded in a more sophisticated understanding of how filth is related to the transmission of disease. The reduction of insect and rodent populations, the maintenance of a clean water supply, the elimination of waste products from living areas, and mass immunization against disease were collective efforts based on the causal explanations of disease provided by medical science. The United States followed the lead of several European countries in the nineteenth century by establishing a public health service to monitor and implement community health efforts. Countries also began to collect statistical data on morbidity and mortality rates. Modern communal health was grounded in empirical science.

The dispute between the Loverros and Stephen Dubansky mirrors some of the differences between the origins and current state of medicine. The Loverros are invoking the oldest and most enduring refrain in healing with their beliefs in holistic medicine, and they claim scientific status for their views. But these beliefs, and the methods of inquiry that seem to justify them, have been abandoned by a Western clinical medicine that is influenced by modern science. In a sense, both parties in this dispute have experienced the historical rejection of holistic therapy that led to the development of scientific medical practices, the Loverros by a court of law and Dubansky in his medical education and training. The Loverros and Dubansky have played out vital historical transitions in a legal setting.

One observation complicates the dispute over Caleb Loverro's medical care. Medicine is not always straightforward, conventional science. Many therapies in recent medical practice require viewing the patient as a complex amalgam of both mind (or spirit) and body. The healing arts in general summon a variety of visions on health and healing, and these visions typically are drawn up from competing accounts of reality within medicine itself. But these different realities often accommodate both spiritual and scientific vocabularies. Moral discourses may be no more than efforts to negotiate differences among these competing visions and to rank them within therapeutic practices.

Determining the proper care of Caleb Loverro is one instance where holistic and scientific vocabularies are in conflict. The contrasts in therapy are more visible and easier to inspect as a consequence of this mutual hostility. But the moral failure to reconcile spirit and body within medical practice only urges a more extensive inquiry into the scope and logic of healing, and the political and legal imperatives following disputes over the healing arts. Also, since it is reasonably clear that moral responsibility varies from one type of discourse to another, attending to the moral roles of the individuals in these disputes must follow an understanding of the forms of reasoning, and ontologies, that separate views on health and healing.

At stake in these disputes is our understanding of the liberal state. The dream of liberalism is governing with neutral procedures, of finding and using those rules and principles that are outside the domain of values specifying the good life in human communities. In conflicts between holistic and allopathic medical values, the state meets the terms of the liberal ideal with regulations that do not depend on the particular worldviews of either community but rather on a set of procedures that are reasonably empty of substance. Like Hobbes' state-as-umpire, the liberal state is not to be a player in the political game. It is to be an institution separate from the partisan views leading to conflicts over health and healing. However basic and comprehensive the reasoning and sense of reality informing the disputing communities, the liberal state must find some high ground independent of these communities of belief if it is to fulfill its own ideals of impartial governing.

2

SCIENCE AND FAITH

Bork: Medicine as Science

Silas Bork is a physician who believes that the empirical realities of science
are the parameters within which therapy decisions are made. He has a private practice in internal medicine, a designation that several of his peers regard as a euphemism for general practitioner. His patients are drawn from a
wide range of social and economic backgrounds. Anyone entering his office
on a typical afternoon might see a local professional or two, usually professors from the university or attorneys, a day laborer, a senior citizen, a welfare mother, and an array of individuals whose social status is either difficult
to fix or simply anomalous.

Sally Dennison, the nurse who helps Dr. Bork and also doubles as his
receptionist, calls patients by their first name in a policy the doctor believes
relaxes individuals. On this fall day, she scanned the chart she was holding
and called out, "Millie," for the doctor's next appointment.

The "Millie" on this occasion was a heavy dark woman who rose slowly
and moved over to the reception desk.

"Miss." The woman signaled to Dennison.

"Yes?"

"Here's what we'll do. You call me by my last name and I'll call you by
yours."

Sally Dennison was aware of a stillness in the waiting room. She looked
her patient over. "You don't want to be called by your first name?"

"Only by those who love me. And I don't know you well enough for
that yet."

Dennison glanced down at the chart. "Mrs. Fleckman. This way please."

Mrs. Fleckman suffered from cardiac arrhythmia and wore a pacemaker. She was seventy-six years old and had been a commercial artist for forty years. Most of her working day now was devoted to making statuettes that her agent shipped to several stores in New England. She sometimes had to remind her daughter that it was at least a living.

In the examination room Dr. Bork listened to the movements in Mrs. Fleckman's lungs and heart with a stethoscope.

"I think we have a problem here," Dr. Bork said.

"We?"

"There is some congestion in your lungs. And I hear some other things. Probably not serious. But I'd like you to check into a hospital overnight so we can run some tests."

Mrs. Fleckman looked at him and rubbed the left cheek on her face slowly. Dr. Bork's voice was crisp. His lips were thin, and he got to the point too quickly from Millie Fleckman's point of view.

"Is this absolutely necessary?" she asked.

"Absolutely. We want to stay on top of things at your age. Nothing left to chance."

"When?"

"Now. Do you have someone who can drive you over to the hospital?"

"My daughter. She's coming to pick me up here."

"Good. Just go to the reception desk. I'll call over and get you a room. Order some tests. Then I'll stop by tonight."

As Millie Fleckman left the doctor's office she looked up, as she always did, at the birch and plum trees lining the back of the parking lot. On clear days, like this one, she imagined the top of the tallest birch tree as a raging woman with cropped green hair billowing in the wind. On this particular afternoon the wind was blowing hard from the south, turning up the limbs of the trees to expose the pale underside of the leaves.

Mrs. Fleckman found no imaginative visuals in the hospital. She stood glumly by her daughter's side as the receptionist checked her in. She did not bother to look at the pastel paintings along the walls of the hospital corridor. She thought instead of the previous evening when she had carried her groceries up to her apartment and into the kitchen. She had sweated mightily. After putting the perishables away, she had slowly stripped off her clothes and prepared a hot bath. She had sat a long time in the water, letting the heat restore her equilibrium while she sipped scotch neat from a glass.

The feeling of weakness she had felt then, when her hands trembled and she felt both hungry and nauseated at the same time, returned to her now.

She touched her daughter's sleeve. "I'm going to sit down."

"Are you all right?"

Mrs. Fleckman shrugged. She settled in the one gracious chair in the room.

A passing nurse stopped and bent over her. "How do you feel?" The nurse touched Mrs. Fleckman's forehead. "You look a bit faint. Are you feeling okay?"

Mrs. Fleckman felt too tired to answer.

"Larry." The nurse stopped a passing doctor. "Here."

The doctor put his stethoscope on Mrs. Fleckman's chest. After a moment he signaled a nurse, who strapped a device to check blood pressure on Millie Fleckman's arm. Mrs. Fleckman's daughter had by now gone to her mother's side.

The doctor stood up. "Betsy. Get a wheelchair. Or a table. Now." He turned to the receptionist. "Alert E.R. that we're on the way. Possible cardiac arrest."

Mrs. Fleckman saw these movements from an area outside of them, a spectator aware of excitement at some point in the distance. She had felt the flutter of her heart, then an interruption of the cardiac function, then more flutters. An alertness had seized her as she realized the gravity of the moment. Now she felt herself turning inward, away from the light and movement surrounding her, like an envelope folded into smaller and smaller squares until the contents cannot be compressed any further.

Dr. Bork saw Mrs. Fleckman fifteen minutes into the efforts to resuscitate her. She had been without oxygen for only a few minutes after her heart stopped functioning. But after a prolonged resuscitation effort in the emergency room Mrs. Fleckman had a blood pressure in the 50–80 range systolic, in spite of having been given a very high dose of dopamine to maintain blood pressure.

Dr. Bork looked at her closely. She had been unresponsive throughout the resuscitation effort, breathing only with the help of a respirator. Early on the emergency team had put in a right heart catheter to monitor pressures. No one was sure from the tracings whether the external pacemaker she had on was working.

During the fluoroscopy, the X-ray part of the procedures, it became apparent to everyone in the room that Mrs. Fleckman's heart was not beating despite electrical stimulation.

"Her heart is refractory," Bork announced to his colleagues. "It is dead."

He called a halt to the resuscitation efforts. Mrs. Fleckman was brought over to an area of the hospital cordoned off by drapes.

In the waiting room Dr. Bork found Millie Fleckman's daughter. He had known her for a number of years, though only through the many crossings they had when Mrs. Fleckman was his patient.

"Sarah. We need to sit down."

Sarah Fleckman stood with her arms crossed stiffly. "Tell me."

"Your mother's heart has stopped. We cannot do anything more for her. At the moment she is on a respirator, which is breathing for her."

Sarah stared at him. "What are you telling me?"

He described in detail Mrs. Fleckman's condition and the treatment. Then he added, "I don't think there is anything more to be done. It is hopeless. I would like to turn off the respirator."

Sarah Fleckman's eyes were fixed on him. Tears slid soundlessly down her face from behind her glasses.

"So." She kept her arms folded. "This is the way it ends."

"I'm sorry. Do you want to see her? Do you want me to call someone for you?"

Sarah shook her head. She touched Dr. Bork's arm. "Do it. Let her go." She covered her eyes stiffly with one hand. Then she turned and sat down.

Dr. Bork returned to the intensive care area. Millie Fleckman was on one of the beds, eyes closed with the respirator tube attached to her face. The regular opening and closing of the respirator was the only sound in the room. A tube extended from Mrs. Fleckman's lower arm to an IV unit by the bed.

Dr. Bork reached over and moved the respirator switch to zero. Then he turned Mrs. Fleckman's pacemaker off. She continued to breath in shallow gasps on her own. He pulled over a chair and sat watching his patient. After ten minutes he took her blood pressure. The reading showed that the pressure was drifting down. Dr. Bork sat in the chair staring at the black tip of the pen he was holding in his hand.

Two nurses entered the room. They moved cautiously nearer the bed.

Dr. Bork stood up, handing one of the nurses the blood-pressure mechanism. "Keep taking Mrs. Fleckman's pressure. She is a DNR patient."

He left the room. When he returned two hours later, the resident on the floor had declared Mrs. Fleckman dead.

From a taped interview with Silas Bork after his decision:

"The lady was dead. We could have let her stay on the respirator and continue the dopamine. Keep the external pacemaker going and sooner or later she would have stopped responding to the dopamine. I rarely use the word hopeless, but in her case it was truly hopeless. The other component is . . . medically, legally to document in the chart that we spoke to the family, explained everything. Because, in essence, with this lady, we did withdraw major support in stopping a medicine that was keeping her blood pressure up. And taking her off the respirator."

Dr. Bork lights a cigarette, a habit he is unable to break but manages to confine to the privacy of his office.

"Actually, in this case, we found later that the external pacemaker was not even pacing her heart. It was doing sort of CPR. The external pacemaker delivers quite a voltage across the chest. It causes the chest to jump and that was probably the only thing that was pumping blood around. So she was truly at the very, very far end of the spectrum."

The interviewer asks Dr. Bork about the religious beliefs of the family and whether these might have affected the decision to discontinue medical support.

Dr. Bork admits to not knowing their beliefs. But he discusses the possibility of a miraculous recovery.

"Myself, I tend to be a rather religious person. But I see very little place for miracles in this kind of setting when the facts are black and white. When they're grey and I share the same kind of hope that the family does, and if that's looking for a miracle, you can look at it that way. If you're looking for just the one percent of patients, one percent of the cases that are going to make a recovery, that's the same thing. But when the facts are explicit, then I think there's no room for looking for miracles. Because I think that simply prolongs the agony for the family and certainly prolongs the agony for the patient.

"That's one thing. I think, after you've been doing this for a few years, interns and residents grow to learn this—that physicians and nurses—the whole system is very powerful in prolonging life and also very powerful in inflicting pain on terminally ill people. I think you have to be cognizant of that and know when it's warranted and when it's not warranted. . . . I think that you have to realize what you can and what you can't do. Doctors just don't work miracles. I think the patient's family has to know that."

Abbott: Spiritual Healing

A typical contrast with scientific reasoning is illustrated by the miracle James Abbott believes his brother experienced after an auto accident. In the time preceding his brother's accident, Abbott had two experiences that complicated and partitioned his understanding of God. The first, occurring two years before the accident, came at the height of an impassioned argument he was having with one of his close friends. The friend, who was studying to become a priest, wanted to hire a prostitute to instruct him in sexual matters before he took the vow of celibacy. Abbott regarded this as immoral, even as a betrayal of the vocational commitment to priesthood.

The argument had gone on for over an hour when Abbott suddenly began reciting the Lord's prayer. During the prayer a presence seemed to enter the room. This presence was so strong that both Abbott and his friend felt it immediately. Abbott was filled with elation. He knew the Holy Spirit was there in the room with them. The friend was terrified. He crumpled on the floor and began crying. Abbott later remembered the experience as divided between serenity and hysteria. His own feelings were dominated by a joy he still cannot express in words while his friend cowered on the floor in terror.

In the days following this experience Abbott was terribly depressed. His friend, no longer contemplating the secular pleasures of professional sex, instructed him in spiritual loss. "You are experiencing 'the dark night of the soul,'" he told Abbott. "You have experienced God's presence and now you have withdrawn back to the mundane world. It is grief that you feel." Abbott accepted this insight and used it successfully to combat his depression. He now had two new beliefs about God. One was an acceptance of the reality of the Trinity, since he was convinced that the Holy Spirit had made itself known to him. The other was a belief, new for him, in an interventionist God, one who does, in fact, enter human experience.

The second experience occurred two months before the accident. During this time he had begun to try to regain a close relationship with God. He was a graduate student then, trying to complete a curriculum in both law and the social sciences, and the daily demands of his work had kept him from extended personal reflections on spiritual matters. The experience occurred at night. He awoke with the realization, the certainty, that his wife, sleeping with him in the same bed, was not really his wife but instead a monster who would shortly roll over to face him with a wolflike appearance and tear his own face to pieces. He was terrified. Everything in the room was absolutely still. He realized that he had to reach out and touch his wife if he was going to escape this nightmare, the threat that he now believed was real. But as he slowly reached over his wife began growling softly, a sound that he knew was no more than a snore but that now was a sign that some malevolent presence was in the room in his wife's physical form.

It was at that point that he understood the experience as a test, a contest of wills. If he managed to overcome his fear and touch his wife he would win. If he did not, if he tried to escape in sleep, he would be diminished spiritually. After a few more moments of silence and prayer, he reached out and put his hand on his wife's bare shoulder. She immediately rolled over toward him, her face normal and relaxed in sleep. He put his arms around her. At that moment in his life he began to believe in the reality of Satan.

Abbott learned about his brother's accident in a telephone call from his mother. She told him in a matter-of-fact voice that Paul, his younger brother by three years, had been in an auto accident and was in the intensive care ward of the state hospital. Abbott immediately drove to the hospital and met the resident physician in charge of his brother's treatment. The doctor was crisp and precise in describing his brother's condition. The car had over-turned at a high rate of speed early that morning and thrown his brother onto the road surface. He had partially severed vertebrae. The attending physicians wanted to operate to repair and stabilize the vertebrae, fearing the obvious possibility of damage to the spinal cord. But they were reluctant to intervene surgically because of the road burns on his brother's back. The skin had been sheared away in large areas around the fracture. The doctors feared a life-threatening infection of the spinal cord if they cut into these areas to repair the vertebrae. They had immobilized his brother's lower body and were administering antibiotics and fluids intravenously.

A number of his brother's friends were keeping vigil near the intensive care ward. Most wore jackets and jeans. One had on a dark blue suit with a red wool tie. This best-dressed friend approached Abbott and took him over to the side of the hall for a private moment.

"I think we should talk a bit. I'm Carl and I want to ask you to do something."

"You know my brother well?"

"We're in the same dorm on the campus. Same floor."

Abbott studied Carl, looking for some familiar sign or gesture that he might use to understand the connection his brother might have had with him. All he saw were stiff gestures and features that appeared fixed. Only the young man's mouth seemed mobile as he talked.

"I know this priest, a monsignor actually." Carl moved to the right and spoke into Abbott's ear. "He is carrying forward the works of Christ. He can heal. Believe me."

Abbott looked at him again. From inches away Carl's face looked flushed at the nose and cheeks. His forehead and chin were as white as exposed bone.

"I don't follow. Are you suggesting that we bring this priest over to the hospital to see my brother?"

"No. The ceremony, the ritual—whatever it's called—can succeed with a proxy. You can go over to the church in your brother's place."

Abbott walked into Paul's room without responding to this proposal. His brother was dominated by the IV unit alongside his bed. Tubes from the hanging bottles ran into his arm. Paul was asleep, under sedation. When they were children, he had tried out mind experiments on Paul. Abbott had become attracted to the mind-over-matter theories so popular in mass circulation magazines. He would take some ingredients from the kitchen and mix them to produce a substance not easily identified. Then he would tell his brother a story that always followed the same narrative lines in each subsequent iteration of the experiment. His brother, four or five years old during this time, would finger a long blade of uncut grass while Abbott spoke to him in the yard in back of their house. There is this liquid, he would say, that gives people the power to jump further. It is magic. I have been given some of it here and I want you to take it. They would first measure Paul's best jump, roughly stepping it off. Then Paul would drink some of the magic potion. He never failed to jump further. He would seem to levitate over the cut grass until he reached the wooded area at the back, laughing and turning over until he was buried from sight in the high weeds and wild plants. The magic always worked.

Abbott came back out into the hall and gestured to Carl. "Let's go. Now."

Carl seemed surprised. "There is a vigil mass tonight. Wednesday. It's starting now. The healing follows."

"Good." Abbott turned Carl in the direction of the exit. "Let's do it."

The Catholic church where the rites were held was located near the center of the city in a Polish neighborhood. The complex of buildings was immense. Abbott and Carl had to park in a lot across the street from the church. A sign over the lot warned users that the church was not responsible for the safety of vehicles. They both walked quickly down an alley between recreational buildings and entered the main part of the church through a side door. The mass was in progress. Carl whispered to him that Monsignor Crossland, the priest who led the healing, was preaching the homily. Abbott stood just inside the door with Carl. They were directly in front of the confessional booths. The altar was set in the front part of the building under a high yellow arch. The lights in the church were dazzling. Every part of the building seemed to Abbott to be ablaze with a white light. No shadows could be seen anywhere.

Monsignor Crossland was holding a copy of the Bible. He talked in a rambling, personal tone, very much in charge from Abbott's point of view.

"Healing is in the Bible." Pause. "Christ placed his hands on the believer to heal. That's important. The laying on of hands." Longer pause. "That's what we're doing here."

Crossland moved to the side and his voice raised suddenly. "You have to understand. He is Lord." He broke into song, urging the congregation to join him.

He is Lord.
He is Lord.
He is risen from the grave.
He is Lord.

Crossland returned to the pulpit. His voice settled into a droning tone. "Let us pray for those with tumors, with arthritis . . . " He continued with a litany of diseases and disorders. Then he started mentioning proper names. "Let us pray for Larry . . . for Grace . . . for Helen . . . "

Abbott mentioned his brother's name in a silent prayer. He also thought, name my brother and I'll be impressed. After a few more names Crossland asked for a prayer for Paul. Or did he? Abbott could not be sure.

After the mass was completed, the healing began. No one had left the church. Two other priests flanked Crossland as he approached the communion rail. Ushers guided individuals to the front of the church. The first group consisted of elderly people, some who looked seriously ill or infirm. One young man had a wire cage of sorts screwed tight somehow around his head. Abbott could not imagine what problem would require such a remedy, if remedy it be. One woman approached the rail with palsy, and left it with palsy. The healing ritual was conducted with no communication between parishioner and priest. Crossland simply put his hand on the forehead of the individual and, to Abbott, seemed to murmur some phrases while staring straight ahead. Some individuals slowly toppled over backwards, caught by the ushers and lowered to the floor. Others remained standing. Some fluttered and collapsed like loose paper as soon as Crossland touched them. The only sound in the church was the shuffling of bodies as individuals fell, got up, moved into and away from the altar rail. Crossland slowly made his way down the rail, administering, touching, staring.

When Crossland had made his way back to the side of the church where Abbott and Carl stood, Abbott decided to move to the rail. The monsignor had said that belief is what heals. Abbott tried to clear his mind. He was not sure what to concentrate on. Stars. He thought of stars fixed in a blue void. When Crossland touched his forehead, Abbott was aware of warmth and pressure. The pressure slowly forced him back to attendant arms, where he was lowered to the carpeted floor. He remembered to think of his brother as he descended. When he opened his eyes he saw an icon of the Virgin Mary high up on a rail at the left of the altar.

On his way out Abbott asked one of the ushers if there was a rest room in the church. The usher took Abbott by the arm and walked with him to stairs leading to the basement. He told Abbott as they walked down that they were renovating the two towers of the church at a cost of $340,000. He pointed out the men's room at the back near a recreation area and left Abbott to his own ministrations.

Carl was waiting outside when Abbott left the church. They did not speak during the ride back to the hospital.

In the morning the nurses removed the gauze from Paul's back. The skin was normal. There were neither lesions nor scabs. The doctors could not explain how the burns had healed so quickly. The surgery proceeded and was declared a success afterwards by the attending physicians.

From a taped interview with James Abbott after his brother had recovered completely from the accident:

"I believe in faith healing, yes, but not necessarily what everyone else calls faith healing. I believe that people can be healed through their faith or through someone else's faith in Jesus Christ. I don't necessarily believe in the people who go around saying that they have some magical gift that allows them to heal you. There are plenty of people who say they are faith healers whom I have absolutely no confidence in and believe to be charlatans. But I believe that each individual, through certain faith in Christ, can heal. And so I've always had a very, very strong faith and that's a part of it."

INTERVIEWER: How does faith healing work, from your point of view?

"How it works. First look at it from a biblical viewpoint. There is good and evil in the world and our good is represented by God in Jesus Christ. Evil, I suppose, is represented by the figure of Satan—whether a physical entity or not is unimportant. But both have control over the world. And when someone is ill, that act of faith in asking for healing—if your faith is true and you really believe—this physical world can be rearranged."

INTERVIEWER: By?

"God."

INTERVIEWER: Would the request itself be enough?

"No. See, someone who doesn't really believe can request—the important part is the belief of the requester."

INTERVIEWER: Is healing bestowed upon those who are worthy of it? Is there some evaluation imbedded in the . . .

"No. There is absolutely no evaluation of the healing or the worthiness of the person receiving the healing. Again, if I went back and looked at biblical script, there were times when Christ was asked to heal third parties and there is no examination of the third party at all. The examination is of the person who makes the request, and it's the faith of the requester that is the critical issue. Nothing to do with the third party necessarily."

INTERVIEWER: If the faith-healing effort fails, is that proof that the belief was not genuine?

"No. Again, maybe a catch-22. Maybe a way out. You know the old saying: 'All prayers are answered. Sometimes the answer is no.' And that's the way it works. In my experience I would ask for healing for the third party if that was consistent with the will of God. If it would fit into his plan, then I ask that it be done. And so I'm asking, not demanding. It is a request. And open in my mind and understood in my mind is the fact that a request can be denied."

From a taped interview with a physician:

INTERVIEWER: You have an elderly woman who wants not to be resuscitated. Or not continue with the ventilator. She judges that she's lived long enough. She wants to die gracefully rather than with instruments supporting her body. What do you do?

"This is her request?"

INTERVIEWER: Her request.

"So it's her request and she's competent and thinks . . . "

INTERVIEWER: That's the question—how do you determine that she's competent?

"Well, how long have I known this person? If it's your own patient that you've seen for a period of time and you know this person—this person talking the way she's always spoken to you—I would probably remove that patient from the ventilator. If she's a stranger and I have any questions with competency, I probably would ask another physician to address that issue. Also probably a psychiatrist. If we both feel that she's competent to make the decision, I would probably go ahead and follow her wishes."

INTERVIEWER: Suppose your patient—you've known her as a very religious individual—believes that God will intervene and take care of her in critical moments. And offers that as a reason for the discontinuation of aggressive medical therapy. Is that a reason you would accept?

"I'm sure your wording is very careful (laugh). Because if she used the same exact wording, my suspicion would there be . . . is this religious ideation as opposed to the reality of the situation? I'm not sure she has appreciated the reality of the situation of coming off the ventilator—that she'll die. I would question her with just that wording. If I know she's very religious and she said, 'God's going to take care of me, meaning that when I die I'm to go up and be in his hands,' then I'd feel a lot more comfortable with that than with 'Take off the ventilator. God's going to come down and bring me a new set of lungs so I'll be able to breathe after that to stay in this world.' I feel a lot more uncomfortable with that type of communication. (Laugh)"

3

MEDICAL TRADITIONS

Alternative Realities

Beliefs in alternative realities and their healing powers are common features of human experience. Yet it is not always clear what is meant by an alternative reality. In many cultures gods, spirits, veridical dreams, and cosmic events are all dimensions of the natural world, no more supernatural than quarks and quasars are to physicists today. Even within scientific traditions the natural and supernatural are elastic terms that vary with different understandings of the range of sensory experience and the boundaries of reality.

The absence of a fixed line between conventional and alternative realities leads to a variety of distinctions between the secular and spiritual in human experience. Often the secular emerges as a rejection of whatever passes for spiritual at that moment in history. A turn to the secular occurred in ancient Greece with the denial of the Homeric gods and the acceptance of conventions as governors of social relations. The belief that nature is objective, a belief found in different forms in all scientific traditions, is a secular conviction that has contrasted with religious codes at various times in Western history. The Marxist identification of commodity value and the reduction of the sacred to a market vocabulary elevates the secular over spiritual beliefs. But this pattern of background rejection and foreground affirmation is eminently contextual. Temporal or material limits on human experience, and the meaning of nontangible or external realities, are fixed by social conventions. The secular in Aristotle's philosophy, for example, is likely to be regarded as metaphysics when viewed from a Newtonian perspective.

Yet within historical or cultural contexts, the distinction between spiritual and secular can rank among the more important issues in human experience. The Homeric vision of the universe dominated early Greek thought. It described a reality controlled by spiritual forces behind objective events, usually gods who played puzzling and erratic games with humans. Nature was charged with purposes and meanings that could be deciphered with the right codes. The rational individual was someone who tried to comprehend a design outside human intentions and powers, often through the interpretation of "signs" and with mental exercises that were thought to expand the spiritual side of human experience.

The spiritual dimensions of this vision were understood best by its opponents. Ionian philosophers regarded the natural world as an objective reality to be studied in a detached manner. Like modern scientists, including Stephen Dubansky, the Ionians sought explanations of the physical world controlled by observation and conjecture rather than simple desire or religious impulse, and expressible in theories that were in some way generalizable. The result is a form of rational discourse that is scientific in the context of ancient Greece. Rules of inference and evidence are applied to a domain of reality experienced by the human senses and intellect, not to a world entirely or in part inaccessible to human inquiry. Homer's gods had to die a natural death, and did.

These two realities, and the rational discourses following from them, have obviously not extended from early Greek thought to the present time. No one today entertains seriously the possibility that Zeus is the source of lightning bolts, or Aphrodite of love, or that Poseidon is the guardian of the oceans. Our libations are directed toward more modern divinities. Nor are the accounts of the physical world developed in Ionian science the kinds of scientific explanations offered today. Experimental science was almost nonexistent among the early Greeks. The lawlike expressions of modern science are not found in these early theories of the universe. The view of scientific theories as provisional hypotheses to be dismissed as evidence falsifies them is also absent. This would not become a part of scientific thought for over two millennia.

But the divergence and mutual hostility between these two views of reality occur (though in different forms) even today. One reality assumes unseeable dimensions and spiritual purposes, and stresses the use of intuition in reasoning to conclusions. The other takes nature as impersonal, with no evidence of a cosmic design that explains and justifies human experience. These differences, even when wrenched out of historical context or cultural limits, help identify competing rational discourses today. They also illustrate the limits of reasoning. Rational discourse is not likely to resolve the differences between Homeric and Ionian ontologies. The effects flow in the opposite direction. Each of the competing ontologies fixes what is rational by controlling the criteria of evidence and rules of inference assigned to observations and concepts.

These theories of reality lead to different accounts of healing largely because they provide rival accounts of the individual and the contexts in which human beings live. In spiritual versions of reality, the external world and the ordinary world of sensory experience and human thought are in constant contact. Humans are the hybrid creatures positioned somewhere between the animal world and the larger cosmos within which all items are located. In some versions of spiritual thought, powerful forces are said to manipulate reality and grant special favors to those fortunate or gifted enough to please the higher forms of life. In other versions, reality is an objective resource for understanding and healing. But in all versions of spiritual thinking the world revealed to the temporal senses is only one entry in a hierarchy of being. The healing powers of this larger reality are said to be considerable, and they work when the individual is understood as a holistic self within a world that exceeds ordinary human experience.

Scientific thought emphatically dismisses the spiritual from its domain of inquiry. The human imagination is vital for scientific achievement. Anyone studying the changes in science from Ptolemy through Newton and then Einstein and quantum mechanics is bound to be impressed with the almost extraterrestrial efforts of the human intellect. But science still views the orderly or random arrangements of the universe as the way things *are*, with no spiritual dimensions behind this reality. The effects of these convictions on understandings of the individual are decisive in health and healing. Humans are seen as discrete *physical* units in a largely indifferent universe. In medical science, body dominates mind, and therapy is conceived as an effort to alter the physical state of individuals who function separately in secular contexts.

Theories of the real finally control the vocabularies of healing, especially when they vary along a secular-spiritual axis. If one could construct a map to negotiate a way through rival beliefs on health and healing, its baseline would be ontology, or what counts as real. From this line a path would lead to the status of individuals in competing realities, then to different understandings of therapy that follow from competing descriptions of the human person. Finally, the moral and political languages of liberty, privacy, competence, and authority would appear. The first position, though, is reality. It fixes directions for the traveler journeying through the languages of health and healing, and provides the baseline references to justify beliefs about healing acts and possibilities.

Park

Joanne Park can remember the exact moment when she began the intellectual odyssey that led her to the study of medicine. Her high school in California had sponsored its annual "college evening" early in her senior year (1970–71). It was the usual affair. Approximately 250 college representatives occupied booths and rooms to recruit good (and sometimes poor) students to their campuses. Park had made the rounds cafeteria-style to sample the wares in as many presentations as possible. She recalls entering one particular room late in the evening in a state of combined fatigue and boredom. A college representative, a woman in her thirties, was describing her campus. As she continued talking about the intellectual content of the courses, the ratio of undergraduates to graduate students, the importance of the classical texts in education, Park realized that this was the university she wanted to attend. She stepped back outside of the room to see the sign above the door. It was the University of Chicago.

No such decisive moment occurred in Park's later decision to study medicine. She had always been curious about the natural world. As a child she used to visit a pond near her home to study the variety of life forms found in and near the water. She was intensely, almost pathologically, shy when she was young. Much of her youth was a struggle simply to learn how to talk to people in social situations. She slowly acquired these skills as a member of the high school debate team and by working as a waitress in the evenings after school and during the summers. But the natural world was all pleasure and no impediments for her. She enjoyed watching life forms move and trying to understand the biological mechanisms that explain life. This desire to comprehend the natural world, not to heal its pathologies, dominated her studies through primary and secondary school.

Park's interest and obvious talents in biology led some of her teachers to suggest medicine as a career. She also remembers reading a book, *Intern*, by Doctor X, that glamorized the medical profession in certain ways. But mainly Park was thinking about a wide range of careers that would allow her to continue and expand her interests in the natural world. Oceanography was one possibility. Another, since she was active (and good) in sports, was physical instruction of some sort, perhaps leading to a position as a physical education teacher in a school.

The University of Chicago does not permit students to major in a narrow trade or professional discipline. There is technically no "pre-med" major. The goal of education at Chicago is an intellectual experience that requires the student to master a robust arrangement of subjects in any one discipline. So, for example, a major in art and design includes the usual array of practical courses on visual structures, but also requires attending to history and theory of art, politics, philosophy, sociology—all providing enlightenment on the larger cultural and historical settings in which structures are conceived and built. Each of the undergraduate areas of study is defined in this way so that the student is exposed to a comprehensive perspective in any selection of a curriculum.

Joanne Park entered this system in the fall of 1971 and immediately began regarding herself as a genuine intellectual (though she now thinks she was probably the paradigmatic instance of a pseudointellectual). She was sold on profundity. She studied numerous classical texts in her courses, including Plato's *Apology*, Aristotle's *Nichomachean Ethics* and *De Anima*, Descartes's *Meditations*. She argued epistemology, metaphysics, logic, and method with both her instructors and fellow students. To this day she views the Chicago educational approach as special, introducing her to a life of the mind that she does not think she would have encountered on any other campus, in spite of its disproportionate emphasis on abstract thought over every skill (no matter how useful).

Park did manage to take all of the courses needed to be admitted to medical school. These included inorganic and organic chemistry; a year each of physics, calculus, and statistics; and a substantial number of courses in the biological sciences (sufficient at minimum to understand DNA, microorganisms, evolutionary theory, and the like). Still, she was uncertain. The climate of opinion on college campuses at the time (the early 1970s) ruled out a business career, which she found (like most of her peers) disgusting. For a time she thought about law school, and considered a career in journalism after working on the fiction and poetry staff of the student literary magazine, the *Chicago Review*. At the beginning of her senior year, she still felt that she was drifting, but the prospect of medical school had become more real to her as the result of two jobs she had managed to find during her undergraduate years at Chicago.

She found the first job in order to avoid going back home to California the summer after her freshman year. The city of Chicago had begun to interest her as much as the natural world had earlier, though for its cultural advantages rather than for its biological life. The job was a clerical position in an osteopathic hospital on Chicago's south side. She mainly typed forms and met people from socioeconomic classes she had never encountered while growing up white and middle class in California. Almost all of the patients were on welfare. The interaction between patients and staff was predictably complex, since all of the medical personnel were white and male. They were largely individuals who had failed to get into a standard medical school and had chosen osteopathic training as an alternative to attending a foreign medical school. Osteopathic medicine emphasizes the manipulation of bones in therapy. But the hospital where Park worked was staffed with no-nonsense doctors who used the best of Western medical techniques to treat patients. It was similar to standard health facilities with the exception that the medical staff was more inclined to focus on the whole person in treatment than would typically be the case in a conventional hospital.

One day the medical staff was particularly busy when a woman came running into the hospital screaming. She had her hands over her eyes and was obviously in great pain. The man with her said that she had been on her back porch when a neighbor had thrown a bottle against the wall of the porch. It had broken and its contents had splattered all over the woman. Unfortunately, the bottle had contained a lye solution that was burning up the skin on the woman's face and the tissues in her eyes. All of the doctors were busy at that moment with even graver emergencies, and so Park took the woman upstairs to another section of the hospital. Her one thought was to get the woman's clothes off and get her under a shower. She remembers that the woman kept crying "my eyes, my eyes." Park didn't know anybody on the floor when they got off the elevator, but she started shouting orders to people, get the woman under a shower, put her face in the cold water, then ran back downstairs to talk to the doctors. They told her, "Fine, fine you are doing the right thing, go back upstairs and make sure she gets her eyes open, irrigate them, wash the lye out." She ran back upstairs and finally got the woman sufficiently clear of lye that she was no longer screaming in pain.

Two weeks later the woman was discharged, and Park had a chance to see the results of her efforts and the medical treatment the woman had received while in the hospital. One eye was not too good, but the other eye had substantially healed. Park had the feeling that maybe what she did had made a difference, even though she knew her actions had been on the periphery of medical practice.

The second job was in the emergency room of Billings Hospital, adjacent to Wyler Children's Hospital and, with Wyler, part of the University of Chicago's hospitals. The pay was better, even though the work was very similar, and the area of the city was safer. But the intensive-care medical needs were greater. Often the entire waiting room would be filled, and black people would be calling Park a white honky bitch because their grandmother (or somebody) wouldn't be able to see a certain doctor right away. At other times an ambulance would bring in someone who was near death—a car had fallen on them or something—and a blood transfusion had to be arranged immediately. Park would be the person running down the hall of the hospital, getting the blood supplies and bringing them back to the emergency room.

It was exciting. It was also mysterious. Even though she was working there, a big piece of the action was always going on behind the closed doors of the emergency room. She later described the experience as living a story she couldn't put down, a gut-level attraction to events that was more real than anything she encountered at the University of Chicago. Undergraduate school was the life of the mind, which the curriculum counterpoised to the life of the body. Working in the emergency room was the life of the body. The high it brought on seemed endless while she was there.

Even in slack times she saw the hospital as a realm of very competent, knowledgeable, self-assured people (for the most part). The nurses seemed as good as the doctors. She made friends with many of the staff, dated a few of them, played tennis with some. Then one day she was playing tennis with a doctor, talking to him between sets about his decision to become a doctor. She remembers him looking away and tracing a bead of perspiration from behind his ear down under his chin around the front of his neck. "Look," he said abruptly, "do something else. You don't understand what it means to be a doctor. You'll hate it. Don't go to medical school. I hated it. I hate my residency. I can't stand this even though I want to be a doctor. Think about doing something else."

Park thought he was crazy. She didn't believe a word he said. She assimilated his remarks to the thoughts one of the doctors at the osteopathic hospital had shared with her. "You might as well not go to medical school," he had told her. "Women doctors do not practice medicine. They always wind up getting married and having babies. Then they quit medicine. So why do it? Forget it. Go into something else." Naturally these views simply made her more determined to pursue medicine.

By the end of the fall semester of her senior year, Park had applied to five medical schools—Chicago, Yale, Columbia, the University of California, and British Columbia (because she had heard on good authority that Vancouver was an "absolutely wonderful place to live"). She cannot remember any specific decision she made to become a doctor. Her thoughts, and goals, simply evolved in that direction. Yale turned her down. Chicago and California admitted her. Columbia and British Columbia put her on waiting lists. She decided to go to the University of California. It was a respectable medical school and less expensive than any other school she had considered. Also, four years away from home had mellowed her attitudes toward her parents. She was the youngest child, and her parents were older than the parents of her peers in college. She had no idea how much longer they were going to be around. It seemed like a good time to mend fences.

Medical Practices

The profession that Joanne Park began studying in the fall is regarded by most of its members as an enlightened practice that must be on guard against superstitions originating in a mystical and discredited early history. The "progress" story of medicine is well known. Every nurse and doctor has heard it. Park can recite it almost from memory. It provides the background against which the anomalous and even mysterious events of spiritual healing and nonstandard medical intervention can be measured.

The narrative is most impressive when it offers an account of scientific developments in the twentieth century, after medicine had recognized, and subscribed to, the scientific programs that took it away from earlier orientations toward spiritual healings. Most historians of medicine stress four advances in the first half of the twentieth century that define medicine as it is practiced today: drug therapy, immunization, the development of endocrinology, and extended and more reliable knowledge of nutrition and the effects of exercise.

Drug therapy is so effective in treating bacterial disease that it is now a commonplace, prescribed so often that medicine is unimaginable without it. A German scientist, Paul Ehrlich, was the first to show the selective bonding of some tissues with certain chemicals. His discovery that arsphenamine is an effective treatment for syphilis was based on this chemical theory. Sulfanilamide was later demonstrated to be successful in treating some streptococcal infections. More dramatic, however, was the 1928 discovery of penicillin by Alexander Fleming in London. Since that time, medicine has discovered or developed (synthetically) over seventy-five antibiotics to treat bacterial diseases.

Diseases caused by viruses have been largely untouched by drug therapy. Success in treating viral infections has been achieved largely through immunizations. The current spread of AIDS in the world is incomprehensible to many people, in part because viral epidemics are now rarer, though extremely deadly. The influenza pandemic of 1918–19 killed twenty million people. Vaccinations, however, have eliminated most of the more lethal viral infections. Smallpox vaccine, developed in the late eighteenth century (even before viruses were known), has eradicated one of the deadliest diseases in history. In 1967, for example, two million people worldwide died of endemic smallpox. After a decade of immunization efforts by the World Health Organization, the disease had been completely eliminated from human populations. The last case of endemic smallpox occurred in October 1977. Typhoid, tetanus, diptheria, whooping cough, and measles vaccines have reduced these diseases to minimal levels in much of the world. Many Western doctors regard pediatrics as a dull profession precisely because the serious diseases of childhood have been eliminated through immunizations. Neither immunization nor effective treatment, however, exists for AIDS.

Endocrinology, or the study of the ductless glands (such as the thyroid and adrenal glands) and their secretions, was almost nonexistent before the twentieth century. But it is a field of medical science that has yielded two of the most important therapies in medical history. One is insulin, isolated in 1921. Insulin is a hormone that has been used to change diabetes from a death sentence into a manageable illness. The other is cortisone, a hormone isolated in 1935 and used as an anti-inflammatory agent in treating arthritis and other diseases. A third discovery does not count as therapy, but it is the main instrument of change for sexual practices throughout the world. The study of sex hormones in the 1960s led to the marketing of a drug that prevents ovulation. Sex, risky since the beginning of time, suddenly became separable from procreation. Women could now prevent conception by ingesting pills on a regular basis. More recently, the development of RU486, a compound that prevents the fertilized ovum from attaching to the uterine wall, introduces yet another species of birth control by aborting pregnancies in the embryonic stage.

Twentieth-century medical science has also provided us with wide and accurate knowledge of nutrition and exercise and their relationships to health and illness. Hippocrates sensed the importance of food in health and offered rudimentary observations on the importance of a balanced diet. But diet is a precise science in contemporary medicine. We know the effects of specific products on the body—animal fats, for example, on cholesterol levels (and the effects of these levels on cardiac functions), or the power of certain vegetables and fruits to reduce the likelihood of cancer. The effects of exercise on the heart, lungs, and blood pressure are also well known. Numerous studies have also identified toxic products, like cigarettes, and charted the effects of ingesting such products on mortality rates. Vitamins, a form of synthetic nutrition also developed in this century, are used to supplement the diets of both the needy and those who eat too well anyway.

The macrobiotic diets that the Loverros wanted to use to treat Caleb's leukemia are restorations of earlier strictures on nutrition. George Ohsawa, a native of Japan, is recognized as the modern originator of macrobiotics. In recent years he has attributed cancer (and other maladies, including mental illness) to the ingestion of refined sugar and excess animal protein. His nutritional therapy emphasizes rice, whole grain cereals, and small amounts of vegetables, legumes, and other foods, a regimen he has said can restore harmony between the individual and the evolutionary order. According to Ohsawa, this harmony can cure cancer. Medical authorities are inclined to view these claims as the dark side of medical therapy, pointing out that the "cure" is nothing more than the traditional Japanese diet, which originated centuries ago. More recent macrobiotic diets urge proportionate amounts of certain foods. A standard diet might consist of 50–60 percent whole cereal grains, 21–25 percent vegetables, 5–10 percent beans and sea vegetables, and 5 percent soups. Fluids are to be taken only in very small amounts, since (according to Zen principles) the kidneys must not be overworked.

The use of nutritional therapy, according to proponents of macrobiotics, will cure the patient without need of medicine, radiation, or—of crucial importance—surgery. The macrobiotic view is that cancer is the organism's effort to achieve balance. To remove the tumor surgically would destroy the possibility of equilibrium. Better to treat cancer through the holistic approach of nutritional therapy rather than the barbarous cut of the knife. But to believers in medical progress, the traditional and even anachronistic orientation of nutritional therapy in cancer treatment is most clearly exhibited in the resistance to surgery. The most decisive progress in medical treatment has been made in surgical techniques, which were particularly crude methods in early medical practice. Surgeons believe nutritional therapists ignore this medical progress by confusing the modern operating room and its sophisticated equipment with the clumsy operators of ancient medical practices.

Surgeons were often barbers in early medical practice, and it is an open question which skill most benefitted the patient. Hindu physicians in 800 B.C. were equipped (or armed) with twenty sharp and 101 blunt instruments. A modern doctor in a satisfactory hospital has considerably more resources. The surgeon performing gallbladder surgery today, for example, has 139 instruments on hand. A hernia operation typically will be carried out with 103 instruments in the operating room. A wide selection of technological devices has dramatically reduced surgical risks, including X-ray machines, cautery equipment, electrocardiographs, O_2 and CO_2 monitors, mass spectrographs, pulse oximeters, anesthesia machines, monitors for urine output and body temperature, arterial and venous lines, esophageal monitors, IV units, and more.

One of the crucial improvements in surgery was the prevention of infection by asepsis, a set of techniques designed to free the operating room and its occupants of all pathogenic organisms. Though the stress on hygienic treatment can be traced to early Greek and Roman medical practices, aseptic techniques were systematically developed in the late nineteenth century. These methods include the now familiar routines of "scrubbing up," sterilizing instruments, and wearing sterile rubber gloves in surgery.

Unfortunately, many physicians resisted modern hygienic methods through the early part of this century. The tardy adoption of even general cleanliness and hand washing led to deplorable outcomes in some areas of medicine. When physicians replaced midwives in birthing practices, epidemics of puerperal fever occurred simply because physicians refused to take even basic antiseptic methods seriously. Forceps were particularly deadly instruments of bacterial contamination. In New York City during the nineteenth century, maternal mortality increased to rates far beyond those found in midwifery birthing practices until physicians accepted rudimentary (and well-known) methods of cleanliness for preventing infection. (This acceptance occurred, ironically, at about the time antibiotics were developed to combat bacterial infections.) The unfortunate truth is that scientific developments were sometimes introduced successfully to early medical practices only after prolonged, and sometimes tragic, delays.

Two of the greatest obstacles to successful surgery—pain and shock—have been overcome with modern medical techniques. Spinal block and general anesthesia have replaced crude drugs like alcohol in shielding the patient from pain in surgery, so that surgery today causes the patient little pain or even discomfort during the operation. Shock was a phenomenon little understood until recently. All that was known in the past was that the body frequently reacts badly to physical trauma, including surgical interventions, and sometimes the result is a severe drop in blood pressure and rapid depression of vital functions. Death can be the unfortunate result. Shock was successfully treated with blood and saline transfusions. Few operations are performed today without a supply of blood products in the operating room.

Surgical intervention is widely used today to treat illness, from relatively simple removals of appendixes and gallstones to the excision of cancer and the correction of major physiological defects. The most frequently performed surgeries in a typical hospital identify the remedial complaints of civilized life. Those performed on an outpatient basis are myringotomy (treatment of the ear), dilation and curettage (D&C), and cataract removal. Among the more frequent surgical interventions that require at least an overnight stay in a hospital are total abdominal hysterectomies, cholecystectomy (gallbladder removal), scleral buckle with implant (retinal repair), transurethral prostatectomy, appendectomy, vitreous removal (removal of vitreous fluid from the eye), intervertebral disc excision, and mastectomy. (Notice the concentration on eye surgery in medical treatment today, an intervention particularly barbarous in earlier medical practices.)

Perhaps the most theatrical of surgical interventions is cardiac surgery. Damage to the heart, whether from congenital defect, disease, or injury, was first successfully repaired in the early nineteenth century. Recent cardiac surgery, however, has exceeded the ambitions of even the most imaginative expectations of medicine. Surgeons now treat heart disease, especially clogged arteries, by constructing bypass vessels. In 1967, a South African surgeon, Christiaan Barnard, became the first person to transplant a human heart. The locus of the human person (in some philosophies) had been transferred from one body to another. Surgery has clearly exceeded the mystical powers of spirits in early medical beliefs.

It is the poor historian who imposes a progress mentality on historical data. But it is difficult for medical students to avoid the conclusion that much, though not all, of the history of medicine is an evolution of understanding and treatment from erroneous beginnings to enlightened states. Physicians in the Western world today no longer regard securing health as simply an intuitive exercise, or dependent on the well-being of gods. The gurus of health, a wide assortment of types, are secular practitioners who rely on scientific knowledge. The lay individual, in turn, can have an understanding of medicine, nutrition, and exercise beyond the conceptual reach of even the most sophisticated physician of the distant past.

Health and Disease

A subterranean story of medicine also invites our attention. It departs from the enlightenment accounts at two points. One is the bizarre and sometimes compelling paths taken by deviant medicine, especially where those medical practices that died a natural death in history were still more humane and reasonable for brief periods of time than "enlightened" practice.

The tradition of homeopathic medicine is an instructive case study. In the late eighteenth century Western physicians practiced what has been called "heroic medicine." Treatment of almost every ailment consisted of bloodletting, often accompanied by large doses of mineral drugs and various purgatives to cleanse the body. Benjamin Rush urged his medical students at the University of Pennsylvania at the turn of the century to stay the course on bloodletting, stressing its therapeutic benefits while scoffing at the possibility of bleeding patients to death (even though an empirical study of bleeding in the 1820s, conducted in a Paris hospital, showed no beneficial effects from the practice). Bloodletting was effected by opening a vein and allowing small and sometimes quite large amounts of blood to escape from the body. Leeches were used for more modest removals of blood.

George Washington, afflicted with a severe sore throat on what turned out to be the last day of his life, was bled three times during the single day of December 14, 1799. The first bloodletting removed a pint of blood. The second, a few hours later, let another pint flow from Washington's veins. By mid-afternoon, a consultation among three physicians led to the removal of a further quart of blood. The president died that evening between ten and eleven o'clock. His medical care was at the highest level of quality for the historical period. One is not certain who is heroic in such therapies, the doctor or the patient.

Homeopathy was conservative by contrast. It was founded by a German physician, Samuel Christian Hahnemann, in the late eighteenth century. Hahnemann encouraged natural cures from diet, exercise, and fresh air rather than the heroic measures of conventional medicine. In a series of controlled experiments he arrived at two principles that later defined homeopathy. One was the law of similia, according to which disease is cured by drugs that produce the symptoms of the illness in a well person. The second was the law of infinitesimals. This law stated that the smaller the amount of a drug ingested, the more effective it is as therapy.

Homeopathy flourished as the main rival to mainstream "allopaths" (Hahnemann's term, which stuck) in the United States through most of the nineteenth century. Homeopathy colleges were formed, and a profession of homeopathic medicine grew steadily through the first half of the century. Much of the success of this deviant alternative was due to the excesses of conventional allopathic medicine, and many of the early homeopaths were regular physicians defecting from the standard therapy of bloodletting and purgatives. Homeopathic principles and practices were more effective in those conditions, such as the cholera epidemic of 1849, in which the patient was better able to combat infection if blood was not released from the body. Also the law of similia was a rough facsimile of the physiological principle underlying immunization. Mainly, however, homeopathy was more humane in its harmlessness, fulfilling at least the ancient Hippocratic maxim requiring the doctor to do no harm to his patients.

Joseph Loverro accepts homeopathic philosophies and techniques. He believes that, with exacting standards and reasonable care, a "mother tincture" can be produced from the extract of an herb or mineral. The care in preparation extends to the time when the plant is removed from the earth, its physical condition, how it is crushed. He claims that homeopathic methods include the use of liquid chromatography and various other spectral analyses to confirm that the active ingredients sought are in the plant in the correct amounts.

Once the mother tincture is produced, there are two other homeopathic methods crucial to preparing the therapeutic solution. One is dilution (developed by Hahnemann). Loverro believes that the ratio of tincture to the liquid (usually water, sometimes alcohol) fixes the remedy for some part of the body. For example, six parts per one hundred parts of water will be a medicine for the sixth part of the intestine. The second method is mixture. The tincture must be shaken with the water one hundred times whenever it is dissolved. Dilution without mixing the required number of times would not be effective. The mixing is thought to be needed to activate various vibrational forces or energies in the compound. If mixed properly, the vibrational energy of the tincture would still be present even when it is in such small amounts that no molecules of the tincture can be discerned in laboratory tests. It is this energy that is released with therapeutic effects, Loverro believes, even from toxic substances (like spider and snake poisons) that would kill the patient if present in physically significant portions.

Homeopathy declined in importance largely because mainstream medical practice abandoned its heroic measures and devised new practices. Conventional medicine evolved through scientific experiment and technological development while homeopathy remained a static practice that insisted on the efficacy of its two founding laws, even when experiments discredited them. One also should not discount the greater efficiency and specialization of contemporary medicine, which permits the physician to diagnose and treat more rapidly than homeopathy allows. A more effective (and profitable) method for practicing a trade or profession is likely, ceteris paribus, to dominate a more deliberative approach.

The alternative story, however, denies the smooth ascent of medicine from primitive beginnings to enlightened practice. It calls attention to those pockets of time in which therapy later proved to be useless was more effective and humane than the best efforts (and barbarisms) of standard medical practice.

A second departure from enlightenment histories is found in the recognition that contextual limits control medical vocabularies. It is an axiom in medicine that health is a desirable state of affairs at any time and in any place, disease a condition to be avoided or cured. But "health" and "disease" are exceedingly complex terms with elastic features. They are "open textured," meaning that they bend and stretch in different circumstances, and they are embedded in medical practices in multiple, and sometimes overlapping, ways.

One indication of the open texture of medical vocabularies is the variation in understandings of health and disease in Western history. The Greeks viewed health as a balance or harmony within the body, and between the body and the natural and social worlds. Disease, whether caused by nature or divine forces, was any disturbance of this balance. Christianity elevated the spirit over the body, and health was elaborated in terms of spiritual integrity. Physical disease could be viewed as a crucible that cleanses and expands the spirit. The Cartesian separation of mind and body favored a mechanistic view of health, analogous to a well-functioning machine. Disease was accordingly a disorder in the mechanisms of the body that could be repaired only by mechanical intervention. Statistical studies of illness in modern medicine lead to a concept of health that relies on an average, the condition of a typical individual in society. Modern medicine tolerates both health and disease as natural conditions occurring within a range of bodily states.

More recent understandings consider health to be the normal state of the body when it is free of disease. Disease is a deviation from the normal state caused by some reciprocal action between an external agent (for example, a virus) and the internal regulatory mechanisms of the organism. Contained in this view is a concept of the body as a living organism capable of homeostasis. Disease, in turn, is traceable to the effects of pathological agents on this homeostatic system. A more comprehensive definition of health can be drawn from the rights languages of current political societies and the high expectations medicine has produced. In the words of the World Health Organization, health is "a state of complete physical, mental, and social well-being and not merely the absence of disease or infirmity."

One way to begin exploring these (and other) understandings of health and disease is to identify single statements that are consistent with all medical beliefs. Here are some candidates: Health is a condition predicated of living humans, not dead or hypothetical humans. It is an enabling or instrumental good in the sense that it is needed for other goods. Put simply, being healthy is usually helpful in acquiring other desirable items (like education, love, freedom). Health is a mixed good: it is both moral (depending on what we do to and for ourselves) and nonmoral (a natural state that can be beyond our powers). Health is also intrinsically individual, not a predicate assignable to groups or collective arrangements. Finally, health is, all things considered, what traditional philosophy calls a good in itself. We notice when it is missing, we would normally prefer its presence to its absence, and it gives us benefits (good feelings, surely) in and of itself.

Accepting these basic statements, however, does not avoid the open texture of both health and disease. Here are some complicating thoughts: Health is not the goal simply of medicine; other practices also aim to produce and sustain health. Nutritionists of all varieties provide advice on how to secure health; few are medical doctors. Marginal members of the medical profession, like chiropractors, devote all of their professional energies to the health of their clients. Of even greater importance, an impressive range of nonmedical associations help individuals to get and stay healthy. Alcoholics Anonymous is one of the most effective of these groups. The success of AA in restoring health to individuals at the lowest points of their lives is well known. Yet AA is not a medical profession (though it has treated numerous physicians for alcohol abuse).

Nor do physicians have as a singular goal the restoration of health or the elimination of disease. Sometimes a doctor's patients are in splendid health. Obstetricians treat pregnant women whose pregnancies are often testimony to their youth and vitality. Sports doctors administer to athletes who may be paradigm specimens of physical health. Hospices have evolved in modern medical settings as arrangements to care for the hopelessly sick and dying who have no prospect of regaining health. In these practices, physicians simply provide comfort by helping to relieve suffering. Plastic surgeons restore or confer beauty on their patients, not health (except tangentially). Then there are the multiple services that doctors perform in any society that have little or nothing to do with health, such as confirming death and signing death certificates for the legal system, communicating information to the police (reporting on bullet or stab wounds, communicable diseases, child abuse), screening candidates in a variety of practices by administering physical exams. Doctors also teach, consult, serve on panels, make money, and sometimes doctor for state purposes, which occasionally includes assisting in capital punishment by supervising and even carrying out executions.

More interesting is the web of relations between health and disease, and the mixed connections of either concept to individual well-being and success. Some diseases do not immediately or directly compromise the functional effectiveness of individuals. A high cholesterol count, for example, is what might be called a laboratory disease. It may or may not lead to later heart trouble, and it need not subtract from an individual's sense of well-being in the present (unless he or she worries about it). Sometimes social values assign importance and even high standing to disease. Epilepsy was the sacred disease of the pre-Socratic Greeks, so that a grand mal seizure could be celebrated as a sign of spiritual intervention. Tuberculosis was romanticized in eighteenth- and nineteenth-century Europe as an expression of sensitivity and intelligence. In his novel *Love in the Time of Cholera*, Gabriel García Márquez describes a city in which the water in the cisterns was honored as the cause of scrotal hernia. His character Juvenal Urbino, when in elementary school,

> could not avoid a spasm of horror at the sight of men with ruptures sitting in their doorways on hot afternoons, fanning their enormous testicle as if it were a child sleeping between their legs. . . . but no one complained about those discomforts because a large, well-earned rupture was, more than anything else, a display of masculine honor.

Later, as a physician, Dr. Urbino encounters resistance to his efforts to enrich the water supply with minerals "for fear of destroying its ability to cause an honorable rupture."

The most intriguing dimensions of disease are those that connect it to the capacity of individuals to act. Artists are often described as having thin psychic membranes, porous shields between the self and the larger world. This unsettling absence of protection may be a physical or psychological defect necessary for artistic insight and achievement. Similarly, megalomania may be an important, perhaps vital, condition for success in some areas of public life (politics, perhaps). Some forms of severe neurological disorder seem to provide the conditions on which strange (and usually worthless) talents thrive. The idiot (or autistic) savant is a classic example of a neurological disorder whose special manifestation includes an uncanny ability to master sequences of numbers. Oliver Sacks, in *The Man Who Mistook His Wife for a Hat*, describes an autistic artist whose selective and eerie depictions of concrete scenes on canvas were in part representations of his neurological deficits. The very absence of a capacity to learn verbal skills had permitted an extraordinary development of visual-spatial skills.

It is too easy to press the functional aspects of disease to unpleasant and distorting levels. Most diseases are dysfunctional, which is one reason why we so value health. But it is also important to note the occasional mixed blessing of disease, not so much as a challenge that might inspire inordinate and admirable efforts to succeed, but as a simple condition for a range of valuable gifts. Newton's irascible and eventually crippling temperament may have been an integral part of his powerful intellect. But in paying homage to the darker sides of genius it is also probably helpful to remember the seamless good spirits of other extraordinary individuals, like Einstein, whose genius seemed unencumbered by either psychic or physical disorders.

If we view health as the primary end of medicine and accept a minimalist definition of health as the restoration of individuals to a positive state of organismic functioning, then we must also accept a wide assortment of secondary aims in medicine that can vary with cultural differences. But the crucial consideration is that the terms "health" and "disease"—even as minimalist concepts—are dependent on historical conditions. What it means to be in a state of physical functioning can change as time and circumstances change. Disease itself is not always a negative physical state in all times and places.

The effect that this more complex view of health and disease has on the enlightenment story of medicine is itself complicated. The simple linear account of progress cannot be maintained. If an area of human experience is said to be getting continuously better, then the terms that mark progressive improvement must be reasonably fixed. A medical improvement that increases longevity, for example, can be regarded as progress only if a longer life span is always valued over briefer lives. But that fixed quality is precisely what may be missing in any realistic history of medicine. Even the value of a long life is rated according to a variety of other conditions, such as whether a culture accepts the reality of a life after death, or what kind of material conditions are reasonably assured over the time needed to live a human life.

The contextual quality of medicine is also put into relief. The language of medicine seems to be relentlessly subjective, not an explanation of reality so much as a set of linguistic background influences. According to the subterranean view, medicine is embedded in culture, not its external measure of progress. The signal that medicine is constructionist rather than fixed and universal is the elasticity of its controlling vocabulary. If "health" and "disease" admit various and sometimes contrary interpretations, then medicine itself must be within the social discourse of time and place, not somewhere outside of it.

The errors of antiquity that were later corrected by medical science are primarily in the areas of diagnosis (including both recognition of disease and understanding its origins) and therapy. Yet there is still dispute over the actual causes of disease and its treatment, most famously generated by religious communities engaged in folk medicine or faith healing. The main disputes in the history of medicine, however, are conceptual, centering on the meanings of health, disease, and perhaps even medicine itself.

Professions

The practice of medicine is a profession, not a trade, labor, occupation, craft, or job. A profession is, ideally, a way of life, often linked to vocational commitments (or callings). Most definitions of a profession identify it as a special activity that promotes discrete goods serving some deep and enduring need of society. Professionals are specialists who claim to know more about the good that is being promoted than members of other groups do, and, as a consequence of such specialized knowledge and the skills needed to implement it, supervise themselves.

The relationship of most professionals to the state, and to other professional associations, is a negotiated one. The profession controls the criteria for what counts as specialized knowledge and skills, the standards that define the level at which professional services will be rendered, the education needed to perform the services, and the ethical principles governing the profession. The state, in turn, licenses professionals and, in doing so, separates genuine from bogus practitioners. The general test of due process is typically the only requirement the state imposes on the discretionary authority of professionals to recognize and monitor their own activities.

The education that medical doctors undergo in most parts of the Western world today is prolonged and demanding. Almost all medical schools stress a kind of empirical training that combines theory and practice. Observation and reasoning from data on the basis of established knowledge are the guiding rules of modern medicine. A pre-med undergraduate who typically takes courses in physics, chemistry, and biology is preparing for extended work in anatomy, physiology, biochemistry, and pharmacology in medical school. Each of these latter courses usually contains laboratory work designed to allow the student to practice scientific methods of reasoning.

The medical school curriculum, traceable to Galen, is traditionally organized in terms of the structure of the body, usually requiring work in anatomy and also including histology (the study of normal tissues) and embryology; the functions of the body, represented by courses in physiology, biochemistry, and pharmacology in addition (often) to a course or two in biophysics; and the agents of disease and their effects on the human body, studied in subjects like bacteriology, immunology, pathological anatomy, parasitology. Courses in public health, medical psychology, biostatistics, and (more recently) medical ethics are also usually part of the medical curriculum today. This curriculum requires four years to complete and leads to an M.D. degree.

Clinical education follows the completion of course work. Doctors in the

United States must spend at least one year working in a hospital as an intern after conferral of the M.D. degree. The newly minted doctor almost always follows this internship with two to five more years of residency training in a medical specialty. This clinical education allows the doctor to apply the theory gained in course work and more important, to learn inductively, from experience with actual cases, what the practice of medicine is all about.

After completion of residency training, the doctor must secure a license to practice. Licensure is controlled by boards in each state in the United States. The state boards administer exams that a doctor must take to obtain a license. If successful, the licensed doctor is considered prepared to enter medical practice, either as a private physician alone or (more common now) in group practice, as part of a national or state health system (as in the United Kingdom), or in some other medical role, such as teaching in a medical school, working for institutions like college infirmaries, the military, insurance companies, the state, and so on.

The professional standards of medicine are designed to ensure both competent and ethical practice (and frequently the two are one, for an unethical physician is usually not acting competently). The ethical foundations of medicine were first set out in the Hippocratic oath, much referred to today and probably infrequently studied. It bids the physician (among other things) to benefit rather than harm the patient, to prescribe no deadly drugs, to refuse assistance in abortions, and to maintain confidentiality with patients. At least one of these provisions, the proscription of abortions, is regularly violated today, and two others—the ban on deadly drugs and the maintenance of confidentiality—are open issues. The first provision is addressed in ongoing discussions of whether passive and even active euthanasia can be justified in current medical practice. The second has always been qualified by the state in various ways, for example, in the physician's legal obligation to report gunshot and knife wounds as well as diseases quarantined by the state. The debate between social need and confidentiality has been reopened recently in the context of the physician's responsibility (or not) to inform an AIDS patient's intimates of the disease.

But the restricted scope of the Hippocratic oath does not indicate ethical impoverishment in medicine. A code of ethics informs medical practice in all of its variations. Physicians cannot doctor to kill or generally aim to harm their patients deliberately. Nor can physicians engage in practices other than medicine with their patients, for example seduction. Physicians are also bound not to use relationships with their patients for financial gain only, nor to break any of a number of conventional moral rules, like promise-keeping, truth-telling, and the like.

The most important ethical features of medical practice, however, may be found in the areas where ethics and competence intersect. A physician lacking certain virtues, for example patience, may on that deficiency alone be incompetent to diagnose illness with reasonable accuracy. The physician who has not acquired adequate knowledge or skills is also incompetent to practice, and in trying to practice medicine would be acting unethically toward his patients. There is often, in short, no distinction between ethics and competence, for ethical practice requires competence from the practitioner, and competent practices require the presence of certain virtues.

Park

Joanne Park did not do well in medical school at first. She took a part-time job in a microbiology laboratory immediately upon entering the University of California. The combined work load of a full medical curriculum and the lab job was too much for her. She failed three of her first four exams, and got a "C" grade on the only exam she passed. She hated the school and the study of medicine. At a meeting with the male dean of the medical school, he tried to interpret her difficulties (she cried during the meeting) in "female" terms, asking her if she needed to see a good gynecologist.

She quit her job at the lab and began taking her courses more seriously. Medical school, after the lofty abstract work at Chicago, seemed to Park like a glorified mechanics school. Students had to learn about all the moving parts of the body, how this part goes up and down, what makes parts turn around, how fuel goes into the machine and what happens when the fuel lines clog up. Memorization dominated the early work. Park was particularly bad at pharmacology. At Chicago she had worked out a mnemonic system for remembering things. It required thinking about the first letter or couple of letters in a word, then reconstructing the word from its beginnings by recalling the syllables attached to the opening letters. The system did not work in pharmacology because there were so many drugs with the same prefixes and so many different chemical reactions that she couldn't systematize what followed the opening letters of anything. She discovered that her intellect was primarily synthetic, which didn't help much during the first two years of medical school. Students had to sit down and cram information into their brains, simply memorize the material segment by segment.

She remembers the experience as being awful. For the first time in her life she became a real student, meaning (to her) a drudge. During the week off before exams she would read and study all day until about eleven o'clock in the evening. Then she would put the books down by the side of the bed on the floor, go to sleep, get up early the next morning, pick the books up and read for two hours, get out of bed to start the coffee, get back into bed, read and study some more, finally get dressed some four hours after awakening. She would follow this schedule until the exam, then come back to start all over for the next exam. The only relief she gave herself was watching "Saturday Night Live" on weekends. She began passing her courses, though the only "A" she got in the curriculum of preclinical medicine was in the mechanisms of disease (the first course requiring students to put information together in a causal chain, in this case from symptoms to disease to therapy).

Once Park began clinical study she found the work both more interesting and (at first) awkward. The medical students talked to real patients, interviewing them and conducting physical exams. She found it difficult to be comfortable while doing all of the private investigations that doctors do, routinely making patients get naked for physical inspection. Nevertheless, the ward work breathed intellectual life into her brain. She became a kind of detective. Diagnosis was conducted on conditions of risk, sometimes uncertainty. Information was piecemeal, always a composite of facts from different sources. An abdomen would feel a certain way, a patient would react to something—all of it was an effort to put data together in some organic whole that expressed the patient's condition. The part that Park found most real was trying to go outside of herself and enter the mind of another person. She tried to think like the patients she examined, asking herself what the patient felt and how she could make the patient comfortable. The experience was completely different from the first year and a half of uninterrupted course work.

Diagnosis seemed to Park to be a mysterious fusion of theory, observation, and intuition. She slowly began to trust her instincts. Once, during the year she was an intern, she was examining a woman, standing there reciting the facts of the case to the attending physician (a respiratory specialist for whom she had the highest regard), and neither one of them was able to figure out what was wrong with the woman. She had just delivered a child, had pneumonia, and Park remembers that she spoke only Spanish. The woman's symptoms struck Park as unusual, unlike any other pneumonia she had seen. Suddenly she turned to the attending physician and said, "I think she has TB." Park had never seen acute tuberculosis pneumonia, had not looked at any cultures from the woman, and so had no reason to make such a diagnosis. She simply knew, without knowing why. The physician looked at her and said, "No, I don't really think so." But it turned out to be a correct diagnosis. The woman had TB.

Park began to appreciate the subtlety of the signals the body sends. At times it seemed to her that patients' responses were almost subliminal, the connections between doctor and patient a kind of psychic symbiosis. She decided to specialize in a field of medicine requiring precise readings of stimulus and response, that of anesthesiology. She admits to an attraction for crisis-management medicine, therapy that deals in calculated risks for the patient. The emergency room once more was like a drug to her, a physical rush when the stakes were high. In anesthesiology, she was in control of what she regarded as an induced coma. She divided the practice into takeoff and landing periods. Putting someone under was takeoff, a time when the physician had to be very alert. Bringing someone out of anesthesia was landing, again a time requiring maximum alertness. She was attracted especially to neural anesthesia and critical-care medicine. It was fun (her word) to be there making decisions, acting quickly and correctly, or someone would go down the tubes right in front of one's eyes. She wanted and found the visceral feelings of life on the wire.

But also throughout her residency she tried to cultivate the skills of "extended sympathy," the ability to enter the minds of her patients. Once, as a resident, she was called down to the emergency room in the middle of the night to do a preoperative evaluation on a woman who needed immediate surgery for vaginal bleeding. The woman was psychotic. No one could get her to do anything, even the simplest actions. The nurses were ready to place her under restraints. Park sat down with the woman and began talking to her in the softest, most even-toned voice she could muster, repeating over and over, "Listen to what I am telling you." She was trying to get the woman to concentrate on just her voice, to tune out everything else and cut through the whirling that Park imagined going on in the woman's brain—just concentrate on one thing, listen to the voice speaking to you. After ten minutes, Park felt a connection to the woman. She knew they would get through the induction of the anesthetic satisfactorily.

Park's next concern was what would happen when the woman woke up in the recovery room. The psychosis would still be there, probably worsened by the effects of the drugs administered during surgery. Park talked to the woman again in the same tone of voice. She explained to her what would happen, that she would go to sleep for a time, and then, when she woke up, "You will hear me again. You will hear my voice again. I will talk to you just like I am talking to you now and I will explain to you everything that happened." When Park brought the woman into the recovery room she had not yet emerged from the anesthesia. She instructed the nurses to summon her the moment the woman started to come around. They did, and Park immediately went to the woman's side. "Hello," she said. "You remember me. I was talking to you right before you went to sleep. Everything went fine." She continued to talk to the woman until she was ready to leave the recovery room. At that point the woman reached over to Park and said, "I'm not afraid. Thank you."

Park couldn't explain, even to herself, what she was doing. She only knew that she was following her gut reactions. The communication she had with some of her patients was almost telepathic at times. Sometimes the effects it had on her patients seemed close to hypnotism. The cues she picked up from patients and their families became important to her. She began to appreciate fine distinctions in examination techniques. One doctor might press more deeply into a patient's abdomen than another, touch the patient differently, and gain different information on the patient's condition. The sensitivity of patients to pain, their fears and expectations, became for her part of the data of diagnosis in addition to standard clinical signs of health and disease. She became sensitive to the person she was treating rather than the case she was treating.

Medical practice began to appear dualistic to her. Reasoning in medicine was linear. Established rules of evidence and inference were in place in medical discourse and transmitted to medical students. Theories and facts were in the standard reciprocal relationship found in science: some theories had primary status and were difficult to dislodge, but all medical theory was at least in principle falsifiable by data. The practice of medicine was also strongly inductive in allowing the physician's observation of cases to control the application of theory. Yet the facts were intelligible only on the basis of a long history of medical research on health and disease. Medicine was science in practice. It relied on a technological base that provided doctors with impressive diagnostic instruments and therapeutic powers.

Yet something else was going on in medicine. Nurses seemed to sense it more than doctors did. In critical-care units a patient could be comatose, nonresponsive, yet the nurses would talk to this person as if the individual were conscious. They would tell the patient what was happening, what they were going to do and why, while the patient lay there in an inert state. Park began to doubt two things. First, she wasn't sure anyone understood what consciousness is. She was puzzled not so much about whether patients were conscious or not in a variety of conditions, but about the reality of consciousness itself. She began to believe that consciousness was not linear, not in accord with the methods of reasoning taught in medical school. Second, the scope of the unknown in medicine began to appear more extensive to her. She began to believe that medical research, perhaps all empirical research, was an extrapolation of huge visions about what the world is like from some small percentage of available data and an even smaller fraction of what could be known in principle. Medicine seemed more and more like an imaginative exercise to her, a set of conjectures about an enormously large reality (mostly unknown) from a very small base of information.

Park completed her residency in anesthesiology and then accepted a fellowship in critical-care medicine, still working in the University of California medical school. But she did not complete her work. Near the end of her fellowship year she collapsed from prolonged abuse of alcohol and drugs, and had to enter a treatment center. She simply stopped functioning as a doctor, and as a human being.

On one level, the life Park had been leading was a familiar one. Her emotions had been repressed. They then found release in the multiple possibilities Western society provides for alcohol consumption, for being boisterous and wild during leisure hours. The internship was the crippling experience. Park worked 120 hours a week alongside other interns on similar schedules. Not enough time to eat, nor even sometimes to go to the bathroom. Always taking care of everyone else instead of the self and regarding that as normal. Park found the worst and most vulnerable parts of herself, and fortified them—that she was worthless and always had to prove herself. The world was black, hopeless. She wanted to die.

It is easy to see, without putting too fine a point on it, that any simple account of Park's breakdown has precedents all over the Western world. What made Park's actions striking and tragic at another level was her aggressive introduction of drugs to cope with these problems. She began taking higher and higher levels of a variety of substances she stole from the hospital laboratory. By the end of the fellowship period she was unable to work and was contemplating suicide. Conventional psychotherapy was proving useless in solving her drug problems, and both her friends and colleagues were distressed at the likely loss of a gifted doctor.

Park's physical condition is described in medical textbooks as chemical dependency. We know more about the effects of drugs on the human brain now than even fifteen years ago. Addictive drugs seem to mimic various neurotransmitters. They fit into receptors in the brain that have evolved for chemicals made by the body, and they also both stimulate and suppress these natural chemicals. Narcotics enter receptors for endorphins, for example, and cocaine enhances dopamine and noradrenaline. An addictive drug produces a feeling of well-being normally not available without the drug by artificially stimulating certain centers in the brain. Physicians believe that the memory of this experience initially drives the individual to use the drug again.

Repetitive use of drugs creates physical dependency far beyond memory inducement, however. The central nervous system enters a state of depression when an addict stops using drugs. The reason is that the body has not only become tolerant to the drugs, but the parts of the brain that produce the natural chemicals replaced by the drugs have shut down. The individual enters withdrawal, a painful and sometimes dangerous experience of irritability, tension, anger, anxiety, and panic. This experience is often intolerable because the brain cannot produce the needed chemicals for normal stimulation until the body is free of drugs for a period of time. The usual result is a strong, often compelling, urge to reintroduce drugs to the body. Sometimes nothing can stop the addict from taking drugs again.

In the early stages of her therapy, Park was the classic drug addict who does not recover. She did not take treatment seriously and continued taking drugs even while undergoing drug therapy. She was also a member of a class of addicts especially difficult to treat. Physicians who abuse drugs present special problems in therapy for a number of reasons. It is not easy for physicians to admit drug abuse, for the admittance cedes a power to the therapist that the physician normally reserves for the self. Professional identity is threatened by the recognition that a habit is both damaging and out of control. The role reversal in therapy is sometimes so stunning that physicians continue to deny dependency past all reasonable points at which nonphysicians would surrender to treatment. Therapists contribute to these problems by using stereotypes of drug users that rarely extend to physicians and by recommending more moderate courses of therapy than prescribed for nonphysicians. Joanne Park was not the first physician in history to conceal a major drug addiction while working for an extended period of time in a hospital, and then continue to abuse drugs even while therapists tried to help.

Ignorance among Park's colleagues about the causes of her collapse did not help matters. Medicine is a high-stress profession, and its practitioners have access to drugs. But precipitating factors like work pressures and availability may mask deeper flaws in the personalities of drug users. No one is sure why some individuals use drugs and others do not in the same circumstances. All the doctors in the hospital knew with reasonable certainty was that Joanne Park was about to die.

L U K E

For most of my life my body has viewed its own vessels as hostile territory. Things simmer inside, occasionally erupting into open warfare. This means fever, disrupted coordination, energies dissipated and bled out like steam into open spaces, a sustained feeling of lassitude.

Once I inadvertently triggered a session of autoimmune reactions with a penicillin shot. It was my sixteenth birthday, and a dog had bitten me while I was out riding a bicycle. After the obligatory confinement had been arranged to check the dog for rabies, the doctor decided to give me a precautionary penicillin injection to protect against infection. Later, while sitting in the shadows of a late afternoon sun, I felt my throat slowly start to swell. My eyes and ears began itching terribly. Everything around me seemed tinged with red and all I could hear was the buzzing of bees high in the limbs of the oak tree near my bench. I sat perfectly still while the swelling continued until my breathing just began to be impeded. Then the reaction seemed to lose energy, it paused at some threshold point of real trouble, and then just as slowly receded until my face and throat were normal and the foliage was rich with green again. It was my last penicillin shot ever. The doctor said that another such injection would probably kill me.

The spectacle of the body against itself was a constant source of puzzlement to me. Which side was I on? Is there an "I" that can legislate the adversarial forces of a single body? Most of the time I simply rode it out, spectator to diminished capacities brought on by my body's inexplicable failures to recognize its own features as friend rather than foe. I was being attacked by me, not as a suicidal impulse but as a form of self-defense that was destructive to the self. And I (in some form) knew this but was powerless to prevent it.

The times I remember feeling closest to being one unified self was when my wife and I made love. "Made love"—the phrase always struck me as at once quaint and insightful, as if couples were artisans who produce some ornament called "love" during their sessions together. Yet we did, my wife and I, invent love and come to believe in it as a tangible presence. I was one body, one with my body, with her body, during those hours. Time itself could not be tracked, sensed, except within the flow of bodily movement. We sought pleasure together, and found it as separate bodies joined to each other.

We were not one person, as the writers say, in those intimacies. I was one person, she was another. But we were, or seemed to be, holistic within ourselves. It is a law of physics that the strength of the forces holding constituent elements together is stronger as the particle is smaller. I seemed to be like an expansive nucleon (or quark) in lovemaking, my bodily integrity bonded by the strong force.

The rest of the time I felt like an occupant in my body, sometimes welcome and many times not. Like some inert but fragile substance, the atoms of my chemistry, of me, seemed always on the verge of decomposition, perhaps annihilation. I was an arrangement of parts maintained by the weak force of gravitational attraction. Occasionally, especially when I was struck low by a virus infection, I would have vivid dreams of restoration. One I remember with special clarity. I was led into a medical clinic and placed on a table for some kind of physical examination. The doctors who conducted the exam seemed preoccupied with my upper respiratory tract, and at one point sent a probe up my sinuses into my brain. Some moment of clarity and disjunction followed, accompanied by a promise from the physician to replace the mechanisms where needed. Then I was standing outside in the sun near an automobile. An accomplice was helping me place a casket in the trunk. The casket contained my discarded body. I awoke without fear or uncertainty, half believing that I occupied a new body that would give me a fresh start.

The problem was that I could never get a fix on what it was that survived one body to be placed in another. Even language failed me. I would think, I cannot settle this in my own mind, as if some ego, some sense of me, owned my mind. In my worst moments I would view myself as a soul composed of antimatter, an antiquark carrying the opposite charge from that found in the terrestrial particles of my body. Yes—my soul with the dispositional capacity to explode on contact the sinews and bones of my physical self. Death would be the disappearance of spirit and body in a burst of light energy.

Yet there would be moments of such intense and concrete familiarity from time to time. I would look out at some physical setting, sunlight through mist, everything seeming to be in place and my soul at rest. My parents' house, where I grew up with my sisters, has a single oak tree in the backyard and terrazzo floors in the family room. In this scene my father is chewing gum and talking to me.

"Let's all take our blood pressure," he tells me. "I bought a new device and I want to show you how it works."

He takes out a standard device to measure blood pressure while I watch.

"Come on over to the table. Just sit here. Good. Let me just strap this on your arm. Roll up your sleeve."

My blood pressure is 130 over 70, which my father pronounces as normal, even excellent.

"Now you take mine," he tells me. "Your mother can't hear the pause in the heartbeat. We're both going deaf together, but she's going faster."

I strap the instrument on my father and listen. "You have, according to what I hear, 260 over 90."

My father is silent.

"Here, let me take it again." I pump up the band on the arm, shift the lever on the gauge and listen as the air hisses out. "Definite. I heard the change clearly. I get 260 over 90."

My father doesn't answer.

Now my mother appears suddenly on his left. "That's high," she tells my father. "You didn't have that reading yesterday. You've never had a reading that high. Let me take it for you." She takes my father's blood pressure. It's only 140 over 70. She looks at me.

"I'm all right," my father says. "There's nothing wrong with me."

The memory of this scene makes me feel inexplicably sad. Now a different memory, though seeming to blend with this first one. I am on a boat with my father. We are drifting, the motor is off. No waves disturb our movement. The air and the sea are both calm. The water is soft glass, reflecting the high white clouds in the sky. It is hot. I have my shirt off. My father sits with just a white sweatshirt on. We do not speak to one another. The boat sends slow thick circles expanding out in the water as it drifts. We must be inland, perhaps somewhere near the Everglades. I look at my father, at the square face and body. He looks back with no trace of uncertainty in his features. A thin smoke from some fire drifts up in the sky.

Now I hear something. A dog barking in the distance? A radio playing? My father is talking about a suit he has returned to Sears, Roebuck.

The size is not right. They keep making adjustments. Finally he gets the suit for nothing. He explains it this way, that finally it would cost them less to give him the suit than to try to correct any more of their mistakes. He sits on the other side of the boat, taping shut the ice chest with strip after strip of masking tape. The sun is very bright on both of us.

A third memory. I am in the backyard with my children and parents. My older daughter, Rachel, is taking pictures of my mother and father with an ancient Brownie camera that she has gotten from someplace.

"All right," she calls to my parents. "Don't move. And please smile."

They pose for the camera. My mother squints behind her glasses. My father pulls back his mouth in a silly grin. He is clowning. Yolanda, my younger daughter, laughs.

"Come on, Grandpa," Rachel pleads.

He gets serious again. This time his look is kindly, grandfatherly.

"Better," Rachel announces. "Now hold it."

The scene freezes for the camera. No one moves. I have watched it all from behind my younger daughter: the shade cast by the oak tree, the sun glinting in on the lawn through cracks in the coverage the leaves provide, the sound of dishes being set on a table in the house next door. I examine the thought now like a photograph, looking for emotion, meaning, trying to feel the origins of what I see. In stasis, timeless, the scene is balanced and serene. I can be at home, one with the others. In movement, when time starts up again, the figures and surroundings fade, recede, like dreams on waking.

I am remembering these events now, in bed at night, passing slowly over a state between sleep and wakefulness. I can never describe this state, even to myself. The room is quiet, except for my wife's easy breathing. I feel—what? My own existence like a small, hard stone. My own sense of myself stretched vaguely to other events. I know my children are asleep in the next room, that the car is in the garage, that the downstairs is still and dark, that my parents are sleeping in their bed over a thousand miles away. I look at the clock on the bedside radio. It is 4:30 in the morning in the month of January.

4

MIND AND BODY

Individuals and Groups

"It is the soul that sees," Descartes tells us, "and not the eyes; and only by means of the brain does the immediate act of seeing take place." Elsewhere Descartes writes that "I am not lodged in my body only as a pilot in a vessel, I am very closely united with it so that I seem to confuse with it one whole." Yet the "I," the self, remained for Descartes only "a thinking thing," a soul without bodily extension. The problem, never solved by Descartes, is how mind and body related to one another if they are separate entities.

To the medical question "What is wrong with me?" the typical modern physician will seek answers in the realm of body rather than mind. Medicine does evolve from early traditions that treat mind and body together, and recent holistic practices in medicine address the health of both. But most of modern medicine comes directly from recent scientific traditions that see disease agents (or their absence) and the related condition of the organism. The body is bound to dominate such explanations and the therapies that follow from them, for the body is physical. The mind is not.

Psychiatry is the most influential exception in medicine to the view that the physical is the domain of illness and health. The thought that the mind is the origin or center of thought, feeling, and behavior is as old as human experience. But Freud, writing in the late nineteenth and early twentieth centuries, appropriated and extended this thought into complex theories on the unconscious in human behavior, the functions of repression and sexuality in both mental and physical problems, and into therapeutic techniques of free association, dream interpretation, resistance, and transference. Modern psychiatry, as a field of medicine aiming to restore mental health through therapy of the mind (empirically understood), begins with this vocabulary and the assumptions on which it is formed.

One of the critical assumptions of psychiatry is that the individual can be addressed as the bearer of mental illness, the site for both the signs of mental disorder and the pathology that society labels as insane or neurotic. At or near the center of this assumption is the theory of the personality. Psychoanalysis in this century ascribed characteristics to individuals, and began demarcating both healthy and emotionally disturbed individuals according to a typology of personalities. The more familiar types include obsessive-compulsive, passive-aggressive, hysteria, passive-dependent, schizophrenia, and megalomania. The patient is typically entered in one of the categories on such a list. Emotional disturbances are often tracked directly back to personality traits.

The theory of the personality is a variation on modern traditions of social theory that regard the individual as the locus of meaning and value in society. Classical social philosophy is distinguished by its celebration of the group as the primary unit in human experience. Individuals are residual categories, derivatives of collective life. In seventeenth-century contract theory, this priority is reversed. The individual is primary, the features of collective life derived from descriptions of individuals and the hypothetical choices they make of social arrangements. The concept of a personality extends this sense of discrete and even atomistic individualism to a spectrum of types. Individuals are distinct from their social contexts as personalities and from each other according to differences among personalities.

Mental therapy typically begins with the history of the individual in social life. Every version of psychotherapy assumes that individuals need some form of social life, at least minimal connections to other human beings, in order to develop. The nature of such connections over an individual's lifetime is important in understanding mental disorders. Included in the theory of the personality is a sense of the whole or complete individual. Many disorders are explained in terms of arrested development, incomplete or skewed personalities resulting from flawed affiliations with other individuals. But the connections between social life and mental well-being or disorder do not lead usually to social reform. Few psychiatrists treat social disorders, even when these disorders are the causes of individual dysfunction. The individual as such is the focus of study and treatment in psychiatry.

The burden is clear. The mental well-being of individuals is the aim of treatment in psychiatry. Body is not ignored. All psychiatric practices recognize that organic diseases can cause mental disorder, and drugs that affect the physical organism are used to treat a variety of mental disorders and can themselves bring about mental disturbances when abused. But a psychiatric intervention is effective only as it conduces to the restoration of a healthy mind. The individual acquires a set of beliefs that permits him or her to function in social contexts.

Duncan

Paul Duncan is a psychiatrist who treats patients in the morning and teaches at a university in the afternoon. He is not sure exactly when he decided to study medicine, though his concern for healing goes back to his childhood. He recalls an experience when he was eight years old that seems now to his trained intellect to be important in explaining his later life. His mother was a social worker. She used to go into the country to visit her clients. Often she took him along. On one trip he found some small rabbits whose mother had disappeared. He brought them home and, in true rational fashion, sought all kinds of advice on how to care for these creatures. He wanted them to grow up under his care and then be released back into their natural habitat. It was not to be. As happens in nearly all such projects, the rabbits quickly died in captivity. It was traumatic for Duncan. He remembers their health and liveliness, his care and attention, and the resulting failure. He is too good at his craft to assign a simple pattern of influence to the experience, but feels that in some complex way this early failure moved him in the direction of medicine.

His first ambition, however, was to go into the foreign service. He grew up on a street in a town in upstate New York where three former secretaries of state had homes. But a rational investigation of the conditions and opportunities of diplomatic service revealed to Duncan a melancholy fact—you had to have money to go into the foreign service (or at least that was what those in the service told him). The only girl in town who did have enough money to support his ambitions was not someone he cared for, so Duncan was left with his own modest resources. Not enough for the foreign service, he concluded.

Like many who study medicine, Duncan was good in science. But Duncan also had access to an unusually wide range of literature in high school. His father had an avocation for psychiatry and philosophy, and especially admired the European thinkers. Duncan read books by Gordon Allport, Karen Horney, and various continental philosophers, including a try at Husserl (whom he found, in the company of other readers, impenetrable). He became interested in the study of human beings as such and began to regard medical school as the place to go to study humans, a kind of eighteenth-century view of education as the "taking of degrees" in medicine, law, history to secure enlightenment. He also began to feel the heat of the Korean conflict, a negative incentive that sent many males toward medical and law schools, and graduate training in general, during the early 1950s.

Duncan's interests in therapy moved from the academic to the real in his senior year of medical school when he was given clinical authority to write orders. When he saw the therapeutic effects of his own efforts, he began to think that he had a calling to assist people who are in poor health, infirm in some way. He also was drawn to those who were mentally ill. An early experience seemed to him to explain this preoccupation with mental infirmities. He remembers being with his father in a rural farm village, maybe five or six years old at the time, and noticing some men who were talking in a language unintelligible to the young Duncan and urinating on the village green where he and his father were sitting. Duncan recalls being very interested in this scene and asking his father who these people were. His father explained to him that they were just crazy, meaning mentally off center and harmless. Duncan came away impressed with the possible range of human actions.

At all points in his youth Duncan was aware of professional alternatives. His father was director of guidance and curriculum in a city school system. He helped high-school seniors select colleges and occupations, in effect decide (if possible) what they wanted to be in life. Duncan remembers spending many hours in his father's office going through literature on professions, occupations, colleges. He was concerned with arcane strategies on preparing for a field of study or work, with the kinds of people, levels of income, and satisfaction found in different occupations. He never felt that he was guessing what things would be like in medicine, that he was just picking something out of a pool. Duncan arrived at the profession of medicine with a level of deliberation probably unprecedented for most teenagers. He knew with reasonable certainty that medicine would combine his therapeutic interests with his intellectual needs for some larger understanding of the human community. It would also make it unnecessary for him to marry for money.

He considered two fields of medicine. One was neurosurgery. It addressed the mental side of human experience that interested him. But the clinical outcomes of neurosurgery at that time were so depressing that he turned his gaze toward psychiatry. He saw it as a field that seemed to address problems of health linked to the kinds of lives people led, the beliefs they had, the cultures they had acquired. Duncan has always viewed psychiatry as a profession that studies and tries to fix the problems that cause mental disablement, the tensions and uncertainties that make the minds of this kind of creature—human beings—fall apart. He has never regarded psychiatry as a substitute for religion. It was precisely as a medical field that he was drawn to it, one that addresses the mental health of humans in secular terms.

Duncan considers psychiatry as an eminently pragmatic field of work. He approaches patients inductively, armed with a bookish knowledge acquired from more than thirty years of intensive reading in relevant literatures, but also keenly aware of the need for creative efforts tailored to the particular case. He prides himself on his craft, admitting to a problem recognized by Sir William Osler's dictum to spend time with both human beings and books: a conflict between love of the patient and love of the craft. Occasionally Duncan will admire his own skills even when the patient does not benefit from them. But mainly he achieves satisfaction when a patient he has seen intensively for two to three years is profoundly altered for the better.

The methods Duncan uses to benefit patients seem to be an open set of items. In one famous (and apocryphal) story related to Duncan, a patient has an obsessive compulsion to tear paper. Years of depth psychoanalysis produce no benefits. In desperation, the man's family takes him to a short-term therapist, who receives him and is seen following him around the room talking quietly into his ear. After the session the man returns home and never tears paper again. The family rejoices and months later asks the therapist what he said to the man. The therapist responds: "I told him, 'Don't tear paper.'"

Duncan's response to the story is, fine, if it works then it is a proper inclusion in psychiatric methods of therapy. He sees the end of psychiatry as a restoration of the patient's sanity. From Duncan's point of view, the best treatments are those that are the safest, shortest, and least costly. He has had patients who respond to snap-out-of-it therapy. But he has also encountered problems that are impervious to short-term solutions. Some of his patients never get well. They remain seriously disabled in all aspects of their lives no matter how much therapy is applied, or what kind it might be.

Sometimes psychological problems have physical causes. Drug abuse is currently a common cause of a wide range of mental disorders. But even some of the classic mental illnesses, like schizophrenia, are now linked to chemical imbalances in the brain. Duncan admits that the mind may be an epiphenomenon that is dependent on the body. The difficulty he sees in reducing all of psychiatry to physiology is that mental illness is determined by observing the behavior of individuals (including their beliefs). He knows of no physiological test that will reveal that someone is mentally ill. There simply is no algorithm that leads one to conclusions about an individual's mental state from descriptions of his or her physical state, with the exception of extreme cases of brain damage.

One reason that mind-body connections are loose, neither axiomatic nor even reliable, is that what counts as mental illness differs from one cultural and even social context to another. Even therapy for the body varies on different interpretations of the "same" conditions. Duncan allows that physicians from all over the world would agree on the treatment of, say, a broken femur (though the nuances of therapy may differ even here). But more complex diseases yield disagreements over proper treatment of even universally acknowledged ailments. Mental illness is in yet another category. It is discontinuous with physical medicine in that the behavior regarded as insane (the most extreme category) is culturally, historically, and economically conditioned. Duncan points to the history of madness to make his point. The mental problems of some neurotic women in Salem, Massachusetts, in the seventeenth century were labeled as witchcraft. Therapy included burning and drowning the sufferers. In general, the mentally ill throughout Western history have been either banished, killed, starved to death, or put away in attics or jail cells. Diagnosis and therapy of mental disorders seem especially sensitive to the dominant beliefs of the times.

Duncan holds the widely accepted view that the logic of mental illness makes it much more vulnerable to cultural influence than physical medicine. The laws of physics seem to govern all empirical reality no matter what its cultural base may be. A sodium atom is a sodium atom at both the north and south poles and everywhere in between. But human behavior has no comparable anchor. It seems relentlessly contextual, a construction of time and place with no physical compass to stabilize its meaning. Madness is manifested in the presence of cultural norms that specify sanity. The assertion that a femur is fractured can be confirmed or falsified with an X ray of the relevant bone. No such direct test exists for the presence or absence of a mental disorder, since the reality of the disorder is the product of social beliefs.

It follows for Duncan that psychiatry is predominantly a set of theoretical constructs designed to respond to the diverse facts of madness. Therapy is controlled by efficacy—whatever works to restore sanity in a given context. If a therapy works for Duncan in his practice, he wants to know how it works (in part to use it again successfully in the future). But he is convinced that the main problem in sorting out therapies is not that so few things work but that almost everything works sometimes. No one is sure why, except that a belief in the efficacy of treatment is one important reason for its success.

One consequence of Duncan's view of psychiatry is that therapy can be exceedingly diverse. If success depends upon utilizing the beliefs of patients, then treatment must be able to accommodate a wide, perhaps open, range of idiosyncratic beliefs. Duncan agrees, and as proof of this range once actually sponsored an exorcism in his practice. During the 1950s Duncan served in the armed forces, and for a time was the head of psychiatry at a Strategic Air Command base. One day he was called in by the head of medicine to see a chief mechanic on one of the B-52 bombers. The mechanic had sought medical treatment for abdominal pain. The internist in charge of the case had run a series of tests looking for ulcers. The results were all negative. During his third visit to the clinic, the mechanic had seized the internist, forced him into a closet on the ward, and confessed that the real problem was to be found in the presence of evil spirits in his body. "I'm possessed," he told the terrified internist.

Duncan was able to calm the mechanic down and get him into an office. Then he began therapy with the usual exploration of the individual's history. The combination of traumatic experiences and religious beliefs was an intriguing expression of religion and modern psychology. The man had been seduced as a youth by one of his mother's male boarders. The religious beliefs he had at the time made it impossible for him to discuss this homosexual episode with anyone. This event, and the fears and worries it engendered, mixed in classical (psychological) ways with his upbringing, his relations with his mother, and uncertainties about his sexuality. The devils the man believed in completed the explanation. They had seized control of his body's physiology, causing the pain in his abdomen.

Duncan supervised a series of exorcism rituals in the hospital that the patient arranged. He also saw the patient in psychotherapy three days a week for three months. (Duncan spooked the chief of pediatrics by getting him to attend one of the rituals in his office one evening.) The effect of the sessions was to mobilize the evil spirits, freeing them to move about in the various organs of the man's body. At the end of the three-month period, the devils had settled in the man's genitals (where, of course, they belonged). It then seemed appropriate to the man that he seek an authoritative exorcism from the bishop of his religion. Duncan arranged a leave from the military so that the man could go and see the bishop. A proper exorcism took place that expelled the devils entirely from the man's body. He returned to his post cured, and resumed fixing B-52 bombers in America in the twentieth century.

Duncan believes that psychiatrists should take the patient as he or she comes and not legislate on the legitimacy of beliefs. The goal of therapy is to maintain or restore the patient's sanity. Duncan does not view this effort as helping the patient adjust to life's circumstances. The issue for him is sanity. Sometimes sanity is achieved by adjusting to institutional norms, and sometimes it can be achieved only by opposing those norms. So to the question of whether a psychiatrist should recommend, for example, the dissolution of a marriage if the marriage is the source of the patient's mental problems, Duncan answers no. He sees the psychiatrist as helping to bring the patient to a state where alternatives are clear to him and he is able to make a choice. The purpose of psychiatry for Duncan is not to make patients adjust to circumstances, or even to find happiness in life. Therapy is designed simply to enable individuals to be sane.

Once Duncan had a patient who was a hit man for the Mafia. He came in for therapy not because of remorse or guilt about his profession but because he was having problems in his relations with his wife and children. In the course of the therapy it became clear that his chosen line of work was affecting his family life, and not simply in incidental ways. But the patient's profession did not become a moral issue in his therapy. It came into the sessions in the same way that any work habits would—as grist for the psychiatric mill. The moral issues found in murdering for a living were not addressed as such in therapy, but only as the profession (among other variables) was creating problems in the patient's connection to his family. Duncan views his own profession in restricted medical terms. Like the orthopedic surgeon who might fix the hit man's broken leg without saying to him that he ought not to use the mended limb to walk to his homicidal appointments, Duncan does not attempt moral reform. For the record, the hit man benefitted from therapy and continued pursuing his profession (though presumably in a more settled frame of mind).

Michel Foucault speaks of the physician's gaze and how different historical conditions are implicated in restructuring the subjects of visibility. For Duncan, the psychiatrist's gaze focuses on the personality of the individual and the capacity of that individual for action. It is an angle of vision that must include more of the social context than the gaze, say, of a surgeon. The fact that one is a communist is remote from what the surgeon will consider in preparing someone for an appendectomy. The psychiatrist's gaze will include political (and all other) beliefs as material to effect a cure but not as candidates for reform. Duncan recently had a patient whose psychosis was almost certainly caused from living with her mother. The goal of the therapy that Duncan administered, however, was not to order or prescribe the patient's separation from her mother. Rather, he tried to get the patient to see certain connections and decide whether or not to live with mother. It is the individual and her beliefs that constitute the focus of visibility in Duncan's gaze, not the social conditions with which the patient must contend, and the autonomy of the individual is inviolate in all of the therapy that Duncan negotiates. Not making value judgments on ways of life seems to be a controlling virtue in Duncan's understanding of psychiatry.

Social Conditions

On what conditions is Duncan's view of psychiatry coherent? The question is not hostile. It merely asks for an identification of what must be in place in the world for this common understanding of psychiatry to be intelligible.

One condition is that social structures have on balance a benign rather than a corrupting influence on individual mental states. The history of race relations in the United States is one among numerous case studies of malevolent social structures illustrating this requirement. It is widely acknowledged that blacks (or African-Americans) have been an oppressed group in American society. One consequence of oppression is self-hate among the victims, a loathing of the self caused by forced subordination. James Baldwin stated what many have observed: "Negroes [note: Baldwin is writing in 1962] in this country—and Negroes do not, strictly or legally speaking, exist in any other—are taught really to despise themselves from the moment their eyes open on the world." In conditions of institutional malevolence, an adjustment of the individual to the world through psychotherapy would amount to complicity by victims in their own extinction. The appropriate response is to change the institutions that create the mental disturbances, since it is morally impossible for psychiatry to be practiced in a world where adjustment to reality is morally questionable.

A second condition is that the individual have primacy in society. A collective state that regards individuals as subordinate to groups is unlikely to find social space for a profession that is focused on individual distress. In the People's Republic of China, there is currently little resembling psychotherapy for individuals. One explanation for the absence of psychotherapy is that the group rather than the individual has primacy in China. Self-determination in medical care is virtually nonexistent. If the family, work unit, or team of doctors feels that an individual is ready to enter or leave the hospital, the individual by definition is ready to enter or leave. There is no system of negative rights that would allow the individual to enter adversarial relations with others or with the state. The individual is defined within a complex communal web of relations that is conceptually and temporally prior to the self. There is technically no self in China that can become the subject of introspection, no official recognition of separate individuals with distinct mental problems.

The individual in Western traditions, by contrast, is the locus of value in society, the source (however indirect) for governing rules and basic principles. Tolerance in psychotherapy for the individual life-styles of hit men quickly follows such an unclouded assignment. But psychiatry also respects individual values for pragmatic reasons. Successful therapy requires working with rather than against the patient's values. A communal society that elevates social goals over individual sanity, and even dismisses the possibility of disorders located entirely within the individual, will not even recognize individual values in mental pathologies.

A third condition is a nonintrusive state. Psychiatry, like many professions in liberal societies, requires the nonporous shields that establish negative liberty for practitioners. The psychiatrist must have discretionary authority to administer therapy without political regulation (save for equity and due process guarantees) by the state. If the state dictates the terms of mental health and therapy, then the individual autonomy and professional authority so vital to psychiatry are both lost.

These three social conditions—benign social structures, individual primacy, and a nonintrusive state—have been core features of Western traditions in the last several hundred years. They can be found in a package of concepts familiar to any student of democratic thought: the importance of negative liberty and individual autonomy, the elevation of individuals to controlling positions over their own lives, the denigration of coercion and paternalistic intervention in individual lives. It is no exaggeration to see psychiatry as an eminently liberal profession in accepting and extending the concepts that so profoundly respect individual beliefs.

It also follows that at least some of the problems of liberalism are also found in psychiatry. One can be called the black hole of liberalism: the paradox that occurs when the toleration of diversity includes destructive beliefs as an entry in the tolerated set. Duncan practiced psychiatry for a brief time in rural parishes of Louisiana just before the civil rights movement. He opened his clinic to blacks. This caused a great deal of consternation in the community, not least because it suggested that blacks could have problems like whites (when the prevailing wisdom was that if blacks had mental problems they were simply crazy like horses were occasionally crazy). Duncan left town early a number of times for his own safety.

The problems presented by beliefs like racism is that they simultaneously can cause mental disorders (in both racist and victim) and constitute an interventionist threat to the practice of psychiatry. Suppose, for example, that mental disease can be tracked back to social oppression like infectious disease can be traced to polluted wells. Restricting psychiatry to individual therapy then would miss the cause of mental disorder inherent in the structure of society. Also, suppose a belief is hostile to the foundations of psychiatry, the fascist, say, who goes the hit man one better by attacking the individual liberties on which psychotherapy depends. The paradox is well known. Treat the man and encourage conditions damaging to the profession. Refuse to treat him and compromise the tolerance of belief needed for successful therapy. Like democratic practices trying to accommodate a referendum to do away with elections, psychotherapy comes up against the limits of tolerance in addressing values that aim to destroy tolerance.

Individual Identity and Competence

One regulating question in psychiatry is: *What* are the individuals who are the subjects of treatment?

The self, or ego, can be a complex unit in therapy. Divided selves (split personalities) are among the more dramatic cases of individual diffusion in psychiatry. Some individuals seem to present a number of personalities that come and go at will. Most of these cases were reported between the years of 1840 and 1910, leading some critics to judge that they represent a transition between demoniacal possession and more recent theories of disassociation. This explanation relies on the acknowledged power of therapists to elicit symptoms in their patients. The Victorian inclination to assign identity to mental processes and to ignore repression would naturally have encouraged patients to produce different personalities to suit new ways of thinking resulting from analysis. But whether attributed to disassociation of the personality or to repression, the rare spectacle of multiple selves in the same body creates puzzlement over what exactly an individual is.

Split-brain surgery also complicates individual identity. Such surgery does not reduce the self to two identities, but many of the functions attributed to one identifiable self in a single body are divided into separate non-overlapping spheres. Perception is bifurcated. Objects felt by one hand cannot be matched to similar objects held in the other hand. The right hemisphere cannot express itself in speech, though it may "know" what cannot be uttered. The left cerebral cortex can produce descriptions of its experiences. Functions that are important in defining persons are separated and distributed within independent zones. Other results of this (rare) surgery include greater awareness of the special powers of each hemisphere. The right side of the brain seems better at comprehending the structures of experience (including topological forms like faces), for example, while the left field commands language. In patients with severed cerebral hemispheres, many activities of consciousness, like feelings and intentions, are generalized to the "entire" person through the brain stem, but the idea of a person as an integrated self is at least complicated by the effects of split-brain operations.

Ordinary life (outside the domains of psychoanalysis and neurosurgery) also yields experiences of multiple selves. The most legally and morally troubling are produced by the influences of cults. A typical scenario finds a young man or woman alienated (sometimes temporarily) from family and loved ones who is taken in by a loving and well-organized group of friends. Social suasion bends the individual toward the life of the group. Reinforcement techniques that are both benign (songs, discussion, affection) and malevolent (deprivation of protein in the diet) lock the individual into a membership so tight, without possibility of disaffection, that the individual's identity seems transformed. The spectacle of a divided self appears when parents (or others) recapture the individual and forcibly subject the young person to the sustained influence of a "deprogrammer," usually in some isolated area. Sometimes these alternative influences do not have any effect and the individual returns to the cult. But often an identity is restored or a new identity is forged. The questions raised by these contrary efforts are deeply troubling for accounts of human identity. They seem to suggest that identity may be a function of circumstances, and, like the coloration changes in immediately adaptable insects, all that we ascribe to individuals may be directly traceable to the external conditions in which they find themselves.

These general doubts about an independent individual nature are shared at different levels by many social theorists. Marx, for example, saw powerful reductionist forces in social structures and, for this reason, urged the eradication of capitalist institutions. He believed that authentic individuals could then emerge from the installation of economic equality with its resulting political liberation. But the cynical view is readily at hand. Individuals so malleable by institutions may never be genuine, or even real. They may simply be extensions of their social contexts.

The spectacle of Odysseus strapped to the deck of his ship, both wanting and not wanting to go to the Sirens, is a theatrical example of such possibilities, suggesting that opposed selves exist in different settings. Not all contradictory preferences suggest multiple selves. An individual may simply be loosely integrated, making decisions that do not meet accepted standards of consistency. But where fundamental and irreconcilable values are expressed as preferences, and where multiple realities occupy the social landscape, it may be difficult to identify the "real" individual. The well-known example of the young man disinheriting himself to control his own future self, and the older man then later fighting to regain the inheritance denied to him by his early self, is a case of serial selves at odds with one another.

Plato asked how a single individual could be in two volitional states at the same time. His answer is framed in terms of a three-tiered map of the individual soul, replete with an authoritative self to govern the other two (lower) parts of the soul. Liberal thought, lacking the integrated hierarchies of classical philosophy, provides the more discursive response. Wittgenstein observed that, since any action can be regarded as consistent with any rule, we fix consistency by descriptions of action. Whatever people do sets the rules of the language game. But, if consistency is a captive of conventions, then the temptation is strong to define individuals in terms of their communities as well.

One powerful impulse in liberalism is to define the real individual in terms of competence. The cult member may not be competent, may not be the "real" individual, because of the unusual collective pressures of a coherent and well-designed effort at control. The problems that this view has in accommodating the counterpressures of the deprogrammer are self-evident. But judgments on mental competence are still made on the thought that competence tests can be used to sift through contradictory selves and recognize the individual who meets tests of mental competence. It is far from clear, however, that there is a definition of competence that can be generalized across competing systems of belief.

One of the more venerable distinctions in psychiatry is between affective and cognitive disorders. An affective disorder is a disturbance in the individual's emotional state. Mood problems like depression are affective disorders. Cognitive (or thought) disorders are defective understandings of reality. Schizophrenia is the classic form of a cognitive disorder. Like most venerable distinctions, this one blurs in practice. Affective problems, like severe depression, can distort reality; and thought disorders, like the inability to distinguish real from unreal, can be sources of serious emotional problems. But the distinction represents the long-standing recognition of emotive and cognitive dimensions in human experience.

The primary instruments used to determine an individual's mental competence are tests of cognitive disorders. Perceptions of, or beliefs in, phenomena that are not real are usually taken as signs of serious mental problems. The emotionally disturbed individual who is able to distinguish the real from the unreal is generally considered mentally competent. Reality testing is always a matter of degree, and the set of beliefs about reality that indicates sanity or psychosis can be, and probably is in most senses, both wide and heterogeneous. But all societies regard some beliefs about the world as unacceptable. In contemporary Western societies, the individual who persists in believing that Martians are communicating with him through the fillings in his teeth, for example, is not likely to be viewed as mentally competent.

One way to administer tests of mental competence is by relying on acceptable ontologies (organized beliefs about what is real, what is specious). Individuals are typically expected to share in conventional descriptions and relations among events. In *Department of Human Services v. Northern* (1978), a woman who refused to recognize that her feet were gangrenous was found incompetent by a Tennessee court. She could not "see" the obvious facts of her physical condition, what her physician defined as the reality of her situation. As a consequence, she was judged mentally unable to make decisions on her own well-being in the case. In *Department of Human Services v. Hamilton* (1983), both the Court of Appeals and the Supreme Court of Tennessee ruled that a twelve-year-old girl suffering from cancer must be treated medically, even though her father opposed treatment on religious grounds. The courts, in effect, rejected the possibility that God might cure the girl, in spite of her father's belief in such possibilities. The intervention of God did not accord with accepted relations among events.

The problems with such tests of competence are legion and go to the center of disputes in liberal societies over the reality of faith healing. It is one of the acknowledged features of human experience that both the real and the unreal "occur" in some sense. Another venerable distinction—between an illusion and a hallucination—illustrates the scope of this truth. An illusion is a false experience occasioned by some real external cause. Visual illusions are the most easily understood. The well-known Müller-Lyer diagram in which two vertical lines are perceived as being unequal in length can be explained in terms of the effects of the arrowhead angles on the retina. A hallucination, by contrast, is a sensory perception without an external cause. Individuals isolated for periods of time—skiers lost in blizzards, for example—will often "see" figures that do not exist. All individuals experience illusions from time to time, and even sane individuals can hallucinate. The sign of mental competence is the ability to recognize the difference between such experiences and reality.

The interesting issue is how such recognition occurs. It is obvious that perception alone cannot settle the question of what is real, for perceptions are notoriously unreliable and can even be contradictory. The famous example of a stick partially submerged in water demonstrates both the point and the preferred solution. The stick looks bent and feels straight. The conflict between visual and tactile sensations is arbitrated with a theory of optics that instructs on the refraction of light and urges an acceptance of the tactile experience as real, the visual experience as illusory. Hallucinations can also be explained (on the whole) by causal theories, for example the influence of drugs, various neurological disorders, and the like on perception. In such cases, internal conditions account for the perceptual distortions. Theory, broadly conceived, is the instrument that demarcates the real from the unreal by providing a map of warranted empirical relationships.

In some technical or specialized domains, a conventional map of human experience helps to identify cognitive disorders. Recent work in psychiatry has suggested that alterations in the structure of reality are strong, perhaps universalizable, indicators of psychosis. The acceptance of time's arrow in ordering life is an especially important condition for sanity. Individuals who distort time are usually mentally incompetent in all species of discourse. Theoretical maps establish competence in a wide range (perhaps all) of human experience. Scientists routinely use theory to define and order sensory data, and members of the scientific community who dissent from the established views of reality fixed by such theories are obligated to furnish alternative theories or risk censure. Even the most ordinary understandings of the surrounding world are informed by shared ontologies. Members of the flat earth society, for example, have long been consigned to the eccentric and even mentally suspect category by those subscribing to the Copernican worldview.

But it is a mistake to think that theoretical maps can always offer clean and precise devices to identify reality. First, theory itself is vulnerable to error and contradiction. It is helpful to recall that the Ptolemaic system was accepted for centuries as a correct account of the solar system, and that even now substantial disagreement occurs among specialists about the adequacy of basic theories of physical reality. Also, paradoxes are surprisingly common features of theories. The visual contradictions exhibited in the drawings by Lionel and Roger Penrose and in M. C. Escher's paintings can be explained conceptually (though we continue to "see" the contradictions). But Newcomb's problem and Arrow's theorem continue a long tradition of theoretical contradiction going back at least to Zeno's paradox. Such problems suggest breakdowns in the abstract languages offered as resolutions to perceptual flaws, and therefore urge humility and caution in using theory to arbitrate among perceptions.

It is also abundantly clear that ordinary (or nontechnical) experience yields a variety of conflicting theories about reality with little hard evidence available to adjudicate among them. At a prosaic level, what competence means is settled within the language games that individuals play with one another. Those competent to drive an automobile, for example, are not necessarily competent to vote, and competent witnesses in a trial are judged by criteria different from those used to ascertain the competence of a defendant to stand trial. At a more significant level, different realities can also be jurisdictional. The father who accepted the possibility of God's intervention in *Hamilton* (1983) was expressing a belief that would be impeccable in most religious communities, but it was a sign of incompetence (in legal terms) in medical understandings of reality. Many forms of mental disorders are severe enough to cripple the sufferer in any social context. But marginal problems are also more or less dysfunctional depending on the community where the individual has membership. (Were this not so, a change in social venue could have no therapeutic effects.) Mental competence is at least in part a variable of community standards.

The jurisdictional nature of mental powers (or their absence) is important in Western societies in large part because of the range and diversity of jurisdictions. In the healing arts communal logics differ dramatically, and these differences often are explainable by competing ontologies. Evangelical preachers have a set of beliefs on healing that draw upon understandings of God and the possibilities of divine intervention not shared by doctors in conventional medical practice. But beliefs vary even within religious movements. Pentecostalism abandons traditional Catholic and Protestant views on healing. Christian Science has no use for modern medical techniques that are regarded as helpful complements to religious healing in traditional Christian churches. Liberal philosophies tolerate and respect diversity, so that pluralistic beliefs are natural expectations. But even nonliberal beliefs in absolute truth invite diversity, demonstrating again the endless elasticity of belief systems. A skeptic might conclude, in company with P. T. Barnum, that people can believe anything in the right circumstances and, in the more refreshing company of philosophers, that a theory is always available to support the belief.

The presence of multiple conceptions of reality and the resulting disputes over competence raise questions that suggest a dilemma for human identity. Are individuals also just a product of some set of conditions, and does individual identity vary with changes in these conditions? Suppose that, like the identity of Theseus's ship, individuals take on identity only in context, with no self constant across communities. Holistic therapies often maintain that healing requires abandoning the discrete self and accepting an identification with a reality outside human conventions. The irony would be fine indeed if there were no fixed sense of human identity in secular practices to give up.

Spiritual discourses assert a contrary view. In these contexts human identity resides in the individual spirit or soul. This identity is defined as invariant across the pluralistic span of social life and capable of extending to a reality that exceeds secular limits. It is this alternative reality that is said to be the source of genuine healing. This view provides therapies, including psychiatry, with individuals separate from their bodies and their experiences. But it is not clear how such individuals are to be regarded, especially since many of the beliefs attendant to this view of the self, such as talking with God, are technically symptoms of a cognitive disorder from a secular perspective.

From an interview with a psychotherapist:
"Personally I have come to the conclusion that there is no clear boundary on what is psychotic. I have seen too many examples of people who were considered psychotic but who when viewed in another context were no longer considered to be. When I worked in the state hospital there was a black man who was diagnosed as a paranoid schizophrenic. He had all kinds of delusions of being in contact with the Lord. One day about fifty of his followers came and demanded that he be released. They regarded him as a very significant holy man. And he was released and built up a large following and became a very important religious figure in the black community. While he was in the state hospital and only had a few adherents, he was regarded as a crazy man. As soon as he got several thousand people to believe in what he believes in he was a revered figure."

Park

In the two efforts Joanne Park made to clear her body of drugs and restore her mind to sanity she had time to reflect on how she came to the brink of losing everything of value in her life, including life itself. The *why* she has never been able to explain. The *how* she believes she now understands. Both of her parents were alcoholics. She was extremely shy as a youth, ashamed of her family but without the verbal resources to discuss and perhaps exorcise her shame. Her only brother, the oldest of the three children, was born with minimal cerebral palsy. He had occasional seizures and some problems with his gait, especially when he tried to run. He was also slow mentally, which set him up for endless grief from the other children in the neighborhood. Her brother's problems, which included institutionalization when he was eight years old, increased the tensions already present at home.

The curious part of Park's history is that she was successful at everything she tried as a youth. Sports came easily. She was on every team in junior and senior high school. The year was a comfortable progression from hockey to basketball, to softball and track, and then fencing and bowling during the summers. She was also an accomplished scholar, finishing at or near the top of all of her classes with little effort. But her most vivid memories are of depressions, moods so low that even in junior high school she thought of suicide.

Once, when she was a sophomore in high school and walking home after basketball practice, she impulsively almost killed herself. It had not been a good practice and the coach had shouted at her for most of the session. Park remembers hearing a car approach from behind as she trudged home along a country road. The thought occurred that she might pleasantly end her depression by jumping out in front of the vehicle. She even leaned over the road in some classic flirtation with oblivion as the auto sped by. The thought that prevented her from jumping was the simple conviction that she would bungle it, that she'd end up in a hospital badly injured, not dead, and her mother would be standing there asking her why she had done it.

Why has always remained the enigmatic question for Park. Her unambiguous memories are always factual, descriptions of experiences without explorations of motives. Her home was a shambles with two alcoholic parents and the older brother with minimal cerebral palsy. Coming home with friends was always risky, since she could never be sure what melodrama might be waiting behind the front door. One *why* she accepts is the obvious one: she was depressed because of her family, and she began taking drugs to escape, to blunt her experiences. But she also entertains an even darker possibility. She may have begun her decade or so of drugs because she wanted to kill herself, and she did not have the courage to select more rapid means. But she cannot be sure.

Alcohol was the predictable first drug. While in high school, she would go out on Thursday evenings, and on weekends, and get so drunk she could not drive home but somehow always did. She did not just sit down and socialize with people over a few drinks. She wanted to socialize and drink— drink to effect, to get drunk. Driving home required special expertise, an equilibrium of craft that guided her car slowly through the California night air while she reckoned and negotiated the relationships of the auto with the street, curb, other cars, pedestrians. Her concentration on those evenings was complete. She never had an accident.

In front of her house she would gather her wits and energies to practice walking a straight line across her lawn. She would then walk into the house, sit down in the living room, watch television with her parents for five minutes, announce that she was tired and was going to bed, walk into her bedroom, and pass out on the bed. She still managed to excel in sports, even while drinking, and ended up being valedictorian of her high school class. The saving grace was that the drinking was episodic, not the chronic and dominating habit it became later.

No one helped her, or even recognized a problem. Her friends also drank, and they made excuses for each other. It was considered normal to get drunk at parties. Park reached out to one of her coaches, a woman who seemed to have an empathy rare among friends and acquaintances of the time. Her mother, "in her infinite alcoholic wisdom," decided that the coach was a lesbian trying to recruit her daughter, a logic impeccably grounded on the premise that since no one else was friendly with her daughter some sexual motive must be the inspiration. Park broke off the friendship to protect the coach's reputation.

In college there were many affairs, a few boyfriends, one person she convinced herself to fall in love with, and one with whom she did form a profound attachment. This last connection was real in one important way. At a time when she and her friends were sleeping around and passing it off to a liberated consciousness, this attachment was exclusive. They both practiced fidelity because it seemed right. He was even jealous from time to time, which Park found refreshing. She remembers those moments as better than getting flowers. Hormones and trust—the combination was as good as she was ever to have. They split up when Park went to medical school at the University of California.

The drinking increased in college. She began to combine the alcohol with marijuana at parties, and then in private moments as well. In medical school Park continued to drink and began using LSD from time to time. Occasionally she snorted some cocaine. She expanded her use of drugs during her residency. She began using LSD more frequently and also started taking a variety of substances that included Valium, codeine, morphine, Demerol, halothane (an inhaled anesthetic), versed (an injectable anesthetic), and more. Most she stole from the hospital. Her depressions became worse and more frequent. She kept sinking deeper into what she now views as her disease.

Park's tolerance to all drugs built up quickly. In the space of one memorable year she found that one bottle of wine did nothing for her, one six-pack of beer was not enough. She had to have two bottles of wine, two six-packs, for an evening of recreational drinking. Eventually alcohol itself could not make her drunk. By the third year of her residency she was freely mixing various other drugs with alcohol. She had married just before starting her internship and it was not working at all by this time. She began injecting drugs directly into the veins on her inner thighs.

Immediately after separating from her husband she used versed for the first time. It is a disassociative drug that allows the user to talk to people, move around and so on, but come away with no memory of the experience. A bit of film chronicling one's life is snipped out, leaving a memory hole where one was yet, inexplicably, conscious. The discontinuity is distinctly unsettling. Park claims always to have remembered experiences with LSD, though the effects of this substance may be gauged by one private measure: she decided to marry her first husband while under the drug's influence. But with versed she would find herself in places with no knowledge of how she got there. It was scary at new levels, and very unpleasant. Yet she continued to use the drug, again and again.

The effects of the drugs on Park's brain seemed to be an intensification of a malevolent sort. She was a fluid person, prone to depression but active and interested in all kinds of experiences. The drugs restricted the range of her consciousness, transforming her into a person whose sensory fields were contracted. She became narrow, repetitive. Her brain's focus, its range of activity, was concentrated within smaller domains. Some see creative chaos as vital to neurological activity. Park believes that this chaos was tightened and reorganized by the drugs. She became rigidly coherent along a very limited dimension.

Yet Park managed to function as a physician during these years, mainly by partitioning drugs and work. She would carefully gauge the active period of the drug she took. At times she would leave the operating room for lunch, use short-acting drugs, and then return to duty. Or she would take a break, disappear from the medical unit, find a bathroom somewhere, and simply shoot up for the short term. The problem was that she began dosing herself with short-acting substances at such levels that they began acting like longer-term drugs. She was (rationally) terrified of being caught. During her first year of residency one of the members of her group had been caught sniffing nitrous oxide out of one of the machines on a weekend when he was on call. The medical authorities had canned him so fast that he was never seen or heard from again by members of his medical group. Still, Park kept using drugs. She also began stockpiling them with the thought of killing herself.

One day during her fellowship year in intensive-care medicine, Park went down to the call room adjacent to the operating room and sat down. One of the attendants unexpectedly appeared and began asking her questions about a medical chart. She responded and her words began slurring. He did not have to ask her if she had a problem. It was obvious. He reported her to the head of the department, who came downstairs from his second-floor office and led her into one of the prep rooms off the operating room for a conference. Was she doing drugs, he wanted to know. She was convinced that her whole career was on the line, that a yes would transform the department head into the Red Queen, who would shriek "Off with her head." So she lied and said no. Then he asked her if she was thinking about committing suicide. "Of course I am," she responded. "Wouldn't anyone in my situation?"

These magic words brought her an escort up to the department chair's office, where he summoned an acute intervention team. Park was taken off medical duties and assigned to lab work. She was regarded as clinically depressed, not as addicted to drugs. Part of her therapy was a required visit to the staff psychiatrist once each week. The psychiatrist began prescribing therapeutic drugs that acted on the central nervous system, an intervention that amazed Park given her addictions. The therapy sessions went poorly. At the first session the psychiatrist asked her if she thought frequently about killing herself. Yes, Park answered. Well, the psychiatrist continued, have you been making any plans? The problem was that Park, like all medical students, had been through a psychiatry course during her first year of studies. She knew the sequence of questions. She also knew that the killer question was, are you making any plans? So she looked at the psychiatrist with the blandest expression she could muster and said no. She knew a yes would get her a quick bed in the mental therapy ward of the hospital, and that would get in between her and her plans. The imperative was evident to her. If she were serious about her plans to kill herself, she had to lie to the psychiatrist.

Her behavior became more, not less, bizarre in therapy. She would come into the hospital on weekends, get dressed up in OR garb, and steal some drugs. Then she would go down the hall to a bathroom and flush all of the drugs down a toilet without using any. Then she would turn around and steal more drugs, again flush them down the toilet, all within the space of twenty minutes. She couldn't stand not having the drugs, yet she was engaged in a tense internal struggle with herself over using them. She knew that if she were caught stealing drugs she was finished. Still she continued to use drugs during this time, though not as regularly as before. At times she would manage to go as long as three weeks without drugs. On other occasions, two hours would be her limit. She tried going back to physical activity, working out at the gym with an intensity that worried her friends. Nothing she tried got her to a point where she could control her habit. The psychiatrist was completely ineffective, even counterproductive. Park knew drugs were wrong, that they were destroying her. But she would take drugs with this thought as her last rational consideration before mainlining.

A friend got her into more rigorous therapy. She was living with a man she loved and trusted. He came into their bathroom one day and caught her shooting up. No words were better than the ones he used in reacting to what he had discovered. "Just because you use drugs," he told her, "doesn't mean you are a bad person." Simple. Almost a cliché. But the effects on Park were transforming. She broke down and cried for two hours in absolute, unqualified gratitude. She swore to him that she would stop using now, this minute. He calculated finely. "If you use again, even once, you agree to enter a treatment center." She agreed. Three days later she used drugs again. But, true to her pledge, she entered treatment.

The first treatment center was like a minimum-security prison. The ward was locked. Through a glass in the door, Park's group could see the adjacent ward where psychotic patients moved about slowly. Her first night, just after settling in, Park was given an entry interview. An attendant asked her, why are you here? Park said, "Because I need to stop using drugs and cut down on my drinking." The woman gave Park one of those looks that can penetrate through to the ventricles of the brain and then nodded, "Right, okay." Park was put in a room with another patient, a twelve-year-old girl. She could not remember feeling more ashamed of herself.

Each of the patients was responsible for her room, for making her bed and keeping the area clean. The idea was to introduce structure into the lives of individuals who had lost control, to get them to act responsibly about little things as a way of acquiring wider responsibilities. Room inspections were conducted every day, including searches for drugs. Breakfast was at 8:00 A.M. and attendance was mandatory. Doors had to be unlocked to allow the group of patients to go over to the dining room, relocked when they returned for therapy. Manual exercises and arts-and-crafts sessions were part of therapy. Park felt like she was in one of those psychiatric wards depicted in old 1950s movies, where the patients are locked up and controlled by benign but absolutely fixed rules. Everything sharp was locked up. You checked out your razor to shave, your needles to sew. Park felt like a criminal. She had no idea what the therapists were trying to do.

Patients earned increments of freedom. The psychiatry offices were across a lawn near some trees and an intervening driveway. Each patient was escorted to these offices for therapy during the first two weeks. Then, if you had behaved well (followed all of the rules and tried hard to be a member of the community), your first reward was to be allowed to walk over to therapy by yourself. The lesson was that you could be trusted to return. The therapy was also dosed liberally with verbal confrontations. Therapists wanted to get the patients to acknowledge their feelings, so insults that brought tears were common.

Park used drugs twice during her stay in this first treatment center. Once, late in her stay, she was permitted to return to the hospital where she had worked in order to discuss prospects for a renewal of her fellowship. After a promising discussion with her department chair, she walked down to the laboratory, stole some drugs, and used them in a nearby bathroom. The center gave her a urine test when she returned. When the results came in, she promptly lost all of her earned freedom and had her stay extended. The second time was during a visit to her home over the Thanksgiving holidays. Everyone in the family was drinking heavily except her. One of her brothers had back problems at that time and was taking codeine. Park was sitting at the kitchen table late on Thursday night while everyone was in varying degrees of alcoholic stupor in different rooms in the house. The bottle of codeine number three was on the shelf. She opened it and stole most of the tablets. For the rest of the holiday, her high was competitive with her family's alcoholic binges. This time she was street smart about the urine test. She brought a sample donated by a friend to the center, hid it, gave it to the lab people. It was clean, so no problem.

After seven weeks of this type of treatment, Park was released with instructions to attend AA meetings. She stayed dry over the Christmas holidays at home. Then she returned to the hospital to resume work. All of the pressures returned. She lasted ten days before resuming the pattern of stealing and using drugs. She would take a chair into an empty bathroom and shoot up or inhale. Usually she would pass out in the chair and topple over backwards onto the floor. After two weeks she had a ring of bumps and abrasions around the back of her head, like Christ's crown of thorns she thought at the time, only confined to the rear of her head.

Stories went around the hospital until eventually the professors in the department organized a classic confrontation meeting with Park. "You cannot continue work in this condition," the leader of the confrontation group told her. "You have to decide to seek treatment again." Park had an idea this time where she wanted to go. One of the residents in her group had just returned from the Ridgeway Center in Atlanta for substance-abuse treatment. Park had immediately dubbed the center "Syringeway," but in talking to the returned resident she quickly realized he had something that she didn't have. She didn't know what it was, or how to get it, but she knew that it made all the difference in the world and that she wanted it. So she asked the group leader if the hospital could place her at Ridgeway. The group broke up with a promise from her department chair to see if the Atlanta center had room for her.

Park drifted out of the conference room and started walking down the hospital corridor. She felt absolutely alone, one of those moments of solitude so complete that she might as well have been in a hermetically sealed bubble. In her room at the hospital, she had an inhalable anesthetic that would arrest respiration if breathed in at 100 percent strength. She put it in her pocket along with a face mask used to administer anesthetics. In a bathroom just behind the gift shop on the first floor she entered a toilet stall and locked the door. She was going to work some cotton into the mask, saturate the cotton with the anesthetic, and strap on the mask. That would do it. Death in just a few minutes.

Park didn't do it. She inhaled most of the bottle, but she did not use the cotton or the mask. When she woke up, sitting on the tile floor in front of the toilet, she realized that she had not tried to kill herself. To this day she does not know what prevented her from doing so. She slowly got up and went back upstairs to the department offices. In the meantime, while she had been inhaling the drug, the whole hospital had been turned upside down in a search for her. The department head, when he realized she was missing and no one had seen her, had called the police. For two hours he had been convinced that they would find Park dead somewhere. Instead she walked into his office with a simple surrender. "If Ridgeway will take me, please just get me on the plane, fast. I want to go." The Atlanta center accepted her. She left on an evening flight for a second try at rehabilitation.

One last humiliation remained. At the airport, with one of the professors as her escort to Atlanta and with her lover there to see her off, the great love of her Chicago years appeared. He was there to connect with a plane to Denver. It was the first time they had seen each other since they broke off the relationship. Park looked like what she was, a drug abuser on the verge of a complete breakdown. She became hysterical, screaming at her former lover to get away from her. She boarded the plane crying, near collapse, half hoping that they would crash and she would burn to death before reaching Atlanta.

The Ridgeway Center was different from the first treatment center in several ways. No locked doors, windows everywhere, nice decorative touches, even better food. Park arrived on a Friday evening and spent the first few days drifting around trying to figure the place out. On Tuesday at the first meeting, with roughly seventy other physicians present and undergoing treatment, she had to introduce herself and tell the others how she came to be where she was. She blamed all of her troubles on her alcoholic parents and ended up crying. Afterwards others in the group told her that she was the most miserable, self-pitying person they had ever heard. It was as close to cold hard bottom as she would ever get.

In the painful aftermath of the first group meeting, Park began to realize that her salvation lay in abandoning all reserve, depending on the group to help her climb out of the pit that she had entered. At the next meeting she stood up and surrendered. She gave up control to the dynamic of the therapy session, uttering the words "I am an alcoholic" as a direct expression of feeling. She remembers a connection to the words. The utterance was a phonetic sequence transformed into an institutional fact. She *meant* the words, *she* meant the words. Something inside of her shifted in that public declaration.

The conversion process remains a mystery to her. She learned a craft for getting better, not understanding the meaning of the changes she felt but grasping how to accomplish the task of restoration. The critical strategy was the deployment of an image. She remembers describing her problems one day in treatment, asking for a solution. The therapist said, "Close your eyes and think about your hand in the form of a fist. It is holding on to a set of keys. Now hold your arm out at full length and just let go." This image immediately dominated her thoughts. The keys became all of the emotional baggage of her life. She stretched her arm out physically and, in her mind, she just let go of what she was holding.

It helped that almost everyone in the group was there as a last resort. Unbearable stories were the norm. One doctor was a convicted felon (for dealing in drugs). Another had gambled away his entire life's fortune while on an alcoholic binge. Therapists were there as patients because they used drugs while pretending to treat addicts. It was not difficult to accept one's own wretched excesses in that context. She found out, slowly over the long dreamy days in therapy, that she could, in David Hume's phrase, "bear a survey of oneself." She accepted her life, her own deep and crippling flaws.

The metaphor influencing the group was drawn from the surrounding countryside. In the national park in Atlanta, a river cuts across the eastern boundary of the grounds. Park began driving up to the park and hiking to the river, usually on a Sunday afternoon. She would sit on a rock and let the river enter her thoughts as a ghost, an image superimposed upon the perceived reality. In the dream picture she floated on the surface of the water with her eyes closed, just drifting with the current, exposed and relaxed, one with the universe. The metaphor was comfortable for all who heard it. It suggested the total acceptance of life that Park's colleague in the hospital had discovered in treatment.

Park was at Ridgeway for twenty-eight days. After this initial stay she was sent to a halfway house, a three-bedroom apartment with four other women who were also recovering from drug addiction. Each individual was given twenty-five dollars a week for food, so close budgeting was necessary. On the outside Park resumed running (though she couldn't quit smoking until fourteen months after leaving the center). She was required to be a functioning member of the small group in the house, which she was. Outpatient therapy continued every day for five more weeks. Eventually she was assigned medical duties at another treatment center in Atlanta where she conducted physicals on patients, gave lectures on alcoholism and substance abuse, and was the primary counselor for some of the patients. The distal requirement, after the service work in a treatment center, was expressed in written form. She signed a contract to go to at least two AA meetings a week for two years after leaving the center, and at least once a month for the remainder of her life. She still has a copy of this agreement.

The rest of it was just learning how to live a normal life again. Recognizing that one was afflicted with a permanent disease was one of the lessons. But avoiding drugs was not all of it. Park also had to learn how to stop blaming others for her problems, to be honest with herself about everything, to accept herself for what she really was. In all of the therapy, the goal was to extend the self to others, to check out feelings and perceptions with other people. The independent and isolated self had to be abandoned. In its place each individual discovered a self that was filtered through others, that trusted others for guidance and even identity. This involvement of the self with the group was to be permanent, reinforced constantly through AA meetings.

Mirror-image therapy was designed to extend the self. When Park was in therapy during her first few weeks at Ridgeway, she could look around and identify with others who were always as crippled as she was and sometimes were much worse off. As a counselor in one of the centers, she worked with people who had seizures, who went through painful withdrawal experiences, and she could see herself in them. She could put herself in the place of the other, not by becoming the other, but by herself seeing the world through the eyes of the other. The mirror image shimmered with multiple identities that, finally, were the same. You look in the mirror and see the image of the other, but the other is just like the self. All individuals are the same. Everything is continuous.

For Park, the restructuring of her self included a restoration of the child she once had been. She regards her true self as the self of five years old, ankle deep in stream water and bending down with curiosity to see life in its natural forms. She has an almost fatalistic belief now in the powers of the mind and the universe to help her. A conviction that if you just let go, there are powers in the unconscious and in the world that will provide guidance. She has not taken any drugs in five years. The defensive shell of the drug years has been cast away, the machine human replaced by an organic self. She is comfortable in seeing herself as a molecular arrangement floating on the river and continuous with the chemical composition of reality.

Joanne Park was offered a position in anesthesiology at a University of California medical school. At one point in her life she might have offered up human sacrifices to be on a medical faculty. After her treatment she didn't want to go back. She turned down the offer. Instead she went back to the University of California to take courses in environmental science, then enrolled in a graduate program at a Michigan university to learn about public health. She has decided to be a teacher and a consultant on medical insurance practices.

The memories of the operating room remain with her, though in a residual place in her mind. She misses the excitement from time to time, and recalls the successes of intensive-care treatment. But two failures also occupy a place in her memories. One was a young man in his early twenties who was brought into the operating room with some type of pneumonia. He was unconscious, had labored breathing, low blood pressure. Park was trying to clear his airway to insert a tube down his throat when he vomited. Then he started thrashing about even more violently. Park injected a drug that paralyzed him. Then, when she started to insert the tube in his throat again, his heart stopped. They coded him, but he never made it.

The other case was a woman, critically ill, who had to have emergency surgery on her abdomen. Park had three lines in her, one to monitor vital signs, the other two for blood and fluid. The woman began to bleed badly during surgery. Park got all the blood in the room into the woman. But she could not get the blood in as fast as it was going out of the woman's body. She died on the table. Park does not know to this day if putting in a larger line before surgery began would have saved the woman's life. Maybe it would have. But then she may have died anyway in spite of everyone's best efforts.

From a taped interview with Joanne Park:

"There were a lot of things in surgery that I didn't know about because I could see only so much of the patients. Then I don't think I am the prime mover anyway. I never did."

INTERVIEWER: The prime mover is the surgeon?

"No. (laughter) A little higher. Higher and wider and multidimensional."

INTERVIEWER: Tell me about the prime mover and what role the prime mover plays in your life.

"I don't understand what the prime mover is. Whatever the prime mover is, the prime mover's insides do not work like a clock. There is serendipity involved. I would rather be lucky than good, because luck always counts. And I don't know what luck is. It isn't just random movement in the linear universe, because I think the random movement is more important than linear movement. Randomness is not a residual. Linearity is a residual."

Park leans back in her chair, her hair framed against the window at her back. The bright sunlight from outside places her face in shadow if one looks directly at her.

"I was brought up a Catholic. I remember listening to the nuns and they always said 'God is everywhere.' I remember sitting in Saturday religious instruction, which I hated, thinking about God being inside of tree trunks. At the same time being in the bark and being in the air. And being puzzled over that for a long time. The prime mover is not the God I thought about when I was sitting listening to the nuns. It is more like an Indian great spirit—it is not even a force or an energy. It is amorphous, and beyond my comprehension. I don't rely on it. I don't plan my life around it. But I assume it is there. Fundamentally it is good. It has something to do with life and it is good. It is not destructive. Even when misery and destruction happen, these are temporary. It is like a unity that is out there even in misery. Misery allows you to appreciate the goodness. Having been close to death helped me to appreciate life. Having been completely, spiritually void, and remembering what that was like, makes my life richer now that I am not. Because there was always something missing, there was always something that I was struggling with and I don't struggle anymore. I don't struggle. Most of the time I am remarkably happy. I don't worry about tomorrow and I don't try to control because I know I can't. Not only that but it is pointless. Control to what end? There isn't any end."

5

SPIRITUAL HEALING

Mind Transformations

The therapy administered by Alcoholics Anonymous shares with traditional faith healing the conviction that only as the mind or soul is reformed can the body be healed. These reforms often involve a complete regeneration of the self. The body is addressed through the mind, and is often restored to health as the mind achieves peace and stability. Joanne Park's experiences suggest that this mental tranquility is secured by means of beliefs in an alternative reality.

The AA program subscribes to this metaphysical doctrine. Alcoholics Anonymous lists twelve steps as the "spiritual stages that an alcoholic must pass through, one by one, if he wants to ensure his physical and mental regeneration." The first three are the most intriguing. The initial step is the recognition that one has a disease ("I am an alcoholic") and that the disease is beyond one's ability to control it. The second is a belief that some greater power can rescue the individual from the addiction. The third is a surrender to this healing power, which in practical terms usually leads to freedom from the substance abuse but not from the physical condition of chemical dependency (an alcoholic is one forever). The twelfth and final step in the AA credo is an instruction to proselytize, to spread the word to other alcoholics that regeneration is possible.

In traditional AA literature, the power that brings about regeneration is God, though without denominational signs ("however [the individual] may conceive of Him"). Many of the steps between three and twelve urge inventories (confessions?) of sins, prayers to God, meditation, and so on. The basic condition for AA membership, however, is stated in a simple and secular declaration: "an honest desire to stop drinking." Joanne Park is uncertain about God. She believes in a higher reality but is convinced that the human intellect is too limited to know a supreme being or even know that one exists. Most of the members of her therapy group are agnostic. Yet the belief that one surrenders to a higher power is genuine. The controlling thought is that something outside of the self, some external being, is needed for the salvation that AA offers.

Therapy is successful as the individual retreats from explicit or linear forms of thought and begins to rely on the unconscious, on the deep intuitive sense that AA sees as capable of apprehending some external reality. It is not inaccurate to say that the discrete and rational individual assumed in so much of contemporary thought is abandoned, and even on occasion seen as the source of the pathology that AA methods attempt to heal. In its place, the therapy attempts to forge a holistic individual, no longer divisible into mind and body, with an identity extended to the group and even beyond to the whole of reality.

The Healing Ministry of Christ

Spiritual healing, a tradition that AA continues in its attentions to mind, is found throughout the history of medicine in the West. But the most influential versions of such healing are arguably those associated with Jesus of Nazareth. The Gospels of the New Testament that record Jesus' life in official testimonies generally regard all individuals as dualistic, composed of both spirit and physical matter. Individuals are unique instantiations of the divine within the material world. Healing is seen both in terms of divine intervention and the disclosure of the divine within each individual. The healing ministry of Christ fits both interpretations.

Healing in the Gospels follows some Old Testament accounts while rejecting others. The view of God (Yahweh) as arbitrary by human standards, dispensing gifts and afflictions according to criteria unintelligible to humans, is left behind. (This view is expressed in a well-known and striking passage in Deuteronomy 32:39, "I will kill and I will make to live. I will strike, and I will heal, and there is none that can deliver out of my hand.") Also abandoned is the thought that illness is a sign of moral failure, a punishment for sin. Instead, Jesus develops the Old Testament views of healing (after sacrifices are made) as a gift from God, and illness as misfortune or test (as in the story of Job) rather than a divine judgment.

The healing described in the Gospels also draws on Hellenistic traditions that address the body by means of the mind. Plato broke with the Homeric celebration of aggressive values (like courage in battle) by stressing the quieter virtues of social harmony. In political society, justice is an arrangement of classes that are themselves defined in terms of functions. The state is a collective expression of the balance within the individual that represents health. In Plato's philosophy, the healthy individual is in a state of internal equilibrium in which reason dominates spirit and appetite.

The state of health Jesus sought is an equilibrium in which the individual soul is without sin in a body free of illness. But for Jesus, unlike the Greek thinkers, the afflictions of mind and body are not the result of fate or destiny but the product of spiritual forces that can be blunted. Jesus was a shaman, a mediator between the individual and a spiritual reality that was seen as having both good and evil dimensions. He claimed the power to heal as an instrument of the good or beneficent side of the spiritual world. Healing in the Gospels is a restoration of the balance between soul and body that recognizes the individual as a spiritual creature in a material universe.

Human nature is complex in Christianity (due to the influence of Paul's ideas). There is first the idea that human beings are created in the image of God and in this sense are identical all over the world. This image, however, is incarnate, a spirit placed within the physical world. Human beings, as both spirit and matter, occupy the lowest place in a hierarchy of spiritual beings. But this location is provisional. The spiritual in humans permits access in some degree to the supernatural.

This duality—spirit and matter—produces and explains conflict within the self. Spirit and matter obviously can be opposed to each other. The demands and desires of the flesh may be contrary to spiritual needs. But a larger conflict also occurs. Jesus taught that the evil powers of the spiritual world can enter human experience and possess individuals. The will in particular can be controlled, creating situations in which individuals are unable to do the right thing even though they know what it is (a possibility that directly contravenes Plato's thesis in the early dialogues that knowing the good is sufficient to act upon it). Individuals can do wrong to themselves and others because of intervention by demonic or unclean spirits. We are landscapes on which spiritual forces do battle with each other.

One of the central messages in Jesus' beliefs is that these higher, supernatural realities cannot be negotiated successfully by the individual alone. God's help is necessary. The will, even the whole of one's life, must be given up to God in order to find one's true self. The simple organized self of Greek thought, where reason dominates desire, is replaced with the more complex notion of multiple spiritual dimensions in the self. The healing effort is a winnowing among psychic states with the help of beneficent spirits. Plato asks, how can an individual be in two volitional states? Jesus answers, because there are multiple and conflicting spiritual realities that can range over the human psyche. In the Gospels, the truly integrated self is one that has sacrificed some of its parts in order to receive God's spirit. The healthy individual is one who is filled with spiritual goodness and has excluded evil.

The explanation of illness follows this dualistic conception of human beings. Illness does not in itself indicate sin or moral failure. It is certainly not a judgment made by God on the sick person. Illness is thought to be the result of evil in the world. Satanic or other forces escape God's control and harm human beings. One expression of this harm is illness of various types. But the acceptance of malevolent spiritual forces as the cause of illness does not mean that the afflicted individual is malevolent or morally defective. The one exception to this is the weakening effects of sin. An individual who sins invites evil spirits into the domain of his psyche, thus increasing the prospects for illness of some sort.

The type of healing Jesus performed addressed the spiritual dimensions of human experience. He claimed to be the agent of God, the individual through whom God heals. The healing power was psychic; it seemed to involve some transfer of power. In one famous story, a woman touches his garment and is healed. He immediately senses (without seeing her) that someone has drawn energy from him. Yet the Gospels also stress the religious nature of these powers. They are neither secular nor simple forms of magic. They are viewed as vehicles of disclosure and intervention. Some spiritual presence within the individual is brought forth (disclosure), and the grace of God is brought into contact with the individual (intervention).

Two techniques were typically used in healing: one was touch; the other was voice, usually a command. All types of illness were addressed, and the healing described in the Gospels is always complete, not partial or temporary. The illnesses addressed ranged over the organic and mental. The organic problems healed by Jesus included wounds, tumors, deafness, blindness, paralysis of various types, leprosy—in general, the worst afflictions of the time. On three occasions Jesus was said to have brought the dead back to life. Mental diseases that were reported as healed were usually viewed as forms of possession. The cure involved exorcising the harmful spirit from the individual. In no case is Jesus reported to have used even the crude medical techniques of the day. He occasionally used spit (his own in most instances) and mud as material to rub on the ill person, usually in the affected area. But no medicine was used. The healing came about (if it did) through spiritual rather than medical means.

In addition to healing organic and mental illnesses, Jesus also claimed the power to forgive sin. This forgiveness, again representing a higher spiritual power, healed the soul and was considered by Jesus to be the superior therapeutic power. The restoration of the soul to a state of grace is the capstone of the healing approach of Scripture, and completes a healing of the whole person, both body and spirit. All of these healing efforts, moreover, are seen in Christian theology as the fulfillment of a natural order in which human beings have a definite, though not superior, location.

The reliability of the healing stories in the Gospels, and even of the historical existence of Jesus, has been challenged in a number of ways. But as narrative, as an account of events and persons, these stories are powerful influences on Christianity. They form the basis for most of the leading ideas in all versions of Christian thought, since the power of a spiritual or supernatural world to enter human experience and reverse material causality (including illness and death) is vital to Christian understandings of human nature and destiny. The strong influence of these stories on Western civilization is real whether the events occurred or not. This reality—the effects of the narratives—is one key to understanding Christian healing today.

It is also worth noting that the official portraits of Jesus downplay, and sometimes deny, the magical episodes of his life and works. The reason for this is that magic appears to be an extension of the secular, a kind of hybrid craft lodged more nearly in science than religion. A professional magician today typically claims no miraculous powers. Magical powers consist only of manipulations of the material world to create illusions. If Jesus were just a magician in this reductionist sense, then no connection between his life and God could be inferred from the miracles he performed.

But supernatural versions of magic dominated the social world in which Jesus lived. Beliefs in an external reality were widespread. The culture was viewed by its members as thickly populated with spirits and demigods of various sorts. Magic thrived. Miracles were almost commonplace. Conversations with God were as frequent as dreams (and often found in dream experiences, both at night and during the day). Many magicians claimed supernatural powers of prophecy, exorcism, and healing. Jesus was part of this culture, and the Gospel version of his life contains strong parallels to the magical rites and works of the time. These include the Eucharist ceremony, exorcism of evil spirits, healings, and even many of the teachings. Jesus also shared with many magicians of the time a belief in one god at the theoretical level as well as the acceptance of many lesser gods and spirits at the practical level. Even the episodic structure and materials of the Gospels parallel the ordinary texts of magic circulating during and after Jesus' lifetime.

In many ways, Jesus was almost a standard magician of his historical period. He performed miracles, which magicians of the time did. There is evidence (not free of controversy) that he claimed to be divine, and that this claim was accepted by his contemporaries as an explanation for his magical powers. He urged prayer and trust in God, also common among magicians of the time. Much of Jesus' life paralleled stories of magical careers, including the descent of a spirit upon the body during baptism, various visionary experiences, his picaresque existence, and the resurrection and postmortem appearances to followers. Magic was a common activity during this time in history. The professional magician of today would have been at the lowest levels of magical claims in Jesus' culture.

It is when the various background conditions are all in place that the life of Jesus seems to exceed even that of his spiritual contemporaries. The life and deeds of Jesus were supposed to have been foretold in Scripture. He was said to have had a god as a father. He was viewed as acting always from good motives, never from dark impulses or for money. The miracles illustrated moral truths and were not performed just as miraculous feats. Jesus had disciples who primarily carried forward the moral message of his life, not just the magic itself. The most important indicator offered for Jesus' divinity, however, is the expression of a higher level of reality in the miracles. It was not just that the magic was advanced as real in the sense that natural laws were suspended, for many magicians of the day claimed these powers. Rather, it was that the miracles communicated moral lessons said to be drawn up by a singular and overriding God who offered salvation. Jesus was a magician whose claims to connect the divine with human experience initiated one of the most influential religions in history.

Pentecostal and Charismatic Movements

At all stages in the life of Jesus a supernatural reality is claimed as the source for healing. The modern Pentecostal and later charismatic movements (if they can be called movements) are recent efforts to break through to a reality beyond human experience. Modern Pentecostalism began in the early years of this century. Though it is almost always a mistake to specify some historical moment as the origin of any movement, two dates are significant in the beginnings of Pentecostal beliefs and practices. In 1901, Charles Parham, an evangelical preacher, instructed his students at Bethel Bible College in Topeka, Kansas, to search Scripture for biblical evidence of Spirit baptism. They did, and became convinced that the critical datum confirming the presence of the Holy Spirit is glossolalia, speaking in tongues. This conviction found its own reality during a prayer meeting on December 31, 1901.

As Parham placed his hands on a student she began speaking in a language (or so it was labeled) unknown to her or anyone else in the room. The experience was quickly duplicated by other students.

Parham held a number of revivals over the next several years and opened a second Bible School in Houston. One of his most gifted students was a black preacher, William J. Seymour. Seymour also had the experience (under Parham's guidance) of speaking in tongues. In 1906, Seymour moved to Los Angeles and started the Azusa Street revival. His success was immediate. The faithful began coming to Seymour's church to experience an emotional catharsis missing in most of the mainstream religions of the time. These two dates, 1901 and 1906, are enshrined by believers as the beginnings of the modern Pentecostal movement.

Pentecostalism, at all stages in its development, has stressed the emotive or nonrational as a device to break through human experience and come into contact with God (through the Holy Spirit). There is no written theology in the movement, no doctrinal innovations. The decisive component is the conversion experience. Belief and spirituality are proven through a second baptism in Christ that summons the self for redemption. This self is thought to be at least in part below the conscious level of experience. A neurologist, and perhaps even a psychologist, would say that the regions of the brain activated by sensual or emotive experiences are stimulated in the Pentecostal service. But the faithful believe that the stimuli actually shift realities. The individual is thought to come into sudden and direct contact with an alternative reality that touches and transforms the self.

The features of the second baptism are all intuitive or nonrational. They consist of three primary acts: prophecies, healings, and speaking in tongues. These are direct acts, tangible evidence of the conversion experience. They must be manifest, not hidden or obscure. But these externalizations represent an inner, spiritual change. Imagine the self as a template in space and time with both an interior and exterior dimension. The observable physical changes in the individual constitute proof in Pentecostalism that the inner dimensions of the self have been changed. Salvation is a spiritual transformation that expresses itself in physical terms.

The conversion experience is individualistic but occurs in a congregation of believers. When it occurs, the individual has an ecstatic vision of the spiritual world that eliminates all uncertainty and elevates the religious convictions secured through conversion to a preeminent position, excluding the secular and even other more organized religious beliefs. The individual is renewed, transformed, and typically enters into different relationships with others, even with those who shared the most intimate experiences previously. Family and friends who have not had the critical experience often view the convert with a mixture of awe, bemusement, and irritation. These attitudes usually do not undermine the convert's transformation.

The congeniality of the cathartic experience with both scientific and religious explanations is illustrated in especially vivid terms by glossolalia, the dramatic event that begins the Pentecostal conversion. Speaking in tongues is sufficiently common in Pentecostal and charismatic religious services to be regarded as commonplace, not unusual. But by most conventional standards, the event is either a sign of mental aberration (usually temporary) or proof of the presence of the Holy Spirit. In either judgment, it is an extraordinary occurrence. It is also poorly understood in both secular and religious discourses.

Glossolalia can be described easily enough. In certain conditions individuals begin uttering sounds—sometimes vowels and consonants, at other times phrases—that do not resemble the language of the speaker or audience and are often simply neologisms. Most studies of glossolalia have concluded that it is not a language at all. It is a string of sounds that are often simply phonetic utterances. Close examination usually leaves the utterances in their original unintelligible state, or revealed as hybrid sounds borrowed from other (and sometimes multiple) languages. The actual "speaking in tongues" event is almost never a linguistic communication.

On occasion the sequence of sounds in glossolalia will evolve during the course of a spiritual ceremony, sometimes culminating in phrases or sentences that do communicate thoughts to listeners. But these utterances seem to be a form of chorus, repetitive sayings of familiar spiritual phrases to encourage a state of mind, or exhortations of various sorts, rather than true speech. Glossolalia may be pure phonetics. Group leaders in religious practices sometimes offer interpretations of such sounds. But the interpretations follow no common rules, so that the meaning of a string of utterances is almost entirely a function of who is doing the interpreting. (Different interpreters will translate the same sounds in radically different ways.)

There is little agreement on the conditions that produce the sounds heard in glossolalia. For those working within certain religious traditions, "speaking in tongues" is a spiritual experience, required in some Pentecostal churches for full entry into the congregation. The biblical precedents can be found in Acts 2:1–4, where the presence of the Holy Spirit is described in terms of "noise, wind, and tongues of fire." In Acts 2:9–11, the apostles are described as explaining the Gospel of Jesus Christ in many languages on the day of Pentecost (a section of Scripture cited frequently in the origins of Pentecostalism in the early twentieth century). The gift of tongues in such traditions is obviously both a manifestation of a spirit from another world (the third entry in the Trinity) and a linguistic communication of the most profound sort. The conditions producing glossolalia are said to be brought about by a contact between ordinary and transcendent realities.

Secular efforts to understand glossolalia concentrate on the psychological and social characteristics of those who speak in tongues, and the empirical contexts in which the experience occurs. Carl Jung portrayed the experience as a variation on multiple personalities. Some part of the self other than the conscious part assumes control of the speech centers. Other studies have linked glossolalia to a wide range of pathologies, including various types of disassociation, hysteria, catalepsy, epilepsy, and schizophrenia. One project has tracked glossolalia to psychopathology in the homes of speakers, including alcoholism and nervous breakdowns among family members. Other studies have assimilated glossolalia to trances, somnambulism, speech automatism, excessive emotionalism, repression, and hypochondria.

Three problems plague all research that attempts to describe glossolalia with various pathological labels. One is that the experience of speaking in tongues seems to have no harmful effects on the speakers. On the contrary, they emerge from the experience with undamaged egos and often with a stronger sense of self than they had previously. They feel no confusion over the differences between ordinary and what they believe is transcendent reality. A second problem is that more recent studies have demonstrated that "normal" individuals (functional in society with well-integrated egos) have the experience as well. Third, research into the pathology of glossolalia misses the point made by those who employ spiritual discourses—that the experience is a genuine contact with another reality, even if it fails to meet the standards of mental stability applied in contemporary psychotherapy.

Social anthropologists, using a different explanatory model, have viewed glossolalia as another entry in a range of ecstatic phenomena that help to maintain certain religious groups. Certainly the renewal of Christian faith among Pentecostal and charismatic movements is testimony to the restorative functions of ecstatic experiences. Much evidence also suggests that speaking in tongues predates Judeo-Christian traditions and is found in both Western and non-Western cultures. Glossolalia seems to be a feature of many spiritual practices in which ecstatic experiences dominate, especially where possession by spirits is accepted as a real occurrence. In all of these instances, glossolalia is a part of spiritual experiences that help maintain those religious practices that stress emotive connections to an alternative reality (even though glossolalia in secular societies is a deviant phenomenon within the larger society and even mainline religions).

No evidence connects glossolalia to disorganized or fragmented groups. Pentecostalism, as a coherent religious movement, is a more typical context for glossolalia experiences than are disorganized communities. Also, conditions of deprivation do not cause glossolalia. While many Pentecostal members were socially and economically deprived in the early stages of the movement, speaking in tongues has persisted as Pentecostalism moved into the middle socioeconomic class in the United States. The one variable strongly associated with all glossolalia is belief in the experience itself, and in the possibilities of spiritual contact. Those who speak in tongues are more likely to see the world in religious terms and to be strongly connected to their religious faith and to their church.

Some of the more interesting studies in glossolalia suggest parallels to hypnotism. In both experiences a neophyte is guided to a different level of consciousness by a mentor. The initial experience of speaking in tongues is enriched by the need for ecstatic spiritual experiences, which introduces a kind of individual distress that must be relieved. Also, glossolalia occurs within an ontology that is understood (more or less) by the parishioner and completely accepted as an explanation of human experience. But in both glossolalia and hypnotism, a willing subject enters a trusting relationship with a teacher during which the self is given over in whole or in part to an emotive experience. Both glossolalia and hypnotism also occur in an organized setting designed to create an emotional context for changes in mood. This combination of trust and setting allows the individual in both experiences to let go, to open up the self for an emotional release not controlled by the ego. The resulting feelings of euphoria (more intense in glossolalia) are partially explainable in terms of the individual's feeling of acceptance by the religious or secular group. One has made it. One belongs.

Yet neither psychology nor socioanthropology addresses the validity of glossolalia. Even the most accurate empirical explanations say nothing about the claim that speaking in tongues is proof of the presence of the Holy Spirit. Imagine a thought experiment in which all variables accounting for the occurrence of glossolalia have been identified, so that a covering law can both explain and predict the experience as it in fact occurs. Still left unattended is the assertion that the experience is a manifestation of a divine being, that the sounds issue from a spirit beyond human experience.

It would be surprising if a religious movement so oriented toward the individual and the nonrational did not yield contradictory insights and convictions. One advantage of rational discourse is that disagreements can be arbitrated publicly on acknowledged rules of evidence and inference (though, of course, not always successfully). The intuitive experience, by contrast, relies on a truth that is seen directly in a critical experience but that may not be communicable outside the intuitive frame. In simple terms, one either knows or does not, and telling is not much help. The long-standing difficulty with intuitions is arbitrating contrary versions of truth with no publicly accessible rules for doing so.

Even early Pentecostalism was characterized by competing insights and interpretations of the conversion experience and Scripture. Some of the doctrinal disputes are typical of religious movements. Traditional Christianity teaches that there is one God enclosing three persons (Father, Son, and Holy Spirit). Some variants on Pentecostalism hold the unitarian view that there is one God and one person representing God (Jesus). Other variants have asserted that there is one God and three manifestations (not persons) of the Godhead. At a more practical level, there have been disputes over the proper number of works of grace and the sufficiency of grace to achieve salvation. The Wesleyan Holiness tradition stresses three works of grace—conversion, entire sanctification, and baptism in the Holy Spirit—while other interpretations collapse the first two into each other for a "two works of grace" creed. The Full Gospel tradition accepts three works of grace plus divine healing by faith and a belief in the second coming of Jesus. The skeptic may view such disputes as verbal at best, nonsense at worst. But they (and other such disputes) have yielded four principal denominations of Pentecostalism: the Assemblies of God, the Church of God, the Pentecostalism Holiness, and the Church of the Foursquare Gospels—each with a substantial following. Whatever the differences among Pentecostal denominations, however, four features are universal to all versions of Pentecostalism and mark it as a distinct religious practice: salvation through conversion, baptism in the Holy Spirit, an expectation that Christ will come to earth a second time, and a belief in divine healing through faith.

The charismatic movement, in all important respects, is the extension of Pentecostal practices to mainstream churches. In each extension of Pentecostalism, the catalyst was an individual or small group able to create a contagion effect in traditional religious organizations. In the early 1950s, a white South African, David du Plessis, used his evangelical energies to establish a series of meetings with the World Council of Churches to spread the Pentecostal message to established church leaders. A California dairy farmer, Demos Shakarian, joined the evangelist Oral Roberts to introduce Pentecostal beliefs to business leaders through breakfast meetings. The Full

Gospel Businessmen's Fellowship International is now an international Pentecostal organization with members worldwide. The Episcopal church has also proved hospitable to Pentecostalism. Dennis Bennett, the rector of St. Mark's Episcopal Church in Van Nuys, California, was baptized by Pentecostal friends and in 1959 began preaching those ideas to his congregation. The church eventually expelled him, but his exile to the more modest confines of a small mission church in Seattle did not slow his proselytizing efforts. He quickly increased church membership by baptizing willing visitors in the Holy Spirit. Many of these new converts went back to their own parishes to convert other Episcopalians to Pentecostal practices.

The most interesting recipient of Pentecostal practices, however, is arguably the Roman Catholic Church. The contagion pattern in Catholicism is similar to the patterns that have occurred in other churches. In early 1967, a group of faculty and students at Duquesne University held prayer meetings and meditated on the Book of Acts. From all accounts, the experiences of that group over the course of a weekend were extraordinary. Most claimed to have been touched by the Holy Spirit. Prayer, singing, tears of joy, transformation of lives and even identities were commonplace among the twenty or so individuals.

One of the participants in that Duquesne weekend, Ralph Keifer, carried the message of catharsis and redemption to Notre Dame. Kevin Ranaghan, a doctoral student, and his wife Dorothy were impressed enough to form a prayer group on campus that sought and found the same intense experiences of baptism in the Holy Spirit. These charismatic encounters quickly spread to other campuses and to increasing numbers of Catholic parishioners. Over six million Roman Catholics identified with the charismatic movement during the next two decades. In 1981, Pope Paul VI gave an official papal blessing to neo-Pentecostal practices in the Catholic Church, an acceptance that widened the scope of diversity endorsed by the Second Vatican Council from procedural and theological tolerance to an incorporation of emotive experiences in religious practices.

It was through Pentecostal and charismatic practices that faith healing was restored, and in some cases introduced, to traditional Christianity. Some of the most famous neo-Pentecostal preachers showcase faith healing in their services. Oral Roberts, notorious in some circles for the uncanny ability he demonstrated in 1987 to extract money (eight million dollars) from parishioners on threat of being called back from earth by God, began as a faith healer on television in the 1950s. Faith healing is an integral part of all neo-Pentecostal practices. It often includes the "laying on of hands" found in Scripture (though much congregational and electronic healing is attempted with no physical contact between priest and parishioner) and an effort to heal both spirit and body. In Pentecostalism, the aim of faith healing is the restoration of the whole individual, mental and physical, to a state of health.

Pentecostal Ministries: Jamison and Penfield

Faith Jamison is a black Pentecostal minister who presides over a small inner-city church directly in back of a large Howard Johnson hotel. The hotel mainly draws visitors who are in the city briefly on business. It is twelve stories high with a cylindrical design. A parking garage to the left of the entrance completes the architectural layout. When asked to describe the rooms, a recent guest remarked, "Nondescript." The church, by contrast, consists of one white clapboard building directly on the sidewalk. A single sign designates the orientation: "Jesus Christ Salvation Mission." On a recent Sunday afternoon Pastor Jamison is preaching to a very small congregation that is nevertheless attentive to every word she utters. Outside the temperature is a sunny 88 degrees, but in the church the natural coolness of the wood structure keeps the air at 68 degrees. In this temperate atmosphere, Pastor Jamison is exhorting her flock to stay with the word of the Lord.

"We are a house of prayer. Amen. Thank you Lord Jesus for blessing us Lord God to continue our faith in your holy name. We thank you for the spirit and the goodness and the courage to go forward in Jesus' name. And Lord, right here, right now, bless us in an individual way. In Jesus' name we pray, thank God, amen."

Jamison regularly asks parishioners to give testimony. She does this now, and several individuals stand and relate events from their lives as proof of God's guidance and concern. One woman tells a story of overcoming a rival for a man's affection. Another tells how a man who crossed her was brought down the next night by a shooting over drugs. Others tell stories of salvation and revelation in the practical (and vital) dimensions of their lives.

The congregation stands for a rendition of "Amazing Grace" led by Pastor Jamison in voice and piano. Then Jamison gets up and resumes her talk with a kind of testimony on her own ministry.

"I just thank God for coming into my life that He has sanctified me. He gave me the gift of the Holy Spirit, amen. And I thank Him, amen, knowing that He is my life, amen, and that He's given me the strength, amen, to go on. I don't apologize for not having a lot of people. People just don't like to go to church, amen. You know when you have the ups and downs the Lord will see you through and I thank God for His blessing. Praise the Lord. Truly you have a lot of people get wrapped up in crowds, but we know today that Jesus is the crowd, amen. It's not us, amen, it's not me. It's the Lord Jesus Christ who is in me. I can thank God that I made up my mind, amen, that I'm going to serve the Lord. Amen. Regardless of how negative it looks, God is going to bless this church, amen. I have no doubts in my mind that God is going to move in His own way and time. We want to go into the word of God."

Faith Jamison is obviously not happy with the turnout in her church, though on other Sundays (when the weather is less inviting) she manages to draw impressive numbers. Still, she sees the best part of her ministry as ahead of her. She believes that she will be celebrated at some point in the future as the most effective and well-known minister in the city.

Jamison, like many other ministers, was called to the religious life as a youngster. She came to the Lord when she was fourteen years old. Her earliest religious experiences were in a revivalist Baptist church. She remembers always being part of a congregation where individuals clapped their hands, shared thoughts and beliefs, testified, and generally got involved. Jamison's aunt was a minister in a Pentecostal church and still preaches at the age of seventy. At the age of fourteen, Jamison followed her aunt into the Pentecostal practices of the Full Gospel Fellowship Church.

She is not sure exactly why she was drawn to religion while most of her friends entered various areas of secular life, except that she has always felt different from others. It is obvious to her that the Lord chose her. She tried a physical life. She married young. Her husband kicked her and their three children out in the street once after a quarrel. That was when she tried the street life, thinking that if she got out there with him, lived it like he did, that maybe she would make him happy. Maybe she would enjoy the life. She would get totally drunk on warm summer evenings with her husband. But she always felt gullible out in the world. The street life did not work for her. The marriage failed. She and her husband were divorced. In her words now, recalling those times, God did not want her to live that life, so God fixed her life by drawing her to the church.

The call from God took the form of extended reflection and a kind of conversation punctuated by tests that Jamison sets up for God. In her twenties, Jamison became aware of different religions, how people served God in different ways. She felt she had a lot of knowledge about the word of God but did not know how to take the knowledge into her life to serve God. She wanted to be like the people she had read about in the Bible. For example, she read Corinthians and wanted to love like that part of the Bible urged. In those moments she would pray to the Holy Spirit for help. Slowly, little by little, she felt she was succeeding in molding her life after the stories and lessons in Scripture. At the age of twenty-five, the Lord called her to the ministry.

It was then that Jamison contrived another set of the stringent tests she has always used to confirm that it is God's instructions she is hearing. Number one, she told God, I need a husband (she was divorced by then). Second, she had an infection in her ear that she asked God to remove. Third, and for the real sign, she said that if she were going to be a minister she wanted God to tell a particular preacher and have this preacher (who didn't believe in women preachers) come to her and identify her as a preacher.

The first thing that happened was that a voice, an inward voice speaking like a person to her spirit, told her to touch the infection and it would go out. She pressed her ear and the infection went away. She was still not convinced. It could have been her, not God. So she waited.

The second sign, the decisive one, occurred at a church service. Jamison was at the back of the church when the minister she had singled out came by. As if in a dream, he turned to her and said the right words. "Aren't you a preacher? Didn't the Lord tell you to preach?" She was convinced. It was the confirmation she had sought. At that moment she began what turned out to be a five-year training period for the ministry. At the age of thirty she was ordained a preacher in the Pentecostal church where she now practices.

Finding a husband was more difficult. She is convinced that God was testing her with one experience she had. She accepted a date with a "good Christian brother" in another town. He was a musician, but his religious credentials seemed sound given that his father was a pastor. Jamison received a quick lesson in religious heterogeneity between generations. She was ready for love, but he was in a greater haste. At their table in a bar, he spiked her juice with a sedative. When they drove away to find a restaurant she felt the drug start to take effect. As they passed a McDonald's restaurant, she shouted at him to stop so she could use the rest room. Inside she prayed and began drinking water. Then she left by a side door and made her way across the street to a liquor store where she asked the proprietor to call an ambulance. Every time she stopped moving she could feel the drug crawling and advancing in her body. At the hospital she prayed for deliverance from the substance in her bloodstream. She swears today that the contact with God was instantaneous. She felt a chill that started at her face and came down her whole body. When it had swept through her she could not feel the drugs anymore. From that moment on, she had no doubt that God can do anything you want him to do. Her husband, the real answer to the earlier prayer, showed up years later.

The special gift she claims is prophecy, accompanied by impressive healing powers. The previous Sunday a young man had approached her after the services and asked her for healing for a sickness. She had immediately felt in her spirit that he was in a state of sin. She described to him the young, physically attractive woman with whom he was sleeping at the time. "She is not good for you," she told the man. "The Lord is saying to you that you should get rid of her—stop seeing her."

The man was stunned. "Oh my God," he told her. "You're right. This is true." He confirmed what she had told him.

A second young woman came up to her after the same service. Jamison looked her over without a word passing between them and concluded that someone was working witchcraft on her and that she must be very careful. It turned out to be true. The woman was from another church. Jamison found out the following Monday that someone in that church was very jealous of the woman and was trying to cast spells on her.

Jamison uses the healing powers in a more private way. She does not present herself to the congregation as a healer, but she does believe that she succeeds whenever she tries to heal. When she married her present husband, he had problems with sweating. He would get into bed and pour sweat all over her. She just couldn't take it, so she began to pray for him in the name of Jesus, and she says he was healed. He doesn't have that problem anymore. Her husband also had problems with his feet. She prayed those away also. Her son's allergies also vanished when she prayed.

She is attentive to her own body. Since the close call with drugs that evening years ago, she has not taken one pill for any reason. She carries with her a jar filled with blessed olive oil to use if she feels bad. She might have half or a full teaspoon of olive oil and that is it. She rests her health on faith, not modern medicine. She also fasts from time to time to bring her spirit into tune with God's spirit. A bonding with God seems to follow fasting. She finds that this is an effective way to resolve doubt and negative thoughts. Her diet when she is eating normally consists of the best foods—fresh vegetables and fruit, almost no meat. She assiduously avoids junk foods, including all types of sodas. Her goal is to stay clean before the Lord. She believes this purified state effectively shields her from illness. She has not been sick for years.

Faith Jamison is a hairstylist as well as a minister. She worked for years at a beauty salon in one of the largest malls in the county. Now she manages a similar salon at one of the most exclusive stores in a rival mall. She sees herself as a role model for young people. When her customers want to talk religion, she is ready. Most just watch and go away impressed by her managerial style—a combination of no-nonsense treatment of a customer's hair and a breezy dominance of all conversation. Jamison attends classes part time at the local university. Last spring she received an A and a B in the courses she took. Her major is social work.

Speaking to God is a commonplace for Jamison. She describes it as entering a particular zone of feeling that makes her nervous at first. She feels herself "get out of myself and get into the spirit of the Lord." At that point she begins talking at a new level and believing in the words she utters. She calls it anointing, an inspiration from God. The words are hers, but she feels that they arrive to her from outside of herself. She feels herself talking and moving in the word of God. It is precisely during such experiences that she knows she will be one of the dominant citizens in the city in the future. She is now thirty-seven years old and completely convinced of her future eminence.

"You have to move in the word of God, and I walk in the word. That is my strongest point, the word of God. If I stay in the word of God, then I will be strong, and all of the impossible will become possible for me because I am going to trust Him [God] to help me. And that is where the faith comes in."

Robert Penfield is a white Pentecostal minister in a middle-class church in one of the northern suburbs of the city. He was raised by devout parents. His mother was especially religious. Penfield remembers her as full of faith and loving God with all her heart. His father was a high school principal who considered himself as standing for God. Penfield's childhood was marked by readings from the Bible around the kitchen table, frequent personal prayers, and the usual accoutrements of religious family life.

Penfield left college after one and a half years to go to work. He had met the woman he wanted to marry and felt that he should support her. He entered the labor force in a steel mill. Shortly after that, the Reverend Billy Graham came through town in one of his crusades. Penfield attended, and in committing to Christ during the services he sensed a call to the ministry. The following fall he went to Columbia Bible College in South Carolina and then to the University of Oklahoma to study structural linguistics. These studies led to missionary work in Brazil, where he and his wife spent the next five years. He recalls the experience as good but physically draining. He also contracted malaria. On his return to the United States for convalescence, he began graduate work in anthropology (still his first intellectual love). He accepted an offer to teach at a branch of the state university, where he stayed for seven years.

The decisive experience of Penfield's life was the research he conducted for his dissertation. The topic was the Jesus People movement on the west coast. He went to California to do participant observation, figuring that his religious background provided him with the language he would need to understand the movement. He had not counted on his vulnerability to the ideas and emotions inspiring the Jesus People.

Penfield's guiding hypothesis was appropriately hard-boiled. His thesis was that the Jesus People were middle-class American youth who didn't want to participate in the Vietnam War and instead had drifted to California where the weather was warm enough to stay on the beach. He also tentatively proposed that the Jesus People movement functioned as a social conveyer back to middle-class American life—that young people who had lost their parents and financial support, and who were deprived in many ways, were entering middle-class Christian families in the movement to secure emotional and financial support to finish school, go to college, join the corporate world. He sought data to falsify or support these propositions.

Something happened to Penfield on the way to completing the fieldwork for his thesis. He was struck first by the sheer number of people in the movement. At a center located between Los Angeles and San Diego he saw three thousand people baptized. At first he thought that the movement had delayed the event for everyone in the organization who had ever come to Christ. No, they told him, this is just one month. The second thing that touched him deeply was the heterogeneity of the movement. Looking down from the balcony where he would sit observing the baptisms he could see professional people, doctors and lawyers, arm in arm with hippies right off the beach. Since church for him had been a blue-ribbon experience and usually austere, he found the scene remarkable.

He began to rethink his commitments to anthropology and his relationship with God. He and his wife opened their home on Saturdays for fellowship. The Jesus youth came over quickly. Sixty or so would visit on a typical Saturday afternoon, sitting all over the furniture and on the rug. Penfield began acting as a kind of shepherd for these people, providing guidance on a continuing basis. He began to realize that these young people were happier with ripped sneakers and an old mildewed sleeping bag than he was with his big car and professional standing. They seemed to have satisfaction, a joy in life. He began to see himself as an entry on the standard academic treadmill: collecting data, under pressure to produce scholarly works, doing administrative chores. The Jesus People were working hard—on communal farms, learning to do vinyl repairs, setting up bakeries, working in pottery shops. But they were happy, and he was not.

Then on a sunny afternoon when Penfield was conducting interviews for his thesis a young man approached and said, "I have a word from the Lord for you." Penfield was fascinated and turned on his tape recorder. The man said, "The Lord says that you are like a little child outside of a bakery looking through the window at people enjoying good things. But you feel that there is no door for you." Penfield immediately saw and felt the truth of this message. Then the man told him, "The reason that you cannot get in is unforgiveness. There is someone in your past that you have not forgiven."

Penfield knew without thinking to whom the man was referring. He had returned from Brazil with real grievances against the program director, who, to Penfield's thinking, had mishandled his situation. Penfield responded to the Jesus movement representative, "Well, what am I supposed to do?"

The man said, "You are supposed to forgive."

At that moment Penfield bowed his head and forgave and forgot the events in Brazil. The bitterness left his soul. He felt a door opening in his consciousness.

From that point on Penfield was a part of the movement and no longer an impartial observer. He left for Lighthouse Ranch, a large Jesus commune in northern California. There he met and received wisdom from Jim Durkin, one of the movement's influential leaders. His wife quit her job and joined him. They continued to gather data, but he was no longer the academic studying a movement from the outside. When he returned home, he left his academic post and became a pastor in a Pentecostal church. The salary was one-third what it had been at the university, which he did not welcome, but his excitement about the Pentecostal practices helped him to overcome his worries about economic support for himself and his family. He and his wife were brought closer together by what they sensed God was doing for them.

Penfield's experiences with God take the form of communication from outside himself. He will become aware of a higher thinking, a type of cognition that enters his consciousness even though he cannot fully comprehend it. He is not sure how to describe such communications. He acknowledges that they are subjective, as hard to explain as trying to describe a telephone ring to someone who does not know what a telephone is, or the taste of cherry pie to someone without taste buds, or a visual scene to a blind person. He can only say that these unusual communications come from outside in the sense that they are not part of his normal flow of thought. They interrupt, sometimes abruptly, the evolution of his thoughts. These entries are unlike any other kind of input he experiences. He knows that they come from God.

Penfield also believes that when God wants to speak to you, it will be a clear message. According to Penfield, if you cannot read God in twelve-inch letters, God will paint the letters twelve feet high, or twelve yards high, or twelve miles high. "God rings until you either tell him you are not interested, or until you pick up the phone," he says.

The anthropologist in Penfield is still able to frame empirical explanations for the Pentecostal movement. His data point to four possible causes for disaffection with traditional churches. First, his respondents viewed established religions as irrelevant to the needs of daily living. They felt the talk in churches was just not practical, not connected to the issues and problems of real life. Second, the respondents also reported being bored in establishment churches. There was no excitement in the services. Third, many people he interviewed said that they felt terrible, even condemned, when they left their church after services. The negative messages frequently left them asking themselves, "Why do I go to church just to get beat up verbally?" Fourth, Penfield's surveys disclosed a widely suspected complaint: "They are always pledging us for money." All of these explanations accorded with Penfield's own experiences in a mainstream Protestant church and his wife's experiences in a Catholic church.

There is still no explanation in the data for the rise of Pentecostalism, except indirectly as one among many possible effects of dissatisfaction with established religion. The historical fact is that many of those disaffected did turn to the subjective and often highly emotional religious services of Pentecostal churches. Penfield relishes quoting the last part of chapter 2 of Acts, where sharing, giving, teaching, prayer, and fellowship are described and extolled. He believes that the Pentecostal movement, in stressing strong emotive contact among parishioners, addresses a deep human need that the traditional churches ignore. Among those needs is direct communication with God, which parishioners claim occurs as naturally as any other event in their lives.

Penfield believes that his current ministry was described to him by God. He was the principal of a small Christian school at the time and making a salary of $250 a week. He also used to offer classes in religion from time to time. One evening he was returning home from teaching a group of women. He had a ten-dollar offering in his pocket for his efforts, which did not even pay for the gas on the trip, and he was despondent. He kept thinking about what he was doing to himself and his family. He considered quitting outright and supporting his family in more traditional ways. Suddenly he had a vision of some sort. No blue glow, skin crawling, breaking out in a sweat, in fact, no dramatics of any kind, just a communication to the effect, "You are late." Then a "tumbling" (Penfield's word), a recognition of people. Flashes of people's faces, crowds moving, a sense that God was going to raise up a church in the area that he, Penfield, would administer. He felt he was being offered bait, that if he would go on with religious work a bit longer, he would become pastor of a church.

The promise of a church was realized. Penfield was offered a ministry in an area that had not supported a church on three earlier occasions. But he started preaching in a small white building, and the crowds began arriving. Today his church occupies a modern building with every physical convenience, including a full staff and computer facilities. He still keeps the photograph of the small white building in the lobby.

Penfield has mixed views on faith healing. He believes that such healing occurs, but he also is convinced that many faith healers are charlatans. He expresses great disdain for those public figures who come into town, go after bucks, and then leave with people still in wheelchairs, crippled and sick. He views W. V. Grant as such a figure and publicly warned his church about him when the man visited the city. But Penfield does conduct healing ceremonies in his own church. Individuals gather and quietly lay hands on a sick or crippled person, anoint the person with oil, and pray for a recovery. Penfield admits that usually nothing happens. But sometimes the afflicted person will get better. No carnival events, no miraculous transformations. But Penfield believes that faith can make a difference in health and healing, at least on the margins.

Roman Catholicism: Crossland and Brantley

James Crossland and Charles Brantley are priests in the Catholic Church who would disagree over healing if they ever met and had an extended conversation. It is unlikely that they will: Crossland is a monsignor in a middle-class church while Brantley works with the most wretched of our society in a prison ministry. Each heals, but uses different methods toward different ends. Both concentrate on spirit, though Crossland also stresses the healing of the body through spiritual contact with God. Brantley bears witness to internal transformations quietly arrived at without dramatic interventions from outside the individual. Crossland practices charismatic healing; Brantley does not.

James Crossland has been a priest for thirty-five years. One of his brothers is also a priest. The other is a doctor. He dropped out of college when he was young and went to work in a factory. He found the work satisfactory. The routines appealed to him and compensated for the physical demands that working with machinery often brings. He did not marry.

He recalls the day when he was called to the priesthood. It was a Monday following a weekend of no particular importance. He went to work and, as he entered the factory, the machines seemed to be talking to him. He remembers that they seemed to say, "What are you doing here? What are you doing here?" Like a chant repeated without chorus or verse, the question kept drumming into his head throughout the day as the machinery droned on rhythmically. He had never heard the machine rhythms speak before this. He knew before the day was out that God was calling him to be a priest.

He remained a parish priest throughout his priesthood, performing the rituals of his calling with a spiritual satisfaction that the factory had not provided and that he had not realized was missing from his life. He heard confession on weekends, said mass, and distributed the host in communion, visited with families in need and with many who were not needy, organized bingo games, raised funds, went on retreats, prayed constantly for the souls of others and his own as well. He remained faithful to the Catholic Church during good and bad times. Crossland was consistently submissive to papal authority and had no moral problems in elevating spiritual considerations above the calls for social justice and reform that had penetrated some parts of the Church. He was one of the strongest opponents in the community of Martin Scorsese's cinematic rendition of *The Last Temptation of Christ*. That it was a blasphemous movie was to him incontrovertible. He urged parishioners to stay away from the local movie theater that showed the film.

His call to the healing ministry was a surprise both to him and to all who knew him. The sign of God's wishes was mundane enough. He woke one Thursday morning with a buzzing in his ears. It would not go away. He thought of consulting his brother the physician, but for some reason he did not. He began to believe that God was trying to tell him something. That Saturday in his church, after two days of chronic buzzing in his ears, a parishioner came to him asking for healing of a chronic digestive disorder. It was the first time in over thirty years of priesthood that anyone had requested healing of him. Crossland felt lost. He explained to the man that he had no powers to heal. The man insisted. So Crossland, with considerable hesitation and even fear, but with the thought that perhaps this was God's message, placed his hands on the man and prayed. Immediately the man collapsed on the carpet. Crossland continued praying. After a few minutes the man recovered and stood up. He announced to Crossland that he was healed of his illness. He thanked the priest profusely and left the church. At that moment the buzzing in Crossland's ears stopped.

The next day, Sunday, Crossland was urged by friends to conduct a healing mass and invite parishioners to stay for a healing service afterwards. He feared an ignominious failure. Suppose he couldn't help those who petitioned him? He was still unsure that God wanted him for this ministry. But he went ahead on the thought that somehow he should not resist the urgent appeals of those around him. At least a hundred people stayed after mass. Crossland went among them, laying his hands on their foreheads and praying that their afflictions would be cured. Many fell unconscious, caught by the two priests who were accompanying him on his rounds. The claims for success among those touched by Crossland were astounding. Word quickly spread after the healing service that a healing savior was present in the ministry.

Crossland professes not to understand how his powers work. He is a man who appears confident, almost arrogant, in the healing ceremony. In private conversation, however, he is humble. He regards himself as the instrument of God and does not know why he was chosen so late in life to serve God in this way. ("I am nothing," he frequently says. "God heals.") Like the chef who can prepare a grand meal but not tell how he does it, Crossland claims to have a skill without an explanation of that skill. Requests for explanation bring forth shrugs and references to God's will. Even faith is not decisive in Crossland's view. He says he has healed skeptics and even used his healing powers to produce belief. There are individuals his brokered powers cannot reach. He admits this, and says he can tell ahead of time who they are. But he does not know what it is about these individuals that makes them resistant to his healing efforts.

Crossland regards his efforts at healing as carrying on the healing traditions of Christ. They follow a practice of physical touching of the afflicted by a priest or member of the faithful conjoined with prayer. Originally, in early church practice, oil was used as an anointment in healing ceremonies. Crossland follows more modern practices that rely simply on touch and prayer in a context of religious belief. The belief, and explanation generally of the healing, is that God intervenes in the human experience to heal the subject. The priest, or healer, has no special individual powers but is only the instrument of God's power. In Crossland's ceremonies, and in others that rely on external interventions, the act can overwhelm the parishioner, often causing fainting. These individuals are said to be "slain in the spirit," or overcome by the presence of God.

Charles Brantley is a priest who approaches healing with different goals.

He does not sympathize with the charismatic emphasis on cause and effect, where God enters human experience in some dramatic and unusual way. He believes that we have access to the divine through prayer. But the healing he witnesses seems to be a kind of disclosure, an awakening of the divine that is already present in the individual. Healing, for Brantley, is an act of recovery, of finding and bringing forth something with God's help. The individual is healed through the attainment of an internal state of grace, which is a change that follows rather than interrupts the laws of nature.

Brantley's entrance into the priesthood was evolutionary rather than dramatic. He admits to never having had a conversion experience, one in which an event or decision cannot be accounted for except by invoking the extraordinary. He occasionally questions whether God did call him to his vocation. He grew up in a family with deep religious convictions. He loved going to mass when he was a child, loved being around the altar. He used to get up at 6:30 in the morning when he was a small boy so that he could go down to the church. He felt at home there. The decision to become a priest just seemed to evolve from his early love of the church itself and the religious ceremonies of Catholicism.

A powerful moment did occur in his adult life. He spent a day with Duke Johnson, who had been part of the Attica uprising in 1970. Johnson was traveling around New York state trying to get support for the defense of the Attica brothers. Brantley had spoken to prison guards who had been part of the Attica events and had read a lot of published material on the experience. But Johnson spoke to Brantley in ways that went beyond the testimonials and literature. He addressed a group of black and white ministers, calling for them to work together. "I need your help," Johnson told them. "I need your help. I've gone through life with you on my shoulders. I haven't got time to do this ministry in 150 years and I need your help." Brantley remembers the words going through his body like vessels carrying an electric charge. The session seemed to change the very chemistry of his blood. At that moment he knew he would do prison ministry work. And he has done so ever since.

The individuals that Brantley works with are often on the far edges of civilized life, sometimes arriving there through their own flaws and sometimes forced to those areas by a social system that to Brantley seems inexcusably brutal on occasion. He does not believe that the criminal justice system can be redemptive. Among his parishioners are alcoholics and drug addicts who are forced out of their addiction by therapies that first substitute one drug for another, and then wean the addict from all drugs while sustaining the individual medically. Brantley does not see genuine healing in these therapies. He has counseled people who have been forced to stop drinking or taking drugs, and they talk about that as healing. But often missing in their testimonies to Brantley is a joy about their lives. Sometimes these people are miserable. They frequently return to the old ways of doing things whenever they are able to do so. Brantley believes that they lack grace, which he views as a gift of God that cannot be imposed from the outside by the imperatives of law or any other social force.

Brantley counsels addicts with what would typically be considered secular methods. He asks the individual to think about what the drug is doing to his mind and body, and to consider the harmful effects of the addiction on family and loved ones. He might also stress the importance of contributing something to society rather than remaining a negative or dormant individual. But he also goes beyond these methods. His aim is not simply to get the addict to stop taking drugs but to become aware of his intrinsic dignity and value to God. He makes sure that the prisoner understands that he, Brantley, will fight for all of this individual's rights, that he believes that this incarcerated individual, placed in a cage by society, should not be in this situation. Then he teaches the Jesus prayer, as short and sweet as any mantra: "Lord Jesus, son of the living God, have mercy on me." He asks the prisoner to say it over and over again, to allow the prayer to resonate in the cell block, to utter it before going in front of the judge, to use it in situations of chaos or great silence. Brantley finds that this prayer can make a difference for some people. It can heal them from within.

Brantley believes that the crucial change is the awakening of a spirituality present within each individual. The sign that this state of grace has been acquired is a kind of inner peace, an acceptance of life regardless of its qualities. One prisoner that Brantley counseled was tried twice for homicide and acquitted each time. But he ended up being convicted in a third trial on testimony that Brantley knows was manipulated by the district attorney. The man got twelve and one-half to twenty-five years. Angry, he was a wild animal at the sentencing. Then, in prison, he began reading the Bible and praying for spiritual sustenance. Brantley saw him when he came in for the first parole hearing. The transformation was complete. He was able to say, "Whatever this will be, God will use it." Brantley describes this as healing through God's gift of grace.

Brantley does not doubt that a higher reality exists. One of his parishioners was a man who came from a family of fourteen children. He was mistreated from day one and was institutionalized as mentally retarded. Violence was the dominant force in his life. Yet as an adult the man was gentle. A doctor treating him remarked to Brantley that this individual had to have had a previous life, for there was nothing in his present life to explain why he could be so gentle. Brantley sees such experiences as requiring a spiritual frame of reference to make them intelligible. Empiricism is not enough.

Canterbury

The parishioners who believe in faith healing in the Catholic Church take for granted the interventionist powers of God, though they also usually regard as real the medical powers of modern physicians. Two individuals who claim to have benefited from Monsignor Crossland's healing efforts are Thomas and Irene Canterbury. They are a pleasant retired couple who attribute Mr. Canterbury's recovery from heart trouble to faith healing.

Mr. Canterbury has had a long and conventional life as a skilled worker in the American economy. Soon after graduating from high school, he began working as an apprentice toolmaker. He might have drifted from one "apprentice" job to another, as many of his friends did, except that he was assigned to a genuine master of the craft he was trying to learn. His name was Max Basil, and he had recently come from Germany. He knew his work and understood the master-apprentice relationship. It helped that Canterbury had studied German in high school and could communicate with Basil in rudimentary fashion in his native tongue. It was 1936. Canterbury would get up at 5:30 A.M. each day to make the early shift at the plant. Basil would always be there ahead of him, impeccably dressed in some combination of work clothes and a pressed shirt with a brief cravat tucked inside of a vest. Canterbury would shed his leather jacket and together they would fashion solutions to the day's problems of design and assembly.

It was in this plant over the next three years that Canterbury learned about tool design, drafting, calculus, geometry, strengths of materials, types of materials, and techniques for making and producing a variety of mechanical items. He also acquired a sense of craft, a desire to do the job right that would later serve him well and badly. Much later, when musing over the way his life had gone, he understood that subordinating salary and bonus rewards to the desire for correct and accomplished work had cost him enormous amounts of money in marketing his skills.

Under Basil's tutelage, Canterbury progressed from apprentice toolmaker to toolmaker, and then later to tool designer. He left for a job with the Carrier Corporation as a layout and product designer, eventually designing a new line of heater units. He also supervised the construction of the prototype units for the heater and worked with engineers on performance evaluation tests he had designed. By that time, his skills were widely appreciated in a number of industries, and he began an odyssey from one corporate job to another across the country. He helped produce the first television picture tubes at General Electric and developed tools at the Chrysler Corporation in various cities. At one time or another, he worked in Syracuse, Detroit, Kokomo (Indiana), and Bowling Green (Kentucky). He lived in twenty-six different houses during this period of his life.

Thomas Canterbury was sixty-one years old when he had the first of his two heart attacks. He and his wife Irene had been visiting their daughter in Freeport, Louisiana. She and her husband had been having trouble and the Canterburys decided to go see if they could help. The visit had gone badly. His daughter's husband was adamant in pursuing a separation, despite the fact that the couple had two small children. The only saving grace of a situation that Canterbury viewed as simply terrible was that his son-in-law was prepared to give his daughter generous financial support before and after the divorce.

At some point on the Canterburys' drive home, Thomas began belching gas and seemed to Irene to be losing his color rapidly. She looked more closely at her husband and noticed that he was also shaking and turning blue. At that precise moment, she saw a sign along the highway that said "Hospital at next exit." They left the highway and quickly found the hospital. The physician who examined Thomas had a name tag, "Dr. Luck."

Thomas Canterbury was in the hospital for two weeks. He had suffered a partial blockage of one of the arteries leading to the right side of his heart. Some of the heart muscle had been damaged in the attack, but not extensively. Later he and Irene found out that this hospital was the only one with coronary care facilities between Little Rock, Arkansas (where they were living at the time) and Freeport, Louisiana. The hospital was reluctant to release him when they did, but Thomas was insistent. They took him to the airport in an ambulance, forklifted him in a wheelchair onto a plane, and he and Irene flew home.

Thomas Canterbury's second heart attack occurred ten years later. He had been careful in the usual ways with diet and exercise since the first attack. One of his physicians also had urged that his wife keep track of his blood pressure, especially if he began to feel odd in any way. On hearing this Irene had immediately gone out and bought two blood pressure devices, one an old-fashioned manual type, the other one of the newer electronic instruments.

The day of the second attack was the first spring thaw of the year. The snow had completely melted off the Canterburys' lawn. Thomas had walked down the driveway to the street in front of his house. He became impressed with the steepness of the incline on the walk back up to the front door. When he reported this experience to his wife she told him to sit down. She attached the electronic blood pressure monitor to his arm. The sounds of the monitor frightened her. Instead of the usual rhythmic pulses it sent forth a staccato beat, the irregularity spaced by intervals of silence. Thomas Canterbury's heart was obviously skipping around wildly. Irene called the doctor's office and described to the nurse the sounds she was hearing from the monitor. The nurse told her to bring Thomas in immediately.

At the office the doctor examined Thomas and took an EKG. It confirmed the arrhythmia. He ordered his nurse to get a wheelchair and take Thomas over to the intensive-care unit of the hospital. The hospital was connected to the physician's office building by both an underground passageway and a skywalk. The nurse wheeled Thomas over on the skywalk. Irene accompanied her husband as they moved across the street at a point several stories high.

In the intensive-care unit, the attending physician ran another EKG and other tests. They also administered drugs to bring Thomas's heart back into a more normal rhythm. By late afternoon, he had been seen by three different physicians. Irene had called her sister and the two of them were talking at the foot of the bed when Monsignor Crossland walked by in the hall. Irene ran to the door and called him. Crossland turned and came back. He recognized Irene as one of the regular parishioners at the Holy Mother Catholic Church where he presided. Irene explained that Thomas was ill again. Crossland entered the room and listened as Thomas described his condition as an irregular heart beat and maybe more.

Crossland announced that they were going to pray. He suggested that everyone in the room grasp hands and form a circle, including Thomas.

Crossland bowed his head and began praying. Irene and her sister closed their eyes. The monsignor reached out and put one of his hands on Thomas's chest; the other hand he used to squeeze Thomas's hand to maintain the circle.

From a taped interview with Thomas Canterbury three years after his second heart attack:

"And while we were praying, I would say half way, quarter of the way through, I don't know . . . I did feel a warm feeling, flushed feeling throughout my whole body. Not just my hand. This was right from my head to my toes. I didn't say anything to Monsignor or to my wife then. But after Monsignor prayed and wished me luck and left, I told my wife that I did have a very warm feeling throughout my entire body."

The next morning Thomas was taken down to the operating room for a cardiac catheterization. A team of doctors inserted a thin metal line through a vein in his groin and slowly edged it up into his heart. He was conscious throughout the entire procedure and could even watch the progression of the wire on a television screen at the side of his bed. The images of his veins and arteries were dark and vague, but the probe was sharply outlined on the screen. It jerked and stopped by turns as it was guided through the milky substances on the monitor, looking like a plumber's snake clearing a clogged drainage pipe. At the left ventricle a clear liquid dye was injected through the catheter. The dye was injected again into the coronary arteries. Thomas felt a brief sensation of warmth and flushing throughout his body at each injection. The X-ray images continued on the monitor.

The following day the coronary specialist came into Thomas's room and told the Canterburys that "something funny has happened." The coronary arteries on the left side of Thomas's heart were blocked anywhere from 25 to 100 percent. But a new vein had grown from the right ventricle to the left side of the heart. It was supplying additional blood to the heart. The doctor also told Thomas that new arteries had grown to bypass the plugged arteries to the left ventricle. The catheterization had revealed the scar tissue from the first heart attack, but the heart muscle was pronounced strong and effective. It was providing reasonably complete blood circulation.

Ten days later Thomas was discharged from the hospital. He recuperated at home. As soon as he was able, he went down to Holy Mother Catholic Church where Monsignor Crossland conducted his healing services. He began going to the healing masses on a regular basis from that point on.

Thomas Canterbury is retired now, but he remains physically active. He shovels snow, works in his garden, installs appliances in their home (including, in recent months, a dishwasher, garbage disposal, and ceiling fan). Last summer he painted the outside of the house completely. He feels good, strong. He no longer has any pain in his heart. At his last physical exam, the doctor uttered the magic words any cardiac patient longs to hear: "I do not know what it is you are doing, but whatever it is keep it up. Your health is marvelous." The only medicine Thomas takes is a drug to keep his blood pressure down. He is seventy-one years old.

Neither Thomas nor Irene regards their faith in spiritual healing as being hostile in any way to modern medicine. They both continue to consult physicians for health problems and seek the best medical treatment when it is needed. Irene says she prays for her physicians. She wants them to be effective and feels that God might inspire them. But the Canterburys do believe in divine intervention. They believe the healing of Thomas's heart was brought about by God. Thomas prays to the Holy Spirit for healing every night before retiring.

One experience in Thomas's youth convinced him of the limits of material explanations. His mother, at a late stage in her life, had several heart attacks and then a stroke that in effect killed her but the doctors revived her body. The encephalogram showed that her brain was dead. The physicians convened the family and asked if they wanted to continue the life-support machine in these circumstances. Thomas remembers that the children could not decide immediately, even though their mother had asked years earlier not to be put on such machines but to be allowed to die naturally.

The next day Thomas's daughter flew in from Connecticut to see her grandmother. A priest was in his mother's room at the hospital when Thomas and his daughter arrived. He introduced himself as Father Cannon and suggested they pray for "Bocci" (Polish for grandmother). The three of them joined hands. During the prayers—and Thomas is sure he did not imagine this—Thomas saw his mother open her eyes, give him a little smile, and pass away. He immediately noticed the respirator cloud up. He called the nurse. She examined his mother and said that the doctor would have to tell them whether she was dead. Thomas pressed her for an answer "just between you and me." The nurse allowed that she was dead. The doctor came and confirmed it.

This image stays with him. His mother, her brain dead and useless, freeing herself from her body to smile at Thomas on the way to something else. The smile, the thought of his mother's spiritual release from the shell of her body, guides Thomas's faith even today.

Mind Affecting Body

One striking difference between the cures brought about by Alcoholics Anonymous and those attempted through faith healing is in the location of the agents of disease. The alcoholic must learn to stop ingesting the poison that is killing him. The agent of his illness is outside his body; to keep it outside, he must transform his understanding of himself. He must learn to extend the self to the group, relying on a power outside the self to isolate the self from the drug that triggers the illness.

The faith healer attempts to eliminate agents of illness that are within the body of the petitioner. The mystical language sometimes used in faith healing recognizes this in trying to expel evil or unclean spirits. Even the deformations of the body addressed by faith healing—crippling due to congenital defects or illness—are still conditions of the physical self, not agents from which the individual is to be insulated. The distinction is important in understanding the limited success of faith healing. If quarantine against external causes were an effective measure to eliminate or prevent illness, then, in principle, strength of mind could control healing. But if the individual is ill from causal factors already present in the body, then mind would have to influence matter directly in order to bring about healing.

To some degree, mental states can influence physical states. Two prominent forms of medical intervention (each discredited by conventional physicians early on) rely directly on mental causation. Hypnosis, regarded as witchcraft or nonsense at one time, is now widely used to address a variety of ailments and bad habits. Biofeedback, a technique confined to Eastern mysticism for most of its history, is a systematic and productive method that individuals now use with medical supervision to control bodily activities (like blood pressure, heart rate) by entering and maintaining an appropriate mental state. Studies of illnesses across a reasonably wide spectrum show the beneficial effects of attitude on healing. Patients who have had a severe physical injury, for example a serious burn, have a better chance of recovery if they are emotionally resilient. One of the oldest known effects in medicine is the placebo effect, in which a healing result is brought on by a false belief that medicine has been taken into the body.

But some physical states also seem remarkably resistant to mental influence. Physical deformities, disfigurements caused by accidents, illnesses, or genetic flaws, do not yield to mental forces. There are no records anywhere to confirm that faith healers can cause an amputated limb to grow back, a badly burned face to be restored, a dead brain to be revived. Nor are many types of diseases amenable to mental therapy. Illnesses caused by physical organisms, bacteria for example, often resist the most strenuous mental exercises. Human history is filled with the corpses of those who succumbed to bacterial and viral disease in spite of the most powerful prayers, supplications, and mental gymnastics. Religious leaders must bear witness to the inexorable logic of natural laws in placing all of us, sinner and supplicant, under the same causal framework.

Some of the dramatic effects of faith healing can be explained in conventional ways. Many illnesses are misdiagnosed, so that a cure is really only a reflection of underlying health missed on the first examination. Sometimes a religious intervention eliminates the effects of disease through emotive influences of one sort or another without affecting the disease itself. Most diseases are also self-limiting, overcome without medical assistance. (Were this not so, the human race probably would not have survived to its present state.) What passes for a miraculous healing might be simply a spontaneous remission occasioned by the body's immune system. Also, the human organism has its own dramatic coping devices. Every cardiac specialist asked to comment on the new veins generated by Thomas Canterbury's heart responded in the same way: "Of course. The heart often grows new veins to compensate for blood deficiencies. It is a common and natural phenomenon." In other words, what the Canterburys regard as a miracle from God is in actuality a small miracle wrought by the human body's impressive abilities to compensate for deficits in its own organs.

Yet the belief in miraculous cures can transform the individual's perspective on life itself and the meaning of death. Some attachment, a bonding even, is formed with a reality that is said to be outside that human experience fixed by the bounds of secular expectations. Catholic priests who minister to those who are ill provide moving testimony of the redeeming features of such beliefs. As in the experience AA provides, the individual is spiritually healed and connected to something outside of the self. But for the ill person, unlike the reformed alcoholic, the mental transformation may continue to mask the reality of a disease whose effects have been blunted through emotional fervor but whose presence remains a potentially lethal condition.

Skeptics who study faith healing also voice another caution. They urge a return to a more secular (read realistic) vision of human experience on the grounds that belief in external intervention and healing from supernatural dimensions cripples the believer with illusions. One is then vulnerable to those who exploit human misery.

From a taped interview with James Randi, a professional magician who has devoted much of his life to exposing supernatural claims:

"The drawback is that faith healing switches people into a magical mode of thinking in which they are vulnerable to every kind of claptrap, from stock issues to having their driveway paved, if they think there is something magical about the procedure, some way of cutting corners. They listen to the kind of talk that is given to them by faith healers, which often includes phrases like—God doesn't cut on your body with a knife and doesn't put chemicals in your body, but God will heal you with the spiritual—that sort of thing. That is appealing. And one of the reasons it is appealing is because people misunderstand the true function of medical science. That's the fault of medical science.

"Physicians do not make themselves clear. Eighty percent of what doctors actually do is to alleviate the symptoms of a disease that cannot be cured.

This then allows the patient to live a long useful life. Diabetes is a perfect example of this. You cannot cure diabetes. But the faith healers say they can, the chiropractors even say they can, the Holy Office says they can. All of these people say that they can cure diabetes. That's a better answer than the doctor saying, 'I'm sorry, you'll have diabetes for the rest of your life until the day you die, but you can live comfortably with it.'"

The main difficulty in assessing the claims of faith healers is that scientific methods, currently the dominant approach to evidence and inference in the Western world, are hostile to the main assumptions and techniques of unconventional healing. This hostility often emerges at the very start of healing ceremonies when the priest or leader tries to set a mood that is primarily subjective, not rigorously structured to suit the objective aims of science. Music, lighting, and lyrical languages are often used to induce an almost hypnotic mental state among parishioners. The skeptic views these efforts with a combination of disgust and suspicion, since they blunt the clarifying efforts of science to strip emotional fervor from truth. But faith healers do not seek an indifferent or impartial truth. Their aims are the reverse of science. They have already accepted (not tested) an intuitive truth prior to the practice of faith healing.

The hostility between science and faith healing also appears in the effects of healing practices. Faith healers will sometimes say that their success depends upon the presence of believers to the exclusion of skeptics. Scientific inquiry, by definition skeptical, would then compromise and contaminate the healing practice by applying the very methods needed to reach objective truth. Nothing can be more infuriating to the proponents of science than this assertion about effects. And there is no doubt that charlatans have seized on such claims to shield utterly bogus practices from strict (or any other) scrutiny. Investigators like James Randi have exposed such tricks again and again.

If faith healing is to be examined on its own terms, however, one must accept two propositions. The first is that the existence of cheaters and exploiters in a practice does not in itself rule out the possibility of legitimate practitioners achieving genuine success in the aims of the practice. Second, some additional criteria of truth must be added to science, perhaps supplanting science entirely. Otherwise it is impossible to address the claims of those who trade on a reality said to be beyond conventional secular experience.

An additional goal, one that can help interpret the competing methods of science and faith, would be to achieve greater clarity and precision about what is meant by the primitive term "individual" in healing practices. It is obvious that two schema dominate understandings of this term: one divides the individual hierarchically into soul or psyche and physical body; the other separates the individual laterally into self and social context. Neither is satisfactory in providing an account of the spiritual healing that is described both in AA experiences and Pentecostal practices. Neither seems to express the more holistic self that is the desired end of all healing efforts.

From an interview with a psychotherapist:

"Many behaviors that are accepted as highly rational in professional communities are much crazier. Lobotomy as an example. . . . A surgeon heard a lecture at an international conference and decided that the way to cure schizophrenia was to destroy significant parts of the brain. Without any empirical data he then proceeded to do this to thousands of people. And thousands of people died, and thousands were maimed. And he got a Nobel Prize for it—to show you how crazy the whole community is. Then as we began to accumulate real empirical data, we found out that this was ridiculous. This is crazier than any idea that you are in contact with God. You just cloak it thinly with a professional rationalization. This stuff goes on all the time with drugs. The history of the treatment of schizophrenia is the history of nutty people making up crazy treatments and doing terrible things to people—which are far crazier than any of these strange religious fantasies. I find it very difficult to separate one kind of craziness from the other kind."

SPIRITUAL DOMAINS

Medieval Theories

One of the distinguishing marks of liberal political theory is the impulse to partition society into separate practices. The partition that seems to cut most deeply into human experiences is that between spiritual and secular. Theocracies fuse religion and politics, thus eliminating the problem of where and how to separate church and state. But the recognition that *spiritual* and *secular* might indicate different species of thought and action has a distinguished pedigree going back at least to Ionian philosophy.

More influential efforts to identify spiritual and secular domains, however, begin with the growing power of Christianity in the early medieval period. Augustine recognized two worlds—the temporal and that of the Heavenly City—roughly corresponding to the dual nature of human beings (body and spirit). For Augustine, history was a struggle between these two realms, not church versus state but good versus evil. The state's primary function in this framework is to establish peace as a means to make service to God possible.

The political philosophies and homilies of the twelfth through the fourteenth centuries contain a variety of arguments that try to fix the proper roles of church and state. John of Salisbury accepted the supremacy of ecclesiastical over temporal power on the grounds that the prince receives authority from the church, much as the soul directs the body in the good or just individual. Aquinas also viewed political power as deriving from God. The moral duty of the ruler is to maintain peace and order so that priests can guide individuals to ultimate happiness in heaven. It is not surprising that Aquinas prefers monarchy over other forms of government, since it is patterned after a one-God universe. Both Salisbury and Aquinas recognize separate functions for church and state but concede superiority to the church.

Dante drew sharper distinctions between the spiritual and the secular. He looked at church and state, and saw different species of authority. In his vision, both the emperor and the pope have power directly from God, but each is supreme in his respective sphere of control. Dante expresses Augustine's dualisms in independent domains of practice. John of Paris restated the independence of spiritual and secular authority in terms of derived authority. He observed that the General Council, the authority that elects the pope, can depose the pope, but the king cannot. The king can be deposed by the people (and the College of Electors representing the people) on secular judgments that he is a tyrant. The pope has no special privileges in these regards.

Marsilius of Padua offers the most subtle brief for independence between church and state. Marsilius recognized two types of law, divine and human, that yield different types of punishment. The state punishes in this world, the church in the world to come. It follows that the state is autonomous in its secular coercive powers while the church maintains authority over matters related to the afterlife. Spiritual and secular domains are separate and independent because they are concerned with different realities.

It is impossible to sustain arguments like these without distinctions between faith and reason. Typically these distinctions are reflected in claims for the proper relations between church and state. Reason is a complex instrument in medieval philosophy. It is sometimes a form of contemplation that can map from sensory experience back to God. At other times it is more nearly a type of calculative power. But its natural domain is the empirical world. Spiritual thinking by contrast must depend to some extent on revelation (truth about a higher reality revealed in part by God to humans) and trust that God knows more and best. Faith is the only word to describe such thinking. Aquinas located revelation above reason (naturally enough) but nowhere contrary to it. The church, as the instrument of revelation, was accordingly superior to the state. Where faith and reason are autonomous exercises aiming at different realities, spiritual and secular domains tend to be seen as separate and equal. Marsilius's two legal systems derive from different but equally valid ways of thinking about reality.

Machiavelli is remarkable in seeing the possibility of an intractable conflict between moral and political authority *because* faith and reason address different rational considerations. The ruler (in *The Prince*) is charged by his authority to ensure the secular goods of life and property, and to secure the general material needs of his citizens. Ordinary morality is concerned with right actions and spiritual needs. Occasionally the demands of morality oppose the means needed to succeed in the secular world. In effect, morality is contrary to the rational imperatives of power. Machiavelli enters history with his clear solution to this conflict. According to Machiavelli, the prince must be ruthless in carrying out the logic of political rule because it is moral discourse that is absurd when it opposes the needs of the state. Morality, including that instructed by the church, must give way to power or the ruler has failed the rational obligations of his office. In *The Prince*, the state is the token of power and must dominate the *spiritual* church in the sense in which power dominates morality.

These attempts over several centuries to establish proper relations between distinct spiritual and secular domains rest on one important insight: religion and politics are separate practices because they perform different functions in society. Religion is concerned with the spiritual (perhaps mental?) side of the human person. This spiritual side is thought to be part of a reality that is beyond what can be known by means of the human senses and intellect. Religion claims to address that reality in ways that nurture the human spirit. The state, by contrast, is accepted by all theoretical adversaries as an institution within the sensory world attending to secular demands.

The bifurcation of spiritual and secular domains leads to different types of authority. Religious authority is based on a peculiar mix of morality and faith. Religion extends from a certitude unrivaled in other modes of discourse, but the scope of knowledge is severely limited when viewed from God's perspective. Secular authority, by contrast, is more modest in its base of knowledge. In medieval political thought, the state acquires its authority in pursuit of the common good in accordance with the law. No higher knowledge is needed to succeed in such secular pursuits, as the common good is defined by prudential interests in stability, peace, and bodily needs for food, clothing, and shelter.

Any survey of these arguments on church and state shows that advocates of dominance and independence are both comfortable with the reality of separate domains. Like Aquinas, we can accept the triumph of the spirit over the flesh on a hierarchy of God to human, cosmos to earth, soul over body. Or, with Marsilius, we can see the natural divisions of labor (represented in different ontologies, epistemologies, punishments, concerns in general) that invite the distinct and autonomous spheres of church and state informing the liberal political philosophies of contract theory and utilitarianism in the last three centuries.

The medieval efforts to establish separate domains for church and state do not include arguments for religious freedom or freedom of conscience. The religious pluralism of the modern world does not exist in the historical periods dominated by the Catholic Church. In these periods, the individual is a subordinate in the organizational hierarchy of the Church, not a free spirit receiving direct commands from God to the conscience. Church-state separations in medieval thought reflect separate spiritual-secular worlds, not freedom of beliefs.

The separation of church and state in the United States Constitution is driven in part by the same recognition that religion tends to different senses of reality than those found in the political world. Two clauses in the First Amendment famously demarcate the boundaries of church and state: the establishment clause forbids the government from making any "law respecting the establishment of religion," and the "free exercise of religion" clause prohibits the government from restricting religious belief or practice.

These two clauses, especially the second one, are often read today as affirming individual rights of conscience and the appropriateness of religious pluralism. But historical evidence suggests that the framers were more interested in establishing the primacy of religious duties free of state interference. "Rights of conscience" was considered and dropped as a wording for the First Amendment, as was any vocabulary indicating religious "tolerance." Thomas Jefferson championed John Locke's thought that the state must simply be impartial or nondiscriminating, but James Madison and most of the other framers of the Constitution did not support this view. One of the driving practical forces behind the First Amendment religion clauses was the evangelical conviction, widespread in colonial times, that *religion* (not just individual conscience) was to dominate a limited government that must be subordinate to a sovereign God. The medieval philosophies of Salisbury and Aquinas, shorn of Catholicism, would be compatible with this thinking.

The other driving force for church-state separation in the Constitution was the conviction that the state should be secular, not religious. This conviction opposed the Republican belief that the government should support religion to promote public morality, a view that stopped short of a theocratic state but nonetheless favored an intimate working relationship between government and religion. The secular view of the state prevailed in the establishment clause, but mainly on arguments that religion should be insulated from state support for the sake of religious integrity.

The concern for religious integrity is evident in powerful arguments from the eighteenth century that summarize Constitutional deliberations. One is the evangelical claim, almost straight from a medieval text, that God is supreme over secular laws and that religion therefore cannot be governed by the state. A second claim, more modern in its orientation, is that religious conscience prevails over secular law and even religious authority. This second argument can be found in restricted form in Roger Williams's strident defenses of religious liberty against church authority (but not civil law) in seventeenth-century Rhode Island. A third argument recognizes a natural conflict between church and state because of the different species of action characterizing each institution. The state, as Jefferson saw clearly, is coercive in nature while religion is based on voluntary action. Allowing the two to become entangled would likely compromise religious freedom. A fourth argument, similar to the two-worlds philosophies of medieval theories, sees the state as concerned with material goods, the church as oriented to the spirit. Church and state must be separated to avoid the inevitable corruption of religion that attends materialistic interference in spiritual affairs.

Debates over the religion clauses in the First Amendment also contain a number of influential arguments that a church-state separation is in the interests of the state as well as of religion. Most are made or endorsed by Madison. One argument is that a barrier between church and state will help the state avoid religious conflict. (Those in any historical period will find this goal eminently desirable once the acrimony and intractability of sectarian disputes have been experienced or observed.) Two more arguments come directly from Madison's writing. The first is that an independent religious domain will likely increase religious pluralism, and this pluralism will increase social stability as religious factions cancel each other out. (The familiar Madisonian equilibrium of balanced factions is used again here.) The second is that splitting allegiances between religion and politics will decrease the likelihood of tyranny, which Madison saw as requiring a total political commitment to the exclusion of all other loyalties, including religious.

If we press these arguments in support of the religious clauses past their client fixations on church and state, more general rules and principles emerge. One is a now familiar argument based on social utility. A separation between government and religion is said to promote the general good by allowing a variety of preferences and values to flourish, and by establishing those conditions that purport to serve the interests of both state and church. Another is a kind of fairness argument. If the state favors one or a few religions backed by the authority of the government, then the claims made by rival churches are at a considerable disadvantage.

It is not always clear how much utilitarian and fairness principles depend on a noncognitive theory of value. Certainly if one religion makes truth claims while rival religions can be shown to be propagating false statements, then neither the aggregation methods of utilitarianism nor the pluralism following impartial treatment of all religion makes much sense. Should one extend lies into the social product or legislate impartially across truths and falsehoods? An appropriate inclusion in the principles favoring separation of church and state would be a view that religious and political statements are not truth functional.

The role of truth in these arguments is further diminished by the third background principle. Separation of church and state is also justified by more general theories of individual autonomy. The main political and moral philosophies of the eighteenth century to the present time celebrate the individual, not the state. Social values on the whole are regarded as derivative products, produced from individuals' choices or from the application of arithmetical composition rules to individual values. This idealistic and almost romantic view of individuals as the primary units in human experience, the rock-bottom base out of which society is composed, requires autonomy. Only as individuals are competent and free from external impediments can authentic social values be produced by their choices and preferences.

Autonomy is not entirely hostile to religious truth. One might maintain that truth is out there, in the world or in God, and that the best and perhaps the only way to discover it is through the exercise of free will and choice. But autonomy is also defended in other terms. Individual autonomy might be seen as indicating a different source for value, represented by the thought that truth is not out there somewhere but within individuals. This defense need not be the extreme view that truth is *only* a matter of preference, for individuals might be said to discover some fixed and universal truth in the landscape of the individual psyche (or soul). But turning to individuals as the source of truth requires that the state not compel choices based on a privileged understanding of truth. The coercive powers of the state are especially abrasive to individual autonomy.

A sympathetic regard for truth in religious practice would hold that the emphasis on individual autonomy means that religious truth must be worked out by individuals and groups, not by the larger society that the state represents. The separation of church and state is justified within a comprehensive theory of individual autonomy built on a deep appreciation of liberty in religious practice, with truth as the product and not the controlling premise of liberty.

The barriers between church and state not only establish separate institutions but also must ensure independence. Two social units can be separate in principle, but one could still control the other. The state, for example, might be separate from a bureaucracy (in the sense that each performs different functions, hires different people, has different goals) but still exercise power over that bureaucracy. The religion clauses of the First Amendment, however, anticipate separate institutions independent of each other.

Two of the most common expressions ensuring independence of church and state are (1) a nonporous barrier (Jefferson's and Hugo Black's "wall") between the two institutions, and (2) state neutrality in religious matters. Taken together, the two expressions mean that the state is to avoid any entanglements in religious matters (for example, no joint ventures) and is neither to enhance nor inhibit religious practices. It is not certain if these expressions can always be maintained simultaneously, however. In many uses of "neutrality" it is impossible to segregate intervention and nonintervention on a neutrality axis. To do nothing is implicitly to condone the status quo (thus, technically, enhancing what already is), to intervene is to endorse a change. Neutrality remains elusive on either pole.

A similar conflict occurs between the two religion clauses in the First Amendment. The establishment clause prohibiting state support of religion is comfortably interpreted by the barrier between church and state. But the full exercise of religion might require the state to support religious practices. Most people today will acknowledge that the shields against taxation satisfying the barrier requirement are necessary for the effective free exercise of religion. From a secular perspective, however, these shields can be interpreted as state enhancement of religion because they provide material privileges not granted most secular institutions. Neutrality is entirely a matter of perspective in such disputes.

The main disputes over barriers and neutrality, however, arise from interpreting the free exercise clause either as impartiality or exemption. On an impartiality interpretation, the state is not restricting freedom when it treats all religions alike *and* treats religions as it treats secular institutions. This essentially nondiscriminatory interpretation of the free exercise clause would place members of religious organizations under the laws of the land like all other citizens. On an exemption interpretation, however, the state is compelled to allow members of a religion to act on their beliefs without interference from the state. This can mean granting exemptions from the law when a religious belief compels an individual to act in a way different than the law requires. In an expression accepted as standard by now, "once a free exercise claimant demonstrates that a state action burdens a practice based on a sincerely held religious belief that is central to his religion, the burden shifts to the state to show that the regulation serves a compelling governmental interest that cannot be served by a less restrictive means."

The government has allowed a number of exemptions under the First Amendment, including, most famously, conscientious objection to military service and, less famously, the drawing of unemployment benefits for individuals who refuse to work on their sabbath on religious grounds. An exemption respects, and perhaps even favors, religious beliefs over secular beliefs and obligations. From a secular perspective such an interpretation is biased because it is partial, while from a religious perspective exemptions are needed to avoid state restrictions on the "free exercise of religion." Again, both neutrality and noninterference can be defined in different ways across religious and secular communities.

One immediate escape route from the localizing forces of these community perspectives is to attempt a justification of state law on independent grounds. A bad or unjust law would then be a proper target for exemptions and even civil disobedience; a good or just law might then compel service to the state. Compromising the escape, however, is the fact that the main criteria for determining good or just rules are located in religious belief for the religious believer (and perhaps for others as well), but are located in secular theories of the right and the good for the nonbeliever. Again, the evaluation depends on the perspective, suggesting that neutrality itself is not a neutral concept.

These problems of perspective go back to the debates over the Constitution and suggest a more intimate relationship between religion and state, conscience and law, than a strict separation between church and state recognizes. Community values, in this case religious and secular, control the instruments normally used to adjudicate disputes and establish separate domains of belief and practice, including the vocabulary of separateness itself, of neutrality, and even impartiality in respecting religious freedoms. The result is that the state must make choices that inevitably favor or deny religious beliefs in ways that contravene the possibility of strict separation between the two institutions. This underlying intimacy never surprises the historian aware of the strong influence of religion on secular laws, or of the ways in which individual conscience values the presence of just laws in a civil society. It should also make us sensitive to some of the limitations in implementing even the more persuasive theories of separate church and state domains.

State Regulation

The first role of the state in the spiritual domain is to define religion. The task is unavoidable. If all possible claims for religious belief were allowed, then exemptions from the law would be a simple exercise in pragmatics: simply assert religious privilege. The United States Supreme Court has given religions wide discretionary powers to define themselves, but if the discretion were without limits, the claims for religious privilege would be empty of merit.

A religion is most commonly defined as a system of beliefs essential to the self-definition of the believer. These beliefs, of course, must be normative in the sense in which all moral languages direct and guide those who subscribe to the controlling principles. But the main feature of religion, one that marks it as a special set of moral obligations, is that it is vital to the identity of the believer. A religion also is a map of reality, and often states the features and structure of reality in terms so detailed that the identity of the individual is fixed in ontological terms.

Perhaps because of the ontological foundation of religion, the beliefs that follow or inform religious commitments are often compulsive. Individuals will consider giving up their lives for the sake of their beliefs, or, if they are unwilling to die, at least will feel extreme remorse at failing those beliefs. The basic nature of religious convictions undoubtedly contributes to the wide support for exemptions, even among nonbelievers. It also highlights the importance of sincerity in religious life, since few scams can be as repugnant as fraud on that which is considered fundamental to human experience.

Recognizing the importance of a definition is no assurance that it will succeed in the real world, however. Although it is necessary to have a formal definition of religion, such definitions allow almost any content to enter as claims, and there is no method that successfully tests the sincerity of claims within a formal apparatus. In general, the legal system is generous in allowing claims for a religion to pass acceptability thresholds if accompanied by a group of adherents. It is a curious fact about the assignment of rights under the First Amendment that the U.S. Supreme Court recognizes few organizational rights for religions, preferring instead to see religious freedoms as inhering in individuals while in general not allowing singular individuals to claim religious rights. Religions are groups or communities under the law but only assert the rights of individual members. Yet all religions, regardless of context and sincerity, must be organized on beliefs that are basic to human identity and reality.

In addition to cautious and benign attempts to recognize only genuine religions, the state also enters the religion sector with a variety of procedural tests of fairness and competence. These include the accreditation of parochial schools, and the application of antidiscrimination laws and fair labor practices to religious organizations. State regulation in these areas seems to follow the logic of generalizable norms of justice and professionalism. The state imposes these norms regardless of the existence of contrary religious beliefs. In this way the state recognizes the preeminence of secular principles in selected areas of human experience.

The state also traditionally concerns itself with certain primary goods that cut across secular and religious communities, especially those of life and health. In general, the state will not regulate the selection of medical therapy, or the choice not to seek medical care, so long as two conditions are met: (1) the individual is legally competent, and (2) the act does not adversely affect the interests of a third party. Jehovah's Witnesses who forgo blood transfusions on religious grounds are allowed to do so as long as they are competent and act for only themselves. But if the individual Witness is pregnant, the courts may legally coerce a transfusion in the interests of the unborn child. When individuals refuse treatment for a third party, acting as surrogate or in some other role, the courts are usually quick to deny the religious belief and require the patient to accept standard medical care. When the patient is not legally competent, as in the case of minor children, the state often imposes secular standards of care in place of the choices mandated by the religious belief. In these cases, the state overrides religious beliefs that compromise life and health.

Long traditions of law and morality support religious discretion in selecting therapy (or not). Medical practice was hostile to individual autonomy for most of its professional history. A beneficence model—roughly interpreted as "doctor knows best"—guided treatment decisions. The practical effects of this model were that the physician not only made the decisions but routinely withheld crucial medical information from the patient. The guiding assumption in medicine was that the superior technical skills and knowledge commanded by the physician required authoritative actions, not patient autonomy or even participation in therapy decisions except at the margins.

But the common law has always recognized individual autonomy, especially over one's body. This autonomy was introduced to clinical medicine in recent years with an emphasis on informed consent. The patient must be provided with the information needed to make an informed judgment about whether to accept or refuse therapy, and which therapy options to select.

Absent informed consent and medical information is liable to legal judgments of battery and negligence.

Informed consent is itself a nexus concept consisting of two principles: competence and negative liberty. The law is chronically unclear (some would say confused) over competence, usually passing it off as the capacity to make decisions without exploring the difficulties in specifying and testing this capacity. But on negative liberty, the law is uncharacteristically robust and interesting, recognizing in the right to refuse medical treatment a fundamental liberty expressed in privacy, due process, and autonomy. The privacy defense is the least well developed in the law, while due process has been used in a number of court cases to protect individuals' liberty to refuse therapy. But the most important expression of liberty is the autonomy represented in informed consent. Assuming that the patient is competent, the doctor today is legally required to secure informed consent before proceeding with treatment.

If autonomy were the only interest to be considered in refusing medical treatment, then the free exercise clause of the First Amendment would simply re-express this interest in religious vocabularies, and religious choices of therapy options would be protected by a shield large enough to extend across both secular and religious beliefs. But the state also has interests in decisions on therapy. The main countervailing interests of the state are (1) preservation of life, (2) prevention of suicide, (3) protection of innocent third parties, and (4) maintaining the ethical integrity of the medical profession. The strongest state interest is the preservation of life, the weakest (in court cases) is the maintenance of integrity in the medical profession. While suicide, in general, is no longer illegal, states still try to prevent individuals from taking their own lives (on the assumption that suicidal impulses are prima facie indications of mental incompetence). The third interest, protection of innocent third parties, is represented in state efforts to require pregnant women to accept medical care and generally maintain their health. Sometimes this interest leads to state constraints on medical choices for the sake of dependent children.

All of these interests, however, can be overridden in the singular actions of a competent individual. The free exercise clause of the First Amendment protects individuals from state interference in decisions over medical care based on religious beliefs so long as the individual is competent and the decision primarily affects only the individual. The thought behind these shields is simplicity itself: if you want to refuse medical care and risk or lose your life for the sake of your religious beliefs, the state will not try to stop you. Both the respect for individual autonomy found in the common law and even longer traditions protecting religious freedoms dominate the state's powerful interests in preserving human life.

Christian Science

One of the more organized forms of spiritual healing recognized in law is found in the Church of Christ, Scientist. Christian Science began in the nineteenth century. Though it is Christian and therefore claims origin in Jesus Christ, its particular interpretations of Christian theology originate with a layperson, Mary Baker Eddy.

Eddy, on any account, was a remarkable individual. As a young widow in poor health with no economic means, she pondered the central questions of theology at length. In a strict circumstantial account, the absence of substantial material goods might explain the early idealism in her thought. She doubted whether matter existed, and her philosophical quest was consistently metaphysical rather than empirical. But a simpler and more useful explanation is probably that she, like so many others in religious movements, was driven by spiritual impulses to explain human experience in terms of categories beyond the knowable.

Eddy's poor health, however, did figure in her beliefs in a decisive way. She suffered from a number of ailments, not diagnosed in terms that a contemporary physician would accept without further examination. The diagnosis at the time was "spinal inflammation," though much evidence in family correspondence suggests gallbladder problems. But no one can be sure. All we know with certainty is that Eddy reported a variety of pains and discomforts that she tried to overcome with the best and worst remedies of the day. These included some of the barbarities of mid-nineteenth century allopathy, and extended to various diet regimes, versions of homeopathy, and brands of mesmerism.

These various "therapies" were not successful in curing her ailments. But she did arrive slowly at the belief that attitude had some causal relation to disease and cure. This belief was elaborated by one of the leading mesmerists of the times, Phineas Parkhurst Quimby. Quimby tried to explain all illness as linked to mind. He applied a therapy that purported to heal the body by altering the state of mind of the sufferer. He believed that he was following the practices of Jesus Christ. Mary Baker Eddy was much influenced by Quimby early in her reflections, especially by his cryptic observation that "there is no intelligence in matter." For a time, she was herself freed of her afflictions by Quimby's methods.

At some later stage, however, Eddy freed herself of Quimbyism. The catalytic event was her successful triumph over yet one more debilitating illness, this one caused by a fall on the ice. During a long period of recovery, she began reading the Bible and "discovered Christian Science." The method was both simple and profound. She came to believe that the life of the spirit, not the flesh, is the only reality. This insight obviously went far beyond Quimby's ideas of mind over matter. Eddy was asserting that mind is the "sole reality," matter is an illusion. She abandoned mesmerism by default. The theology that Eddy slowly developed endorsed mind *in place of* matter.

In this theology, the physical world, including the entire range of social experience and human history, is a construct of the senses (except as revelatory glimpses of the eternal are found in history). The material world is not reality but a false mode of consciousness that the human brain conjures to render sense experience intelligible. Reality is outside of sensory human experience. It is coterminous with the mind of God, not human consciousness. This mind is the realm of the spiritual, which is not abstract but rather tangible and concrete. Christ is the singular figure in history who represents the divine in the temporal world.

The understandings of disease and health in Christian Science follow from Eddy's ontology. Illness is in the realm of the physical, an entry in the domain of the material. It follows that illness is illusory, not real. In one of the most quoted sections of *Science and Health*, Eddy testifies to the spiritual state of being with these words:

There is no life, truth, intelligence, nor substance in matter. All is infinite Mind and its infinite manifestation, for God is All-in-all. Spirit is immortal Truth; matter is mortal error. Spirit is the real and eternal; matter is the unreal and temporal. Spirit is God, and man is His image and likeness. Therefore man is not material; he is spiritual.

The message of Christian Science is that human beings are lifted from the error of the senses by divine love, which can reveal the spiritual nature—and the reality—of humans. This spiritual nature is without illness of any sort. Eddy's metaphysics in this way precede her views on healing. The dispelling of illness is a consequence of the identification of reality as a spiritual domain. Healing is simply a demonstration that this ontology is correct.

The conviction among Christian Scientists that illness is not real but merely an error in perception or attitude is held universally by members of the religion. But Christian Science also recruits and provides practitioners who minister to others. These practitioners are especially valued as advisors in negotiating the passage of a sick individual back to a state of health (as reality). One such practitioner is Bryan Seth, a second-generation Christian Scientist. His family was Lutheran for several generations. When his mother was a teenager, however, she rebelled against what she perceived as the rigidity of the Lutheran Church and found her way into Christian Science. Seth was raised in the beliefs of Mary Baker Eddy.

Seth is an engineer by profession. He earned a degree in electrical engineering before World War II. After the war he did some graduate work part-time with the thought of a Ph.D. and an academic career in mind. But in 1948 when he was a graduate student, newly minted Ph.Ds in his field were earning $3,500 a year. He decided to stay on fulltime with General Electric, where he had been working since the war began in 1941. The problems he was assigned were interesting. He was part of a team of engineers and scientists who helped to develop an early version of Star Wars—missiles that could intercept ICBMs. Seth was in charge of the electronics-detection radar. The study he helped complete demonstrated (even then) the enormous cost of such a system. The project was subsequently dropped, though Seth was asked to complete the development of the new-age computer it had required. He was also part of the research that brought GE into color television, and then later—in the 1950s—contributed to the engineering work on transistors.

In 1963, Seth left the corporate world and became a full-time Christian Science practitioner. This life change meant going from a corporate executive salary to an income, in his first year, of $900. He and his wife had four sons, and Seth had to use all of the money he had saved for their college educations to support the family during the first five years of his practice. Helping matters was the farm he had purchased while still an affluent executive. The Seths were able to raise most of the food they needed and rent some of the land to pay taxes on it. The four children all eventually did get through college, and Seth has not regretted his radical career change.

Christian Science practitioners are not licensed. They are interviewed and officially approved by the church. Also, every three years the church selects thirty individuals from around the world to attend a class in metaphysics. Seth is proud of the fact that he was one of the select group in 1976 and enjoys quoting Eddy's observation that "he who teaches by healing or heals by teaching will succeed." He is regarded by the church as both a teacher and a practitioner. The identification of practitioners is eminently practical. Individuals who sense the call to practice simply try to do so. If they succeed, the church recognizes them as practitioners. Some try and fail. Seth recalls a man who was successful in business and wanted to be a practitioner. He tried and found he could not do it. After eight years of effort he went back into business full time.

Christian Science accepts the idea that practitioners should charge for their services approximately what a physician charges. The reality is usually not even close. Seth's fee is seven dollars per treatment. For that modest sum the patients (Seth's term) receive spiritual guidance on a problem that is usually, but not always, manifested in some physical debility. They call Seth on the phone or visit his house (where he now works since closing his office in the city). Sometimes he finds it necessary to visit a patient's home, particularly when an illness does not yield to counsel right away or the patient is a young child.

The one impression dominating all others in conversation with Christian Scientists is that the religion is what might be called "user friendly." Seth is like all practitioners in stressing the autonomy of parishioners. When he enters a home to teach and minister, he tries to address the entire family situation. Individuals always ask him, "What should I do?" Seth responds, "I will not tell you. That is your business." Instead he provides options, references from Scripture, general counsel calibrated to the needs of the particular family context. He regards himself as a comforter, not a healer. On occasion individuals will feel an imperative to seek medical therapy of a conventional sort. The church does not condemn such individuals. It merely waits patiently for them to return to the fold. Nothing Seth says to patients prevents them from doing what they think is best. He emphasizes again and again that the individual Christian Scientist must be guided by God's directions, not those of the practitioner.

Still, Seth firmly believes the Christian Science tenet that illness is the product of an incorrect state of mind. A man who seemed to have a very serious cold once came in to see him. In working with the man, Seth had the thought that some immorality was the source of the problem. He didn't know how to proceed, so he consulted with a more experienced practitioner. The advice: "Why don't you handle immorality?" Seth did so in a shift in counseling. The man was healed and later admitted that his situation had an immoral component. Seth points out that many mental attitudes have physical correlates. Feeling embarrassed, for example, can produce a blush. The practitioner has to find a way to treat the state of mind that must be corrected to dissolve the illness. "Correction," in this case, means bringing thought into accord with God, or reality. Seth likes to cite Eddy to the effect that ignorance of God produces apparent discord and right understanding restores harmony.

Seth had a crisis of sorts himself shortly after he began as a practitioner. He developed a physical problem that involved substantial swelling in his face and throat. He had no idea what was causing the problem, but he remembers feeling some embarrassment that he, a practitioner, was manifesting such a thing. He went to his son's graduation from Principia College, a school for Christian Scientists (exacerbating Seth's embarrassment, of course), and on the trip home he felt he had reached a point of such discomfort—he could not eat or move without pain—that he could not go on. He recalls that at that moment the thought came to him that God is life and that there was no way that he, Seth, could avoid being the expression of that life. Within a few seconds, an opening of some type appeared on his face and whatever was afflicting him drained away. For Seth that was the end of doubt. He never again felt any unease or fear about physical illness.

He expresses some irritation at the attacks made on Christian Science by those who endorse modern medical techniques. Doctors fail also, he points out, and more frequently than Christian Scientists. But they are not challenged in the way that Christian Scientists are. "We have to be one hundred percent," he observes. When asked why Christian Science cannot simply view modern medicine as the handiwork of God, he replies that Christian Science has a better handiwork. It is a religion that recognizes that there is only one healer, God, whether the individual is healed through faith or medical techniques.

Seth endorses Mary Baker Eddy's wish that all doctors would become Christian Scientists. He believes that then they would be more effective. His point is that Christian Science is a science of being, which medicine is not. Medicine, according to the ontology that defines Christian Science, treats illusions as though they were real. Seth concludes that many doctors do wonderful work in alleviating symptoms and attending to physical ailments, but they do not heal. If doctors realized that, if they could see through the constructs that make up empirical experience, then they would see more clearly into their craft. For one thing, Seth points out, doctors would have a different attitude toward death if they knew reality. Death, according to Christian Science, does not do a thing to the individual. It does not change him one iota. Medicine that accepts such a belief would obviously be different than medicine driven by life-preservation imperatives.

Seth does not have any doubts that reality is outside human experience. In his teaching, he includes the story of Daniel and Nebuchadnezzar. Nebuchadnezzar had a dream that he could not remember and called his wise men together to describe the dream to him. They expressed consternation at the request. The king told them (in the way only kings can) that death was the penalty for failing to carry out this task successfully. Daniel was one of those summoned, and he asked for more time. He retreated from the court to pray. When he returned, he told the king the story of his dream.

The question that is compelling for Seth is, how could Daniel do that? According to Seth, Daniel succeeded because he could read the thoughts of others. Seth sees the same logic at work in healing. "I am able to read the thoughts of others," he claims. There is nothing miraculous in this claim as far as he is concerned. Seth believes that most people read their own thoughts in situations because they cannot escape the conviction that they are individuals trying to read the minds of other individuals. But according to Christian Science there is only one mind, and that is reflected in each individual. If one views only the reflection, then one would conclude that individuals have minds of their own. But this is a false belief. God is one, and in each person. To read the thoughts of others only requires listening to one's own thoughts, which are universally embedded in the one universal mind. Healing for Seth is the revelation of this spiritual reality. It is a natural dispersion of illusion, not a supernatural action, and begins with a natural access to universal thoughts.

Seth believes no one has seen God. To illustrate this principle, he draws an analogy to the sun (which Eddy also used in a slightly different way). We see rays of light from the sun. But the rays, because they take five hundred seconds to reach the earth, can be viewed only as representing the sun as it actually is. No one sees the sun directly. In similar fashion, the human individual is a representation of God. We see God's reflection in each individual if we look at the whole person, but we do not see God directly.

For Seth, the basis of Christian Science is a way of life based on an understanding of the real. Physical healing is only an indication that the individual understands this basis. The goal of Christian Science is to see the truth beyond the misconceptions of human experience. Seth does not believe that this reality must be demonstrated again and again to prove this point. One time through will do it. He is satisfied that the truth he accepts has been demonstrated.

Vecchio

Anthony Vecchio combines the healing approaches of James Crossland and Charles Brantley. He uses charismatic methods while remaining attentive to the primarily spiritual effects of his efforts. He also carries the burden of a restless skepticism unusual in those professing the healing ministry. Vecchio has been a priest in the Roman Catholic Church for over two decades. He was not a deeply religious priest (by his own admission) until he became involved in faith healing. The healing ministry seemed to provide him with deeper involvement in the lives of his parishioners. He claims the gift of compassion—the ability to enter the suffering and tragedy of his parishioners—rather than the gift of healing. Yet he holds six to eight healing services a month. They each last a minimum of three hours and are exciting and draining experiences for Vecchio. He regards himself as an instrument to assemble people in prayer and to touch them in a healing ceremony. What happens after that, he believes, is between God and the individual.

Vecchio grew up with Christian Scientists. For over fifteen years (between the ages of thirteen and thirty) he had a strong bonding relationship with two adults who lived next door to his parents. He did their gardening and took care of their lawn when he was young. They would invite him over to talk afterwards. He remembers their stories of healing as extraordinary tales that influenced him deeply. No superstitions seemed to inform their beliefs. They were simply intelligent and loving people.

Later, as a seminary student, Vecchio met Father Ralph DiOrio before DiOrio became nationally known as a faith healer. Vecchio remembers him as a bright and gifted priest who had a lovely speaking voice. It was precisely DiOrio's speaking ability that started him on the path to faith healing. DiOrio attended mass in a Boston church where Father Edward McDonough, a well-known healer, was having a service. DiOrio was in the back of the church with some of his parishioners when prayer petitions were being placed in a basket carried around by a seven-year-old girl. DiOrio had felt for several months that he was blessed with the gift of healing and petitioned in writing for a healing ministry. McDonough recognized him and invited him to preach on the Blessed Mother. DiOrio was splendid, striking just the right note in a spontaneous sermon that excited the Hispanic congregation, which to observers was ripe for healing, magic, and prayer to the Holy Ghost. Then DiOrio began blessing the people with McDonough. The magic was strong. Individuals began fainting, collapsing, as DiOrio placed hands on them. DiOrio reported later that when he returned to his car, his body was so hot that he burned the leather of the seat when he sat down.

Ten years later Vecchio met DiOrio again, this time on a retreat. They became friends. DiOrio offered to come to Vecchio's church to do a healing service. Vecchio was elated. DiOrio was by that time a star in Catholic healing ministries. Over twelve thousand people came to the local auditorium for DiOrio's healing service. The ceremonies were pure excitement, with some people trembling and fainting in cathartic experiences. Vecchio had never seen such emotional highs as he witnessed that day.

After DiOrio returned home to his own parish in Boston, Vecchio became lost in the mundane duties of his priesthood. Nothing resonated for him. He was impatient, irritable. There seemed to be no sacred qualities around him. Everything was ordinary. He began reading all he could find on faith healing. Tentatively, he began his healing ministry by duplicating the rites followed by DiOrio. He cultivated his looks to fit more neatly with his own images of Christ. He grew a beard, let his hair grow out a bit longer. One evening he looked in the mirror and was stunned by the effect: piercing eyes, charismatic presence. He was a little scared by his own appearance. The effects on the congregation were electrifying. He began drawing crowds. The services seemed to lift everyone into some higher orbit, including Vecchio. In the meantime, he continued to study the literatures on faith healing.

The crowds that began to appear for Vecchio's healing services were remarkable for his parish. His church is in the worst section of the city. Houses in the area sell for $3,000. The crime rate is the highest in the county. Vecchio himself has been mugged three times in his own churchyard. Yet over two hundred people began turning out twice a week for the healing mass. They also put real money into the collection plate—nothing, of course, like DiOrio's collection rates. In three days of work during a visit, DiOrio raised over $35,000 in Vecchio's parish. (DiOrio left with the lion's share, a check for $27,500. He regularly demands, and gets, two-thirds of the proceeds for his healing sessions.)

The main change, however, has been in the attitudes and temperaments of the parish members. Vecchio claims to have seen revivals of faith that defy explanation. One professed atheist was brought to a service by his wife. When Vecchio touched him during the healing rites he collapsed in a trance. Vecchio recalls with amusement the spouse's observation, "There goes the atheist." Vecchio favors 1 John, with its words, "God is love." These three words indemnify for Vecchio his visceral approach to the congregation. He hugs people, cries with them, agonizes with them, in general establishes a deep emotive connection to the people at the services.

He is not sure, however, if anyone is ever healed physically through spiritual efforts. Vecchio once conducted a service in Albany, New York, that culminated with over one hundred people clustered around the altar praying, even begging God to heal a woman with liver cancer. The woman had six children and she was crying, pleading with God to let her live so that she could raise her children. She died a month later. Over nine hundred petitioners came to the Albany service asking for healing. Vecchio is not sure that anyone was cured of anything. He received a number of positive letters from individuals who professed to have been healed. But his critical intelligence will not permit him to accept such testimonies. He wants an agnostic doctor to examine these individuals and provide plausible evidence that an incurable disease has been cured.

Yet Vecchio wants to believe that faith healing is possible. Once he administered to a woman with breast cancer and the tumor in her breast disappeared. It vanished completely. Vecchio was not convinced. He kept asking himself, where did the tumor go? How did it dissolve? He contemplated a causal relationship between word and deed—that his prayers and the petitioner's beliefs had somehow altered her body chemistry in such a way that the woman's immune system successfully attacked the tumor. He thinks that such causality may be possible, that if he uses enough loving words, feels enough compassion, has a Christly look, that something may happen in the petitioner's body to bring about a cure. He psychs himself up before the services with the thought "I've got three hours to make something happen"— create a mood, a mentality, an attitude. He exhausts and drains himself emotionally to get some physiological ball rolling, a hypnotic state in place, to start a healing process. The woman's tumor did go away. But six months later it showed up someplace else in her body. He does not know why God would move tumors around in someone's body.

Only once in all of his years of holding healing services has Vecchio felt something occurring. At one service he suddenly felt a heat that seemed to radiate from a petitioner's body. Vecchio felt that something was really happening for a change and, for the first and only time, he uttered the words "You are healed." The man turned out to have lung cancer. It stopped progressing after the service. The man started calling Vecchio frequently to thank him. Vecchio rejoiced in the man's faith, which was almost childlike in its simplicity. Six months later, a tumor was discovered in the man's spine. Vecchio agonized over the relapse, for they had both prayed so hard and so long for a cure. Before the man died, he believed that the healing, which was in effect a brief respite, was given to him to get his affairs in order before death. He died believing in a benevolent and omnipotent God.

Vecchio believes that healing services can lift people from the ordinary to transcendent moments of pure faith. He ministers to people who are hurting, crying—from broken hearts, broken marriages, perhaps terminal illnesses. He believes he can restore their dreams for a better world. This restoration can extend their lives, conquer their afflictions for a time through will and belief. His petitioners' last words to him are often, "I would never have gotten to this point without you. I would have died with no hope, in misery." One terminally ill individual told Vecchio as he died that he wished he could have been healed for his, Vecchio's sake. Vecchio knows that without faith healing his priestly duties would have been a combination of mundane administrative work and ordinary clerical responsibilities. Now he has the opportunity to enter the souls of individuals who are pleading for help, for more time to live, for healing itself. He is convinced that his efforts can prolong life and restore belief in an afterlife. He does not doubt for a second that spiritual healing can occur.

The issue is whether there is physical healing of the sort found in the Scriptures. When asked whether he believes in the possibility of complete spiritual and physical healing as practiced by Jesus, Vecchio answers that he wants to believe in that possibility, that as a priest he must believe in it. But he also admits that all the remissions of illnesses that he witnesses could be explained as natural occurrences with no supernatural causes. At this moment he is praying intensely for a young woman who has had bone cancer for a year and a half. She seems to be doing well. The hole in her spine has closed. Her doctor thinks that new bone may be growing there. Vecchio and his congregation have prayed on a weekly basis for this woman over the entire course of her disease. He regards her as a test case of sorts. He admits that he would have a hard time dealing with the standard "It's God's will" explanation if the woman dies of her disease. She has begged God for enough time to raise her six-year-old son until he is on his own as an adult. Yet Vecchio knows that the cancer could simply be sleeping, in a state of remission, and could flare up to kill her at any time.

Vecchio also knows that faith healing brings risks as well as benefits to any religious movement. He is careful to separate tests of faith or goodness from healing. A person's failure to be healed cannot, in his view, be regarded as a sign of any flaw in the person. But he admits that chronic failure in bringing about cures could undermine the general faith of parishioners. If nothing occurs, if faith healing is entirely bogus on the physical level, then the revival of religious faith inspired by healing ministries may be compromised permanently. Vecchio does believe that God has a plan that humans cannot know entirely, so that eternal time frames may not correspond to human expectations. He also believes that all prayers are answered with a yes, but not necessarily within this life on earth. Yet he worries that a congregation may dismiss the notion of a divine schedule for healing, for the healing services are devoted to cures in the here and now.

The Catholic liturgy that influenced Vecchio when he contemplated the priesthood as a young man was severe when compared to recent practices. He remembers the priest as authority figure, masses in Latin, altar boys as virtual servants. Now the masses are held in vernacular language, the priest faces the congregation (instead of saying the mass turned to the altar with his back to his parishioners), laypersons read the sacred text and distribute Holy Communion into the hands of communicants, women are in the sacristy. In a word, the mass now belongs to the people. The priest is a mediator, not an authority. Vecchio admits to having nostalgic longings on occasion for those times when the mass did not seem to be a Protestant ceremony. He believes that the charismatic movement in Catholicism and the renewed interest in faith healing represent an attempt to put mystery back into the Church. He would hate to see these efforts collapse on the revelation that faith healing is fraudulent.

There were moments during DiOrio's service in his parish that embarrassed Vecchio. DiOrio would ask the congregation to pray for the departure of the evil spirits occupying the sick person's body. The prayers were sometimes particular in the extreme, such as "Foul spirit of cancer depart from this man's body." Vecchio viewed these rites as medieval at best, witchcraft at worst, and totally irrational. He still feels guilt over inflicting these injustices on his people. He also had to pick up the pieces after DiOrio returned to Boston. Illnesses supposedly cured returned in strength. Vecchio now regards these sessions as classic instances of group hysteria. Yet he retains his awe over the sight of twelve thousand people gathered in prayer.

In his own ministry, Vecchio has tried to cultivate spiritual healing as both an end in itself and a causal influence on physiological processes. He continues to believe that mental attitudes can affect health. He prays with his congregation twice a week for three hours. They meditate together, hear some Latin verses and music, experience a high mass of some sort, and for a brief time leave behind their ordinary lives as they try to experience a transcendent God. Vecchio believes that these ceremonies admit individuals to a higher plane of life that can and does benefit both their souls and their physical states.

Vecchio does not believe that God gives any special gifts to priests or to anyone else. During the four years of his healing ministry, he has read much on faith healing and thought so long about the services he conducts that at times he has become confused about exactly what he is doing. He has refined his answer to that question again and again over the years. Mainly he believes that he is not a healer sent by God, only a priest who gathers his congregation together to find love and faith. The healing that may result from this effort he regards as an occasional indication of the spirit's dominance over the incarnate flesh. But the healing of the spirit is more important to him than physical healing.

From a taped interview with Father Anthony Vecchio:

"I have presided over numbers of them who were not afraid to die. And their last words were: ' . . . I wasn't healed physically, but I was healed spiritually. I felt the presence of God. I'm not afraid to leave my children, my family. I'm not afraid to die.' I'm forty-eight now. If I can get older and remember these words of mortal human beings, then on my deathbed I can say that I interwove my own soul into the lives of hundreds of people who left this world for the unknown and were not afraid. I want God to bring this song to my funeral."

Medicine and Faith Healing

The emergence of modern medicine is marked by several features. First, the human body, and the illnesses that strike the body, are given secular names that identify the visible bases of physiology. The parts and processes of the body as material object are mapped with a detail previously unknown in history. Second, a reliable understanding of the causal relations between the agents of disease and the state of the body, and between the functions of the body and health or pathology, is in place. Third, modern medicine relies increasingly on explanatory laws of physiology that are generalizable across all particular human bodies.

Modern medicine also disaggregates the conditions of the body to discrete units of analysis, so that explanations are tracked from micro to macro levels in fixing the state of the body. The sense of time in medicine is strictly linear, meaning that both health and disease are explained in terms of antecedent events that can be organized in a causal continuum from past to present. Space is in similar fashion specified in terms of standard three-dimensional areas that permit the deployment of physiological terms in mapping sequences. The result is a species of discourse that accepts the visible as a primary influence on vocabularies and subsumes medical explanations under the physical laws developed in the natural sciences, especially those found in biology, chemistry, and physics.

Clinical medicine introduces this discourse to the intuitions of diagnosticians. Physicians vary considerably in their abilities to diagnose illness, and few practitioners of medicine seem prepared to explain this variance in terms that would satisfy the explanatory standards of science. Instead a mystical quality enters descriptions of diagnosis. Successful diagnosticians are presented as skilled wizards, able to divine the unknown from touch and what appears to be second sight. In this sense, clinical medicine is akin to faith healing on an intuitive surface, so long as one appreciates the grounding of medical intuition in an extensive practical and theoretical training in medicine never found among faith healers.

The hostility between medicine and faith healing is generated by the unavoidable overlaps between the two types of discourses. One can imagine medicine and faith operating as separate and autonomous sets of beliefs that never intersect, with one consequence being the freedom of individuals to choose selectively (or categorically) between the two sets of concepts. But such independence is impossible. Faith healers claim healing powers over the body, which is currently the domain of medicine. Healing may be conducted by priests as well as doctors, but the success of the efforts must be judged from within the discourse of medicine as a secular practice.

It is not a universal practice to test the claims of one discourse by another. Religious believers may see spirits in visitation rites, but there are no recognized experts in the secular world to falsify such visions (though they are widely debunked). One might even say that such testing would be unfair, on the grounds that a secular temperament will assign scientific or material tests to any miraculous happening, and this assignment is not neutral. Religious discourse uses inference and evidence differently than secular discourse. Stories may be used to communicate truths not amenable to linear renderings of experience. This is not true of faith healing, however. Faith healers claim that physiological changes must be subject to medical examination. Yet once the placebo effect is incorporated into therapeutic agendas, these examinations usually show no success at all.

A typology might charitably allow causal efficacy for religious beliefs. Here is the exercise: Think of a continuum. At one pole are those diseases with unclear or multiple causes. They respond to different and unusual treatments, and are subject to unexplainable remissions. Included here might be arthritis and certain forms of cancer. At the other polar extreme are those diseases, like meningitis, where the causes are known to be infectious agents, the treatment is a standard and successful therapy (for example, antibiotics), and the disease is serious and often fatal without treatment. A reasonable view might expect faith healing to be aimed more appropriately at the first rather than the second pole. Many faith healers acknowledge this continuum and accept the reasonableness of the view. But others, Christian Scientists in particular, reject the distinctions, preferring to see all disease as the same and uniformly amenable to the efforts of faith and the intervention of God.

Such views, extreme by secular standards, not only question the entire edifice of modern medicine but also require modification in the very secular view of the world that slowly led over centuries to the dismissal of spiritual vocabularies in medicine. To assert the reality of miraculous healings—either through direct suspension of natural laws by external forces or by means of an ontological rearrangement that jettisons disease by recognizing it as a complex illusion—is to give up the recent dominance of empiricism in favor of a reality outside human experience. Both science and magic are abandoned for the sake of the miraculous and all that it implies.

One must be careful to be fair here, to listen to the side that claims so extravagant a view. Certainly it is not fair to dismiss the possibility of miracles using the limits identified by the current state of science. What is inconceivable today, or at any point in the history of science, may be commonplace at some time in the future. If energy and matter, time and space, could be viewed in a Newtonian paradigm as mutually exclusive and interchangeable variables in relativity theory, what appears to be an impossible world today may be a scientific reality not yet discovered. It is part of the history and logic of science to allow for the acceptance of anomalies within the main body of theory, for even the most natural of laws may be bounded by later understandings. So much is clear in any fair use of science.

Yet the central logic of science is set against faith healing. Scientific inquiry is designed to falsify claims with some use of evidence and inference rules. It is one of the main pillars of religion that faith replaces doubt. To accept any kind of falsification in faith healing is to begin negotiating a slippery slope toward no spiritual discourse at all, because even a provisional belief that God does not heal is already a dismissal of faith itself. This resistance to falsification helps explain the ultimate elastic clause in religious discourse when healing efforts fail: God will heal only if it is part of an eternal plan not accessible to humans. Such a clause makes scientific testing impossible, though secular physicians can point out when God has failed to eradicate a disease (for reasons unknown and unknowable).

None of this hostility affects the benign overlaps between medicine and faith healing. If faith healers call spontaneous remissions consistent with medical understandings of disease patterns "miracles," medical and religious practitioners are simply using different explanations for the same phenomenon. Religious beliefs may even help individuals move into a set of patients with a higher probability for a remission of disease. Again, the placebo effect is real in both medical and religious discourses. But the methods of medicine and religion differ, and, in the current state of logical priorities, the therapeutic assertions and outcomes of any discourse are medical by definition and so subject to secular tests.

The dominant consideration in adjudicating the differences between medicine and spiritual efforts at faith healing, however, is the existence or nonexistence of a reality outside human experience. Science does not deny it. Recent physics, in its virtual merger with cosmology, suggests a range of possible worlds rivaling the metaphysical speculations of medieval philosophers. But the religious discourses of Pentecostal-charismatic and Christian Science traditions accept such a reality as the architectural product of a grand designer who influences and ultimately controls human experience. It would be helpful to know when it is reasonable to refer to such a reality in health and healing.

An external reality would obviously affect human identity. However individuals are partitioned—mind-body, individual-community—it is impossible to regard them as being independent of the social contexts that nurture them. The individual is in the social world, the social world is in the individual. No other view can explain the reciprocal influences of self and group documented in all social theory. Now imagine that the human community is an entry in a larger cosmic scheme unknown and unknowable to the human intellect. Such a reality, a sense of community beyond all conventions, would expand human identity to include some dimensions of the supernatural. The social world within each individual would be beyond empirical boundaries. Secular interpretations of individuals would have to be revised, and perhaps abandoned entirely.

Authority and the Individual

Alternative realities both occasion and call into question the social partitions that liberalism favors, even when basic freedoms generate the partitions. In political societies, four separate freedoms seem to establish distinct spiritual domains. One is the freedom to choose religious lives, represented by the basic right to accept or reject the messages that religions attempt to bring to individuals and the secondary right to choose or establish particular religions once those messages have been accepted. Liberty of commitment, the freedom to decide (a) whether to commit to the religious life and (b) how to realize that commitment, seems to express this first freedom in a social context.

A second freedom is that of conscience. Conscience is a compelling force. The individuals interviewed here are not free to accept or abandon their religious convictions. They are driven by those convictions at the most fundamental levels of their existence, which is precisely what we mean by a religion. Freedom of conscience is an entirely negative freedom, preventing the state from imposing restrictions on those individual practices that follow the dictates (not choices) of conscience. It is in fact the recognition that individuals are driven by religious convictions that makes religious exemptions reasonable to grant, even in a society governed by secular principles.

A third freedom is directly religious—the freedom to practice the beliefs that define and sustain religions. These freedoms are not recognized in American law as organizational rights. In spite of the fact that churches do things as organizations, for example, own property, make decisions about theology and ceremony, the courts are cautious in assigning rights to religious organizations. Nevertheless, the freedom of religions, not individual choice or conscience, was a decisive consideration for the framers in writing and supporting the religious clauses in the First Amendment. Like freedom of choice, religious freedom constrains the state to introduce no impediments on the practice of one's faith.

The fourth type of freedom is an anomaly in the package consisting of all four freedoms. It is the freedom to dissent. Freedom of conscience and religion are compatible with authority in one way or another. Conscience is the authority of religious conviction, and freedom of religion can be the freedom to practice according to religious authority. Freedom of dissent goes further. It is the freedom to question and even undermine authority.

One of the remarkable features of dissent is its inertial force. Like some perpetual motion machine, it often appears to have no natural limits on its energy. It can capture and dispose of all impediments, even those offered as conditions for its own rationality. For example, the Catholic Church, like many institutions, distinguishes between core and noncore beliefs. The doctrine of transubstantiation, an obvious core belief, has a different status than the manner in which the communion host is distributed. The Church maintains its infallibility on core teachings but allows dissent on noncore beliefs, which are matters of convention and do, in fact, change over time. But how is the distinction between core and noncore beliefs to be shielded from the critical scrutiny of individual dissent?

The extraordinary range of dissent originates in the simple recognition that the power to draw distinctions is often, de facto, the power to control dissent. One who demurs on noncore beliefs, for example, might be met by extending the category of a core belief to the dissenting target. The potential ubiquity of authority invites dissent to address definitions and classifications, for failure to address basic demarcations risks paralyzing dissent. And why stop at an authoritative division of beliefs? On the terms of liberal political philosophy, institutions are legitimate because they are derived from consent, which inspires the more generalized scrutiny that follows the freedom to dissent—on criteria as well as substance, distinctions as easily as entries.

Only a demonstration of natural and reasonably permanent divisions in beliefs can limit dissent, given the compelling reasons to extend this fourth liberty to the agendas that channel liberty.

The recognition of these four freedoms as religious liberties turns social thought in various directions. The oldest traditions of political theory are concerned, sometimes exclusively, with authority. On what grounds do some individuals rule over others? The divine right of kings, arguably the most ancient of legitimizing devices, grants to monarchs a power that is legitimate because it derives from God. Plato's *Republic* offers arguments for authority based on intellectual skills. Religious freedoms shift authority from political to religious institutions, and in the case of freedom of choice, shift the grounds for conscience and dissent to groups and individuals within religious practice. The result is not only the heterogeneity of religious belief and practice that one might expect with such impressive freedoms, but also a splintering of legitimacy itself. Heresy is incompatible with religious pluralism. It also follows that the state cannot be part of the church so long as such liberties are valued in themselves, for the naturally coercive power of all states, even those grounded in consent, is hostile to the discretion of religions and individuals to follow basic beliefs about human experience.

Spiritual healing, whether religious or secular, poses special problems for liberal partitions. Liberalism disjoins human experience: appetite is separated from contemplation, body disconnected from mind, state and religion are broken apart and redeployed as distinct institutions. Spiritual healers, however, believe in the possibility of two ideals: a fused or integrated self, and a reality that is a seamless web of actions, events, and powers. Complete healing is said to occur only when the individual is properly located within such a holistic framework. The problem is that this framework simply is not found in the fragile and often mutually antagonistic arrangements of liberal democracies, where institutions compete on a constantly shifting background of values and resources. The practical ideal of spiritual therapy opposes liberalism with a world where natural harmonies prevail and the whole unit dominates its own arrangements.

Can church and state be distinct institutions in a holistic society?

All spiritual healing requires a surrender of private authority. The individual transfers autonomy to some more expansive force, whether it be to God, the universe, or cosmic energy. Freedom of will is abandoned as the power to decide is given over to the external force. In some real but not easily understood sense, the individual merges with a larger reality. The interpretive powers and freedoms that provide independent religious domains are extinguished. Equally interesting is the way the individual rejects dualism both within and outside the self in the ultimate stages of spiritual regeneration. Not only are mind and body one, but spiritual and secular are the same. Authority is a resource distributed universally throughout social practices and individuals.

It is difficult to see how church and state can be separate institutions when some of the main arguments for distinct and independent spheres of human experience are jettisoned by the logic of spiritual healing. The holism of such healing does not recognize different spiritual and secular functions since both mind and body, this world and the other world, are governed by the same design. The individual powers that are the source of private moralities and separate religions collapse under a single authoritative voice. Not only are church and state part of the same ontological agenda, but it is impossible, strictly speaking, to distinguish between the two according to the vision that spiritual healing proclaims.

L U K E

My mother called them reveries. Where you are so deep in thought that
you are not conscious of anyone around you. Once, in the second grade, I
remember the nun who taught the class shouting at me, calling my name,
which she obviously had been doing for several minutes without my noticing it. The whole class was staring at me when I came to the surface. I do
not know how long I had been under, only that the entire world around me
had been sealed off while I browsed among my thoughts. While others
called from the edge.

Smoky emblems on trees. Artifacts from another civilization. One
time my cousin was hunting in some woods in upstate New York and came
upon a clearing where a dog was hanging from a tree like a tire. He cut
down the dead animal and wondered what kind of people would execute a
dog by hanging. He did not stay around to find out.

At this moment I can see the neighbor next door mowing his lawn.
His reflection, shirt and jeans, moves back and forth across the glass windows in my porch. He is concrete, a mass of particles, even in glass. His
body, which Scripture says will be resurrected with all other bodies on
Judgment Day, is the locus for his identity. If I lean over outside the door
and he sees me, the body will wave in what conventions call recognition.

Do you believe in ghosts? In disembodied spirits?

I was cured of cancer when I was a small boy. The remission was complete and permanent, at least during my lifetime, which is what makes it a
cure. The doctors treated me with chemotherapy over a three-year period.
No trace of the leukemic cells could be found anywhere in my body five
years after the therapy had been completed.

The woman who claimed a healing ministry, Faith, treated me with prayer. She would recite familiar verses from the prayer books and then her voice would trail off as her eyes closed. When these healings occurred in front of the congregation she would grunt at this point and begin uttering sounds from no language I knew. Consonants and vowels strung together in rhythm from discourses I could only imagine.

My mother believed in Faith. She drew comfort from this black minister of ritual truth just as she was repelled by the modulated voices of the medical specialists who traded in chemicals and radiated the vessels of the human body with invisible light. Chemicals designed to poison and light calibrated to enflame and destroy the remaining cancer cells. My father did not know why my mother preferred Faith to conventional medicine, or why the fallback position was medical practice rather than religion. But he was grateful that they could both agree on conventional therapy while one of them pursued faith healing.

What cancer could triumph over both medicine and prayer? The doctor thumped my chest with delight when the last set of tests came back negative. Faith cried and rejoiced that evening in church. I took it all in stride.

The moment of transformation occurred later, when I was an adult living in Florence. My wife and I had to drive over the border to Switzerland with our two daughters to get our passports renewed. It was the easiest way to extend visas for another six months and the city of choice for most Americans was Lugano. Flee the country by choice, stay the weekend, have the passports stamped again on reentry.

The spell was cast the day before the trip. Near the Ponte Vecchio a gypsy woman approached me asking for money. I gave her five hundred lire and she told me I would have a safe trip the next day. I had made no mention of a trip in our brief conversation. It had seemed like a movie script at the time.

"Take my breath away," the car radio croons the next day as I take the Porsche up to the customary ninety miles an hour on the autostrada. My wife is sitting in the bucket seat on the passenger side with Yolanda on her lap. Rachel is asleep in the back.

My dream of the night before is no comfort. In the dream I am driving alone on a road with trees and farmland unusually close to the shoulder of the highway. I approach a curve to the left at high speed. The car leans to the right and slowly turns over. The last part of the dream, the sensation that is most vivid, is the surface of the road coming up to my face. I can see the dark tar and flat pebbles as I wake up.

Now, in the reality of this day, I punch the buttons on the radio for another station. The late morning sunlight is unbearably bright across the front windshield. Shadows almost blue in their darkness streak the green foliage on either side of the pavement. The contrast in color sliding by outside gives me the sensation of gliding through a corridor with the car. At times I feel like we are falling down a long tunnel.

Yolanda throws her orange juice bottle down on the floor. "Would you like to pick that up now?" my wife asks her.

As we pass three cars on the right I start to pull back into the right lane, which is clear. A highway tunnel is ahead. My hand instead keeps the steering wheel steady. We blow into the tunnel in the left lane at ninety-five miles an hour. In the near darkness I switch on the lights. A nearly stationary truck, going not more than fifteen miles an hour without taillights, flashes by on the right.

"Jesus," my wife says. "Did you see that?"

I say nothing. Instead I think about what would have happened if I had followed my first impulse to switch over to the right lane. In the thoughtful silence Yolanda starts crying for her orange juice bottle. It is a moment when I feel myself located in a natural pattern, an entry in some sequence of recurring events.

My thoughts in the car are counterfactual. I imagine the wreckage back in the tunnel, the luggage and clothes strewn about. But I see the scene now in the car as one I have already experienced. It is embedded in some larger and familiar context, which I know in some way before the events occur.

The disjointed mood continues in Lugano, a city as clean, well appointed, and depressing as I had anticipated. Clerks are careful to check and restore the arrangement of display items after my daughters have left a store, even when they touch nothing. But at night I feel the delirium of a fever taking hold in my body in the midst of this structured society, bacteria or viruses insinuating themselves into me from the clean Swiss order. By the morning my skin is hot and crawling with a temperature of 103 degrees.

We decide to return early. But I insist on fulfilling our plans to visit Milan on the way home to see Leonardo da Vinci's *Last Supper*. It is extraordinarily warm and dusty in the church. The fresco is larger than I thought it would be. But Judas still pulls away from Jesus in mock disbelief at the question of betrayal. The fever makes me feel at odds with my body, a mind inside a physical frame that has slowed to a crawl.

Back in Florence my wife summons the doctor to our apartment. He arrives late in the evening with the traditional black bag, his formed from elegant Florentine leather and suede. He places his hand on my forehead while the thermometer is in my mouth.

"This fever is too high for someone your age," he announces with a glance at the thermometer. "Let's give the virus a real whack right away."

He withdraws a syringe and quickly fills it with a clear fluid. The injection has an immediate effect. I feel sleepy, even my mind is lethargic. The yellow lights overhead seem to penetrate my skin.

The doctor snaps his bag shut. "Synthetic penicillin, vitamins, aspirin, sedative. A concoction I make myself."

"He's allergic to penicillin."

"This is a synthetic. He'll be all right." He leaves a bottle of tablets on the night table. "Here. Follow the directions." He throws a kiss in my direction. "Ciao. I'll call in the morning."

White light. Fixtures that hang down from cathedral ceilings. I glance at the clock radio. It is two A.M. My wife is sleeping next to me. No sound in the room that I can hear. No feeling of my body. I am floating slightly above the bed, drifting up toward the ceiling. I turn slowly and look down at my body, at my wife, the bed with green bed covers gathered loosely at the foot of the mattress. The clock, luminescent on its face. There is no sensation except height. After a few minutes I float back down, back to the surface of the bed.

In the morning I have tactile sensations again. I am in my body and can move its parts. But it is me in my body making the effort to coordinate limbs and a torso that is alien to me. I feel disembodied. My body does not feel like mine.

In the hospital later that day I am examined by neurologists. They conclude after extensive tests that either the high fever or the injection, or both, have damaged critical parts of my nervous system. I have sensory powers, but no muscle or tendon or joint sense—no sense of my body.

The chief of neurology is sitting in a chair near my bed. He tilts his head and looks at me glumly. He places a sheaf of paper on the night table and puts his hand on my arm. I watch the movements like an observer. His hand with two rings on one of the thick fingers. A gold wristwatch protruding from under his sleeve. Resting on an arm extending from under the covers. Thin wrist. Light hair across the back of the hand. My arm.

At this moment the life I now lead begins. Here is the conundrum. If the self that is "me" is nothing but my body, if "I" in some way am identified with my body, then who is the self that is currently occupying the body with which I cannot identify? Who is the soul or ghost in the body that was me before the illness in Florence? Who am I as a disembodied self in "my" body?

I can walk now, after five months of rehabilitation, by carefully steering the body in which I live from one point to another. I balance it like a bicycle pedaled by a skilled cyclist. There is no mastery in this, only a contrived equilibrium that I find and fix from moment to moment. I am disjoined, my life a sequence of segmented events.

In the late afternoon I watch the sky through the glass roof on my sun porch. Sometimes migrating birds fly overhead in flocks of hundreds. They move with a fluid grace that seems to shift the very colors of their plumage as they slide across my field of vision.

Every evening, on the way to bed, I pass a mirror in the hall upstairs. My image is in it, a slim figure with a slight slope in the carriage. When I stay too long staring at the body staring back, my wife calls out to me, "Are you all right?" Lately I have been checking the fixtures and appliances two, three, four times a night before going to bed. I keep thinking as I do this that no one can be sure of everything at once. I cannot even see all of the switches at the same time.

I have facticity. I am here, others are there. My body carries me about in the world. But when my body dies, will I die? Can I step out from that frame and live without physical location?

I am a pilot in a vessel. The vessel is not me. Can you give me the same answers on living and dying that you give to the embodied living?

7

HOLISTIC MEDICINE

Alternative Therapies

All healing therapies begin with the assumption that the individual to be treated is ill or damaged in some way. The healer's task is to find and realize the method or condition that will make the patient better. Any effective therapy requires a response from the patient. Individuals who do not respond to therapy at either conscious or unconscious levels cannot be helped. The body is an obvious target of treatment in modern medicine. But sometimes the beliefs of the patient are more decisive than physiological responses, and on occasion can even control the body's powers of rejuvenation.

These rudimentary observations are as true of the most technological, allopathic medicine as they are of spiritual healing. All therapy helps the person to heal herself, though sometimes medical intervention can be crucial in restoring health and avoiding death. But the methods and conditions of effective therapy differ widely even when these truisms are accepted. Western medicine today relies on a mechanistic view of the body that inclines physicians to regard illness as a malady caused by bacteria, viruses, or organic damage (for example, genetic flaws). The goal of therapy is a restoration of that equilibrium defining the healthy organism. Today this restoration is usually accomplished with modern medicine and/or surgical techniques.

The healing therapies that are regarded as nonstandard or unconventional from allopathic perspectives generally have a different view of the individual, of health and illness, and the range of methods and conditions that can successfully heal. Nonstandard therapies tend to regard individuals in holistic terms. Individuals are seen as singular wholes and as constituent parts of some larger reality. The problem is that an abundance of evidence and argument suggests that individuals are more complex and fragmented than commonly thought. Rival social and intellectual contexts can provide competing definitions of the individual, so that societies often present different selves with no changes in psychic references. Also, the brain seems to be a heterogeneous arrangement that can contain multiple selves within a single physical endowment.

Nonstandard therapy uses a wide and interesting range of justifications to prove that the whole individual is better than the fragmented self, for example that the individual as an integrated whole can respond more effectively to treatment and is closer to a more complete equilibrium extending to both body and mind. Even the duality of body-mind is rejected in most holistic medicine. In its place is a unity of mental and physical domains. The healthy individual is one who is in a state of harmony achieved by subordinating the self to a larger purpose. This purpose meets the enduring interests of the individual. Health, and the therapy that secures health, is as much a matter of attitude as physical condition.

It is the effort to connect the integrated self with reality, however, that most sharply distinguishes nonstandard from more conventional therapy. Traditional faith healing claims interventionist powers for a reality outside sensory experiences. Health is achieved by a healer who acts as an instrument for these powers, primarily by the laying on of hands or invocation of special healing forces by words and thought. Another form of faith healing attempts to realign individuals with reality, a kind of restoration of a cosmic balance between the individual and the universe. Christian Science aims at such a harmony, and a number of recent therapies use various meditative techniques to achieve this comprehensive equilibrium. The result of such an equilibrium is said to be the amelioration of certain pathological states, and on occasion the eradication of illness in its entirety. This latter type of meditative healing joins paranormal experiences with therapy.

Therapeutic Touch

The spiritual efforts found in the Pentecostal and charismatic traditions stress the interventionist type of healing. Practitioners in these traditions heal by touch and prayer. One recent variation on such healing that bridges some of the differences with meditative types of healing is "therapeutic touch." This form of healing is conducted by a healer who attempts to diagnose and cure a variety of ailments by a noninvasive sweeping of the body with her hands. The method is squarely in the tradition of spiritual healings that stress the laying on of hands. The assumptions informing therapeutic touch, however, are similar to those found in meditative healing, especially the belief that the sick individual must be brought back into a natural balance with nature.

Therapeutic touch is based on the belief that a universal life-energy field flows through all living organisms. This energy field flows freely and naturally through all healthy organisms, nourishing all parts of body and mind. Illness is an obstruction or disorder of this energy field within individuals. The causes of such disruption are many, including emotional distress and disease agents (bacteria, viruses). The aim of the therapy is to remove the energy obstructions and restore harmony within the individual and between the individual and the environment.

A typical exercise of therapeutic touch begins with the healer engaged in a private effort to relax and bring her mental powers into focus. When centered—her body and mind at rest—the therapist then assesses the condition of the petitioner. The assessment is conducted by sweeping the subject's energy field, moving the hands over the subject's body at a distance of three to five inches from the surface of the skin. The assessment is done quickly, usually lasting no more than fifteen to twenty seconds. Therapists report that a healthy energy field feels unbroken, exudes a continuous sensation of gentle warmth or vibration, and is accessible to the therapist. The assumption is that a healthy person is engaged in continuous and beneficial energy transfers with others and with the environment, and this vibrant exchange can be sensed quickly and accurately in therapeutic touch.

Illness sends different signals. If the subject is sick, the sweep of his or her body will reveal areas of congestion, deficit, or imbalance in the energy field. Therapists report feelings of heaviness or pressure, sometimes diffuse and sometimes concentrated around an area of the body, when illness is present. A blocked area is described as cold, sometimes empty of energy. The therapist who senses such emptiness will report the area as the site of an illness, for example ulcers in the lower abdominal areas or pneumonia in the lower areas of the chest. Therapists claim to be able to feel an energy depletion in all illnesses. The sensations here are those of drawing or pulling, "as though a stream of very fine water bubbles were being pulled through one's hands." Energy deficits are said to be located under congested areas of the energy field. A sensation of discomfort in the hands, a prickly feeling, or a feeling of disruption or thickness can indicate an imbalance in the energy field. Therapists believe that these sensations suggest that an organ of the body is malfunctioning.

The techniques for sensing illness can be taught through meditation experiences and practice sessions. But some practitioners seem to have more talents than others in these exercises. The workshops in which these skills are taught always include practice seminars in which a subject suffering from some undisclosed illness is assessed by each member of the workshop. Then the assessments are evaluated, using the physical condition of the subject as a baseline. Though sensing illness may be a latent ability we all have to some degree, some members of each workshop will typically surpass the others and some will have only marginal abilities to sense illness. Since the subject's illness may not correspond to his or her own feelings or symptoms, even the gifted individual practicing therapeutic touch is instructed to seek validation of impressions with another practitioner if possible.

The therapy following the assessment is remarkably uniform. Practitioners of therapeutic touch try to clear energy congestion by sweeping it downward (said to be its natural direction of travel) towards the legs and out through the feet. Beginning at the head of the subject and moving down to the feet, the practitioner uses downward sweeping motions of the hands, as if urging smoke or water to move. Sometimes the feet must be "opened" by exerting gentle pressure under the arches, or by massage, to facilitate the flow of energy. The release of congestion is designed to alleviate illnesses (like migraines, colds, etc.) and help rebalance the subject's energy field.

One of the more dramatic techniques in therapeutic touch is the therapist's attempt to transfer energy directly to a subject. In these efforts the therapist consciously tries to be the instrument or conduit to allow universal energy forces to enter her body and go into the subject's body. This method is used if the therapist senses a depletion in the subject's energy field. These deficits are sometimes felt around wounds or injuries, though even local deficits indicate that the whole energy field is depleted. In an energy transfer the therapist leaves her hands near the subject, at the site of the local deficit if one is sensed, and allows energy to flow into the subject's field. Therapists often report a sensation of pulling, of energy flowing through the hands until the subject's energy levels feel whole again and the flow stops on its own or at the subject's suggestion. It is possible, according to therapists, to force too much energy into a subject's field. The overburdened recipient will then feel restless, impatient, or dizzy.

The aim of therapeutic touch is to restore the subject's energy field by rebalancing it, removing congestion, repairing breaks and rough edges by smoothing out the troubled areas, replenishing energy levels, and in general stroking and tuning the field until it is in a healthy integrated state, flowing easily and continuously. The illness is said to be helped, and sometimes overcome entirely, by bringing the individual to a holistic state of equilibrium.

Patients say that they can feel the effects of therapeutic touch. The first response almost always is one of relaxation, often indicated by words like "I feel so relaxed right now." Respiration and heartbeat often slow down, sometimes immediately at the very beginning of therapy. Subjects also feel warmth when the therapist's hands hover over an area of the body. Sometimes a tingling sensation occurs, and sometimes the subject claims that he can feel the congestion of energy being moved down to the area of the feet and out of the body. Sometimes the subject feels nothing during a session and still feels good at the completion of the therapy. Most subjects report that they feel better after the therapy.

Are there physiological effects that correspond to these subjective reports? Evidence indicates that there are. Psychogenic diseases respond to therapeutic touch. Some types of headaches, asthma, and gastrointestinal disturbances (including colic and constipation) are especially responsive. In fact, many patients with stress-related illnesses seem to improve with therapeutic touch. These effects are not surprising, for the strong psychological connections that often arise between therapist and patient would almost surely produce psychophysiological benefits. It is surprising, however, that these benefits seem to follow even when the subject is skeptical of the therapy. The only attitudinal impediments to a successful outcome seem to be denial of illness and a hostility toward the therapist.

There also is evidence that therapeutic touch accelerates healing of somatic illnesses. Pain is alleviated and sometimes eliminated by the therapy. Wounds can heal more rapidly. One frequently cited study introduces evidence that the wounds of mice who had received a kind of laying-on-of-hands treatment (similar to therapeutic touch) healed more quickly than those of a control group of mice who did not receive the treatment. A more recent experiment monitored the healing process of two sets of identical-sized, surgically administered dermal wounds, one subject to therapeutic touch and the other not. The therapist in this experiment was isolated from the subjects and treated only the wound on the subject's arm, which was extended through a hole in a wall to the control room. Subjects were told that their wounds were simply being monitored by instruments in the control room. The wounds treated by the therapeutic touch practitioner improved more rapidly than the untreated wounds.

In both experiments, the placebo effect was nullified, in the first case by the obvious fact that the subjects were mice and in the second case by the use of double blinds (isolation of the practitioner and the subjects' ignorance that therapeutic touch was being employed). The beneficial effects of the therapy seemed to be independent of the subjects' attitudes. Other experiments have provided evidence that the hemoglobin level of subjects in therapeutic touch can be increased. In these and similar efforts, a physiological change seems to be brought about by the techniques of therapeutic touch in and of themselves.

Theory and Practice

The temptation is strong to divide therapeutic touch into two domains, one containing its metaphysical assumptions and the other laying out its practical effects. Something seems to be going on in the therapy that cannot be adequately explained with material assumptions. Thousands of health professionals have attended therapeutic touch workshops and presumably have learned a method of healing that is a clear alternative to conventional medical practice. The outcomes of the therapy do benefit patients, and sometimes the effects are transforming. This practical side of therapeutic touch is widely acknowledged, although it is still disputed within mainstream medicine. It is also important to note that the modern techniques of therapeutic touch originated in practice, apart from theory of any sort.

The genesis story of therapeutic touch is repeated by almost all practitioners trying to explain the therapy. Oskar Estabany, a former colonel in the Hungarian cavalry, was confronted one evening with a problem. He loved animals, horses in particular, and his horse had become ill and did not seem likely to survive. He spent the night with the horse, contriving a cure from his instincts and religious impulses. His efforts included massages and caresses, prayers and exhortations. In the morning, to his astonishment, the horse was well. He used these pragmatic techniques on other ill horses with remarkable success, then slowly and reluctantly expanded them to include humans. When he retired, he immigrated to Canada and joined a research group studying healing. He had no theory to explain what he did. He regarded his ability to heal as a special gift, often referring to himself (in the manner of faith healers past and present) as an instrument or channel for the healing powers of God (in this case, Jesus Christ).

The research group Estabany had joined evolved the theory of healing that later provided the explanation for therapeutic touch. The evolution illustrates a standard pattern of concept formation. The members of the group were studying the practice of healing. The early efforts were inductive. They included observing and cataloging acts of healing, generalizing the observed techniques, and trying to duplicate what they were observing. More than collating the facts was required to explain the practice, however. A theory or philosophy was needed. The key participants in the group drew this theory from a variety of sources but stressed Eastern literatures. Sanskrit, for example, provides the word *prana*, which is a kind of energy roughly translated as vitality and conceptually linked to regeneration. The group members began to accept the Eastern doctrine that *prana* is the organizing energy of life itself and that health is an excess of this energy. They also accepted the notion of a transfer of energy. The healer was viewed as someone with an abundance of *prana* and the power to channel this energy to ill persons.

The vocabulary of this Eastern approach to healing was adopted and expanded to the current view of energy fields in therapeutic touch. The *chakra* (or "wheel") is postulated as the mechanism that modulates and distributes *prana*. Living persons are seen as enclosed in an etheric field extending one to six inches from the body. The idea of an equilibrium explains the simultaneous stability and interactive motion of this energy field. In this philosophical perspective, humans are no longer defined as solid entities. They are regarded as forms of energy in a symbiotic relationship with their environments. It is then but a short step to extend the theory to the healing act, now seen as a successful restoration of a damaged energy field.

There is nothing unusual or perverse in this pattern of concepts. They fit the known facts, and in standard fashion begin to define the facts by influencing observations. But the temptation to divide therapeutic touch into theory and practice is strong precisely because of its pragmatic origins. If it works, it works without introducing the elaborate ontologies that currently offer explanations for the practice. Healing occurred before a theory was attached to the practice and occurs today among subjects who know little, if anything, about energy fields. Further, and this is the case with all explanatory theories, alternative theories and rival philosophies may be equally effective in explaining the causal chains of healing in therapeutic touch.

The one thing we do know is that therapeutic touch can improve the conditions of ill or damaged life forms in ways not explained adequately by conventional medicine. How and why the improvement occurs is open to discussion.

Sulzman

William Sulzman became interested in religious movements and metaphysical problems in high school. In his senior year, he wrote a brief essay on comparative religion. His theme was that there is one God who speaks through many different religions. He was a practicing Protestant at the time but open to the appeals of competing religions. Years later, when he came to New York City after college to study Spanish at the Latin American Institute, he reconstructed these ideas for a conversation exam near the end of his first term. The instructor in the course was a member of the Theosophy Society. She identified the ideas as congenial with theosophy and gave Sulzman pamphlets about the movement.

Sulzman scanned the history of theosophy quickly and easily. The society was founded in New York City in 1875 by Madame Blavatsky, a seer who had traveled extensively in the East (especially in India). Blavatsky, like many Westerners, had become intrigued with the philosophical ideas of the East, in large part because they seemed to combine rather than separate religion and science. They also contained vast stretches of mystical thinking and experiences. Blavatsky appropriated a variety of doctrines and fused them into a complicated system of thought that addressed all of reality. The Theosophy Society was formed to disseminate these ideas to others.

Sulzman began studying the philosophy elaborated by Blavatsky, sometimes spending more time on these works than on his Spanish. In fact, he switched from Spanish to English philosophy publications to make sure he was absorbing the right ideas. His instructor continued to assist him, making sure that he got the more sensible interpretations of theosophy rather than the bizarre offshoots of the movement. He continued studying theosophy throughout his two year stint in the Army. When he returned to New York, he realized that he had accepted the basic ideas, so he joined the Society.

Even a rough sketch of theosophy can suggest how complex the system of thought is. Basically, and without the elaborations found in the major works of the movement, theosophy recognizes a seven-dimensional reality with corresponding individual forms in each dimension. The lowest dimension is the physical, that reality encountered and constructed in sensory experience. The physical body is the individual form located in this dimension, along with an etheric double. The etheric body is the instrument connecting the body to higher planes of reality. It both permeates the physical body and surrounds it as an energy field. It exists in the etheric dimension of reality (consisting of undetected electromagnetic areas).

A second dimension of reality houses the astral body. It is this body that is said to travel in out-of-body experiences. When at rest in the physical body, it can be seen (by those with the requisite abilities) as an aura, a spectrum of many colors that represent virtues and vices. In theosophy, the astral body is the locus of consciousness and the processor of data sensed by the physical body. Higher dimensions of reality are progressively more abstract and distant from the sensory world. The individual's task is to progress to higher states in successive incarnations.

Sulzman believes the most vital parts of theosophy are its unifying powers. It provides him with a view of the personality as a changing unity—feeling, acting, sensing, moving—against a more comprehensive background that fixes meaning on these changes. This larger context allows him to see events from a long-range perspective, not in any way diminishing their importance but calming and reassuring him when bad things happen. His creative energies increase dramatically when he realizes that there is more to existence than this life here and now. He is able to see himself and others within a transcendent reality that guides his efforts to achieve higher states of consciousness.

Sulzman believes that everything is part of a cosmic whole. For him, the highest state of consciousness and the lowest, inert rock are different aspects of one unchangeable reality. Like the violent emergence of empirical reality from a primordial big bang, all of reality for Sulzman derives from some common origin. He points out that water, steam, and ice look radically different from one another but are each manifestations of H_2O. In similar fashion, a human being may appear to be different from an insect, but the two forms of life are expressions of the same reality.

Meditation is crucial for Sulzman in gaining access to the foundations of reality. He has sensed in meditation the truth that all individual humans are processes or waves in a kind of cosmic sea, having existence from one perspective but only parts of a larger whole when viewed correctly. Sulzman does not denigrate human consciousness. Like classical theorists, he regards the individual mind as a transforming feature of the universe. In the absence of thinking and reflection as it occurs through the instrumentation of the cerebral cortex, the universe might be nothing, or perhaps just a passive state with none of the intelligible properties that consciousness recognizes. Sulzman believes that individual consciousness is a remarkable product that focuses reality in unique ways. His point is simply that the goal of human life is to move beyond this state by realizing the transcendent unity of reality within the self.

The fundamental law of the universe in theosophy is karma. This law states that an individual is the result of all of the acts in one's previous lives. One consequence of this understanding is that human action must be seen as an incremental effort set against the inertia of all earlier incarnations. Most people find this thought both encouraging and daunting. Actions must be judged from a time perspective considerably longer than the measure of any one person's life, and the chances of reaching an enlightened state must be measured against the additive consequences of a long history of past lives. *Destiny* is a good interpretation of karma, meaning that life is determined by forces beyond individual control. Yet followers of theosophy, like William Sulzman, believe that the effort must be made to attain this enlightened state, for the whole point of human life is to transcend it by moving to a higher dimension of reality.

Sulzman uses the idea of a connected yet layered reality to explain healing. He practices therapeutic touch. He admits that he does not fully understand how the therapy works. He does know that successful therapy requires that the healer be properly centered. For him this means that the center of one's being is stilled, the emotion and the intellect quieted, a harmony and connection to a universal order carefully set in a place at a conscious level. Then compassion must occur, a feeling for the person to be healed that is not exactly love or sympathy but a reflective concern for the other. Sulzman believes that in this mental state energy can be sent out to another person that will help the healing process.

Sulzman learned therapeutic touch from the originators. He took the early experimental classes organized by Dora Kunz in New York City. Kunz would bring a patient into the group of fifteen or twenty students and ask each student in the class to diagnose the patient's illness. The students would go over in pairs and sweep the patient's body with their hands. Then Kunz would move around the room and ask each student, "What did you feel?"

Sulzman remembers one woman Kunz brought in who looked perfectly normal in every respect. When it was his turn, he placed his hands over the woman's body while she sat quietly in a chair. Something felt different to Sulzman around the woman's eyes. Yet she was not wearing glasses, and she obviously was having no trouble seeing. Kunz went around the room asking for diagnoses, and Sulzman reported, "Well, I felt something around the eyes." Kunz nodded and went on to the next person until each student had offered an opinion on the woman's condition. Most centered the diagnoses on the woman's torso—the liver, the heart, the lungs, and so on. After everyone had spoken, Kunz announced that the woman had glaucoma. Sulzman was the only member of the class who had sensed a problem in the woman's eyes.

Sulzman was able to demonstrate this diagnostic talent in a number of subsequent classes. He found that it was better for him to work in back of the patient. He believes this was because he then avoided eye contact and a lapse into sentimentality. Time after time he and the other students would work on patients under Kunz's direction. Kunz would ask both the patient and the students what they felt during the sessions. Sulzman would get to a certain point on the patient's back and feel this tremendous heat pouring through his hands, often so much heat that later (when he conducted his own healing sessions) he would sometimes touch the back of his hand to the patient's skin to see if the heat came from that direction. It never did. The heat he felt was in his own hands as he diagnosed disease and then, later, began healing. Often in Kunz's classes another similarly gifted student would also feel heat around the same particular site on a patient's body and corroborate the diagnosis Sulzman offered.

The healing sessions Sulzman later conducted on his own were gratifying to him and to his patients. He kept everything simple and never considered himself a professional healer. He administers therapeutic touch mainly to friends and family on a need basis. He enjoys most those sessions with individuals who are skeptical (since he admits that believers could be imagining the cures). On one evening he and his wife were at the One World Festival (they do Scottish dancing) and one of the dancers came in for the performance looking awful. She showed every sign of coming down with the flu and felt as bad as she looked. The only reason she had even appeared was for the sake of the dance team Sulzman and his wife had organized for the festival.

Sulzman went over to her and asked her to sit quietly for a moment. "Why," she asked, "what are you going to do?" He passed his hands above the surface of her body and she immediately started feeling a heat go through her. Sulzman remembers her saying, "My God, this is amazing, what are you doing?" He said, "Does it bother you?" She said no. He asked her to keep quiet and talk about it later. The result was a dramatic improvement in her condition. No cure, no complete healing of the flu. But her energy level went up and she was able to dance without discomfort.

Sulzman sees the main effects of therapeutic touch in exactly this kind of rapid increase of energy levels. He believes that all therapy, conventional and unconventional, helps the body heal itself. He is convinced that therapeutic touch infuses energy into individuals from a higher level, and from this level into the whole person straight down through to the physical body. For this reason, he does not believe that healing works if the healer stays at the surface level of purely personal contact. It is not the charisma of the healer that is decisive, Sulzman believes, but the ability of the healer to address the whole person and release that deeper, more powerful energy that can radiate through the patient's entire being. Sulzman gives special attention to local sites of illness on the patient's body, but he aims his efforts at the whole energy field.

Not everyone accepts unconventional healing. Sulzman knows this. Once he was standing next to one of the male dancers in his troupe when the man complained of back pain. Sulzman spontaneously ran his hand down the dancer's back without touching him and felt a withdrawal of heat at a certain location. He touched the dancer's back at that spot and said, "It's there, isn't it?" The dancer looked at him and said, "You're weird."

But what Sulzman thinks is weird is that the scientific community has been so reluctant to examine therapeutic touch with an open mind. In his ideal world, both the healer and the patient would be scrutinized carefully according to the canons of the best empirical inquiry. Much healing fraud and many gullible patients would be dismissed in such an inquiry. But he believes a strong and broad residue would remain. Somewhere between utter skepticism and complete gullibility Sulzman sees that rock-hard universal reality which is accessible to the human intellect and the source for genuine healing.

Meditative Healing

The goal of meditative healing is an abandonment of the discrete self and a fusion of healer and patient for a brief time during the healing session. No direct healing occurs. Healing is the consequence of the momentary transformation in both individuals. An altered state of consciousness is said to produce therapeutic benefits because both individuals enter a different reality. The healer attempts to bring to the one seeking therapy the healing forces of the larger natural world.

An individual viewing meditative healing from the outside may see nothing extraordinary even when the session is successful in reaching a different state of reality. In a two-person healing session, the therapist and patient typically sit across from one another in comfortable positions, perhaps even reclining in lounge chairs or on a sofa. Both individuals fall silent at the onset of the session and each begins meditating. The goal is to sense and merge with the other in the different reality sought through meditation. Nothing may appear to be happening because the two participants are engaged in mental efforts. The fusion, if it occurs, is psychic, not physical, and may involve no discernible movement at all. At the end of a brief period of time, say ten to fifteen minutes, the session ends and each individual usually relates the experience to the other.

In one session a man and a woman (who is the therapist) sit in her New York City apartment late in the afternoon meditating together in a healing session. The man's thoughts rocket in several directions as he tries to control his psychic energies and escape his physical fatigue. He is extremely relaxed, with good feelings seeming to radiate throughout his body. He thinks at first of becoming one with the objects in the room and tries to enter the inert state of being that is represented by the ashtray in front of him, the large painting of a woman in a leotard, two glass art objects of uncertain lineage, the coffee table. Then his thoughts suddenly jump to Key West, Florida, where he grew up, and then he is in St. Mary Star of the Sea Catholic Church where he served as an altar boy in his early youth. He can feel the Sunday morning heat and movement in the church while mass is being performed. At the corner of his right field of vision he can see the therapist. She raises her arms in a kind of supplication. The man's vision becomes more concrete as he allows the apartment setting to dominate again his meditation. After a few more moments pass the therapist sighs and says, "All right, tell me what you felt." He describes his experience and asks her to relate her own. She tells him that she felt his presence very strongly, though with enough space within it for the freedom of others, and that the two of them did become one during the session. The man is pleased that the session was successful and the two part amicably, almost fondly.

The meditation occurred on a Friday afternoon. That weekend the man had vivid dreams on successive nights. The first provided him with what he is convinced are fresh and important insights into his marriage. The second night he dreamed that he had a near-death experience, one so detailed that in the dream he reached out to crush some dry leaves in one of his hands to test tactile sensation. The sensations were so impressive that he concluded in the dream that he was not dreaming, that the experience was real. Skeptics among his friends offered an empirical interpretation of the dreams. When they heard that he had been suffering from a mild viral infection during the interviews, they explained the vivid dreams as neural activity stimulated by the effects of an active virus. Friends knowledgeable about psychic matters offered a different interpretation. They accepted his report as routine and told him that the meditation freed some blockages in his psyche. The vivid dreams were simply the natural result of his union with the therapist in an altered reality. Again, two incompatible but plausible (in context) explanations comfortably accord with the experiences.

What is the union of individuals that some claim occurs in psychic experiences? What does it mean to say that two individuals are one? Setting aside colloquial uses of language (as in mythical and unrealistic accounts of marriage), the merger of individual identities can mean several things. Arguably, the most common meaning is a transfer of one individual identity to the circumstances of another individual. When we wonder what it is to be another, we usually mean to ask what it would be like to have that person's profession, income, house, perhaps spouse and children. The commonplace attempts of academics and others (including political leaders) to enter the life world of certain classes of individuals fall under this category. The professional, for example, who lives on the street for a period of time to see what it is like to be homeless, or stays in prison to get a sense of incarceration, or tries to live at an income below the poverty line to see what it is like to be poor, or cohorts with rich people to see what being rich is like—any ethnographic or participant-observation experience is an effort to see the world from the circumstances of the other. The merger is largely (perhaps entirely) at the contextual level.

The limitations of such efforts are well known and even standard by now. In addition to the obvious drawback that such experiences are usually voyeuristic, the fantasies of a dilettante, it is easy to point out that even serious excursions into ways of life inevitably miss that which is most distinctive about the experience being investigated—its permanence. Trial marriages, prison visits, and temporary poverty do not duplicate the essential features of these experiences, for by definition they avoid the contextual traps that hold the occupants in their social conditions. Also, the visitor in other people's lives does not tap into the effects the conditions have on the perceptions of others. Try to imagine, as the reader of this book, what your perception would be like if the circumstances of life had denied you the possibility of reading a single book before this one in your entire life. What would you be like?

The main point, however, is that circumstantial identification is not identification with the self. More ambitious efforts are required to be the other. The nearest point away from the self as a discrete identity is the economic exercise of "extended sympathy." Here the individual tries to see the world from the perspective (and the circumstances) of the other. A variety of devices are used in this exercise. Imaginative renditions, as in fiction, are crucial. One individual reconstructs the views of another and tries to transport himself inside the other's perspective. The identity of the transported individual is not abandoned. The exercise asks this question, what is it like for me to be you while I retain some sense of myself?

The difficulty with this interpretation of extended sympathy is finding a balance between the two identities. The task is more or less demanding on different features of the self and the other. One can more easily imagine entering the emotive consciousness of a different other, becoming chronically angry or sentimental, and so on, than taking on the intellectual apparatus of another who is mentally distant. What would it be like to see the world through Einstein's eyes, or from the view of someone who is afflicted with Down's syndrome? It is not easy to see how one's own identity can be maintained while assuming the perspective of another who has the mental endowment to structure reality in radically different ways.

A more radical interpretation of extended sympathy beckons. One might try to become the other without maintaining self-identity in the exercise. Here the same problem of extending self to other occurs. But the effort can be imagined with others who are less like the self, the genius even, or the mentally retarded, so long as the original self can be abandoned completely and the other's mental resources are reasonable continuations of the self (not, say, a species distant from the human, like a hawk or spider). But finding the vocabulary to render the other's mental perspective intelligible is another matter. It may be impossible to translate such experiences back to one's own reality.

Meditative healing identifies this different reality as the site for fusion between healer and patient. The problems of identity that occur in sensory reality are unimposing in a dimension of experience that has already denied the separation of individuals as distinct egos. The key to success, then, becomes whether one can enter this other reality even if translation is impossible.

Edwards

Philip Edwards is a microbiologist with long-standing interests in the paranormal and psychic healing. A few years ago he signed up for a course on meditation given at a local college. One book on the reading list was Lawrence LeShan's *The Medium, the Mystic, and the Physicist*. Edwards read the book and immediately knew that he had to find out more about psychic healing. The instructor in the course turned out to be a close friend of LeShan and was able to steer Edwards into one of the training seminars LeShan had organized to disseminate the healing techniques he had developed. The workshop Edwards joined was taught by Joyce Goodrich, an instructor LeShan had trained himself.

The training sessions were held in an old house in Connecticut that had once been a Catholic monastery. The group of twelve students included a wide assortment of what Edwards considered ordinary people: a couple of therapists, a former priest, nurses, psychologists. They began with simple breathing exercises, attempts at visualization (imagining positive connections between the self and the world), some brief meditations, all interspersed with Goodrich's instruction on changing realities to make healing possible. On the fourth day, the group began deeper meditations, designed in particular to open the heart and generate compassion.

It was at that point that Edwards discovered emotions he had never encountered before. He simply opened up, his feelings flowing out in tears that seemed never to stop. He and the person next to him in the meditations began keeping a roll of toilet paper between them, sharing the tissues in wiping away their tears. By the time the group entered the stage of healing meditations, Edwards felt he was completely receptive to new realities. The instructor stressed that no healing as such was to be attempted; rather, the individuals were to try to move into a different level of consciousness with the other person in mind and then merge with that person in the altered state of mind.

The exercises involved one person in the group acting as patient, a kind of practice subject who would lie down in the middle of the group while the others would try to move into the altered state of consciousness along with the acting patient. The group was instructed to use visualizations. One suggestion was to visualize one's self and the other person as being two trees, and then visualize the root systems under the ground intertwining. Another suggestion was visualizing two streams entering the ocean and becoming one. Those with religious backgrounds were urged to use religious imagery. Edwards had no religious background at all. He used natural visualization, utilizing his early training in physics to imagine persons as constituted by space and atoms and having the possibility of synthesizing with one another.

Edwards reports merging with the others on two occasions in the five-day session. It was, in his words, "a weird experience." He remembers the visualizations as seeming to take on a life of their own, controlling his thoughts and perceptions. He cannot find words to describe the experience, except that he tends to see them as field-effect phenomena where the individual enters a reality that is continuous in all respects. He believes that language breaks up experience into separate items and so is inadequate as an instrument to explain the merger experiences he had.

Edwards also refuses to use his training in scientific methodology to explain the experiences. As a physical scientist, he is used to isolating phenomena and performing experiments on them. But he sees the experiences in the healing workshop as relationships, and he believes that reducing any relationship to an isolated datum would be to deny its essentially connective nature. He also believes that experiences are inadequately depicted in the limited concepts of classical physics.

Edwards does not claim to have lost his identity, even momentarily, in the experience. He says that in two healing meditations he became one with the other person with some sense that he was still himself. He did not feel any contradiction in the experience. There was always a duality of self and other, but he was able somehow "to see how things are from the inside of somebody else." He sensed his subconscious taking over in a group that became like a close family. In his words: "One thing that I did was visualize myself with a person who was the healer. And then, with my eyes closed, at one point we just kind of teamed together and became one entity. That was not something I was trying to do. It just happened. It was a spontaneous merging in the visualization."

It is in this state of individual fusion that Edwards believes psychic healing occurs. One person does not consciously, intentionally, do something to another. It is the connecting in itself, he thinks, that produces the therapeutic benefits.

There was one apparent instance of a dramatic healing in the workshop. It turned out that a woman in the group had been diagnosed earlier as suffering from Lou Gehrig's disease. Both the Hershey Medical Center and Johns Hopkins had confirmed the presence of the disease. On the last day of the workshop, Goodrich told the group what the woman's problem was and asked for a real rather than a simulated healing session. The group went through the healing routine with the woman. Edwards remembers that the session was very emotional, the energy level in the room so high that it was almost palpable. After the workshop ended, the woman went back to both the Hershey Center and Hopkins. Edwards says no trace of the disease could be found. The physicians at both centers concluded that they had misdiagnosed the illness. Edwards stayed in contact with the woman for two or three years after that traumatic session. She is still well and healthy as far as he knows.

Edwards does not practice psychic healing regularly, though he continues the meditation exercises. He did go back for a second workshop, but has not really kept up with the training or literature. The experience did convince him that everything is more connected than he had ever realized, and so consciousness in one part of the system is going to affect other parts. He is also convinced that the healing power of the body can be augmented with meditation. These connections for him are as natural as anything he studies in the physical sciences.

Kaster

Gloria Kaster is a psychotherapist. In the 1960s she was one of many therapists trying to break from conventional methods of treatment. She was intrigued by what she now regards as putative distinctions between mind and
body, in particular by the ways in which the states of the body affect the mind
(rather than the reverse). Her work explored body awareness, or how individuals can have a type of physical knowledge without being conscious of it. In
her therapy sessions, some strange things occurred when she introduced
techniques to make individuals more aware of their bodily responses to the
environment. In one sequence of awareness sessions, she noticed that the
members of the therapy group were picking up on each other's habits. Unconscious mimicry occurred. Some individuals began responding to the
mental images of others. One person would be having trouble with another
person in the group and say she imagined a horrible person, a witch, for
example. The person so transmogrified in the other's thoughts would begin
feeling bad, even without knowing that she was the target of these negative
feelings. Kaster knew that these transferences should not be happening according to every scientific principle she had ever learned. But they *were* happening. So she began trying out a different, more controversial way of
conceptualizing what she was observing. She began thinking that energy
from one body could go into another.

Love relationships seemed especially appropriate for this concept of energy transference. A typical situation would be what the romantic calls love
at first sight. People would be drawn to one another in almost magnetic fashion, often against all reasonable understandings of self-interest. After awhile
the relationship would sour and the couple could not understand why. If the
contact was prolonged, the individuals could end up hating one another.
Kaster would have couples in therapy who would literally become ill in each
other's presence and wanted nothing more than to escape the relationship
and perhaps even destroy the other. This came from people who a short time
before were completely, absolutely in love with each other.

Kaster began using an energy-transfer metaphor in trying to understand
this pattern of behavior. She speculated that in the early stages of a relationship (the love part), each individual was giving energy to the other, which
was absorbed successfully. Then, as the energy transfer continued, the givers
would feel drained. They were made sick by the depletion of some kind of
psychic energy, something lost in the intense love relationship. Kaster recognized that this metaphor sounds like the wildest kind of superstition if intro-

duced as an explanation for any type of human behavior. But then the standard psychological categories could not explain the emotive pattern of attraction and revulsion either. All Kaster knew at this stage in her therapy work was that some kind of tacit response was occurring that the participants could not grasp or even control at the conscious level of the self, no matter how successful their therapy might be in recovering forgotten and repressed experiences.

At about this time, Kaster began exploring the literature in parapsychology to see if any helpful insights or theories could be found there. Nothing seemed relevant in this work. But she did come across an advertisement for a seminar on psychic healing conducted by Lawrence LeShan. She called LeShan and asked him whether the seminar was to be about psychic healing, or was he going to do psychic healing. LeShan answered, "We are going to do psychic healing." Kaster said, "Sign me up."

It was at this seminar that Kaster saw a more refined way to state her intuitions about energy transfer. LeShan described his thesis on Type I and II healings. In Type I healing, individuals meditate and enter that different reality that encourages the body (or mind) to heal itself. The wisdom of the universe and the organism will bring about the proper therapy. All the therapist does in the meditative session is seek a harmony between the larger natural world and the patient. Type II healing is closer to magic. The therapist finds and uses powers that can heal or harm depending on their use. Kaster remembers LeShan warning the group about the danger of Type II healing, even in its more benign forms as the "laying on of hands" of faith healing traditions. It is too narrow a focus for healing, she remembers LeShan telling the class, and can lead to a blowup in other bodily illnesses even when curing the immediate problem. LeShan used her metaphor of energy transfer to explain the danger in Type II healing. Putting energy into one part of the body can cause other vectors and domains of the energy field to go out of balance. At last Kaster had a theoretical reference for her intuitions.

In the weeks and months following her first seminar in psychic healing, Kaster studied everything she could find on the subject. Events in her life convinced her of the truth of these claims for healing powers and meditations. Once she was a member of a leaderless therapy group of therapy group leaders (a kind of therapist-heal-yourself session without anyone to direct it). The group was meeting on the terrace of a sixteenth-floor apartment in New York City overlooking Central Park West. She remembers the setting as beautiful. But the man sitting next to her was feeling very depressed and was more than willing to share his depression with others. It turned out that his wife was very sick with renal failure and he had to get a dialysis machine into their home to treat her. It was a genuinely sad story, and as the man told it he became more and more depressed.

Kaster was distressed over the man's situation and thought he needed to be picked up a bit emotionally. So she began transferring energy to him in the way she had learned in Type II healing. The man kept talking with no awareness of what Kaster was doing, but his demeanor became more cheerful, a note of optimism began appearing in the accounts he was providing of his life. Then he got up from the sofa and went over to stand by the railing overlooking Central Park. By this time he was telling the group how great he felt, so good in fact that he thought he could actually spread his wings and fly across the park. Kaster started pulling back the energy so fast that she felt like she was running across a psychic landscape. The man came down from his emotional high and returned to the sofa with more moderate perspectives on his life and powers. Kaster came away from the session with a renewed appreciation of the dangers in Type II healing.

On another occasion she was in the audience during a performance by one of the Living Theatre ensembles. At the end of the play, the actors gathered on stage and, in a gesture common in the 1960s, invited the audience to join hands with them. Kaster was at the theater that evening with a black judge in the city's judicial system. The man, according to Kaster, was very uptight and wanted nothing to do with tribal superstitions and the like. Nevertheless, he joined hands with her and the others. Kaster knew what was coming. She could feel the energy move from her hands through his body. The judge said (in atypical language for him), "Wow, I can feel it, it's going through me." It was indeed, according to Kaster. Only she was "turned off" by the display of public energy transfer on that evening because she regarded it as exploitive. Real, but also very show biz in that setting.

Kaster believes that there is something in the universe that we do not understand and cannot name. This something, which she calls theos (Greek for god), is for Kaster the energy that heals. In meditation a reality can be reached where theos suffuses everything. In this sense, Kaster believes pantheism is true of the reality known during the altered state of consciousness. God is in us and in everything in that world sought and found through meditation. In ordinary reality polytheism reigns. Theos is distributed as diverse pockets of energy. It can be found in a mountain, in a tree, in a spring, in the stones of the Wailing Wall in Jerusalem, in cathedrals, at Lourdes. Kaster believes that this energy can be owned, packaged, bought and sold, exchanged for other bunches of energy. It is a commodity no stranger to her than nuclear energy, electricity, or gravity. She believes that theos can be used for good or bad purposes (white or black magic) and is the stuff that is stored by shamans and sorcerers to practice their magic. Type II healing depends on pockets of theos used in the therapy sessions. She can feel this energy as a psychic current whenever she touches some source where it has accumulated.

The healing Kaster practices in her therapy sessions is meditative. Her patients do not completely abandon their identities in meditation, though she confesses to a chronic puzzlement over exactly who or what we are in ordinary reality. She points out that individuals sit in chairs that are mostly empty space, congeries of particles joined by forces that are not really understood. Persons are also compositions of space and particles. She sees no insurmountable problem in merging these different compositions with each other, one person with another and persons with their surrounding reality. She sees no individual identity that will resist fusion with a reality that is, after all, continuous with persons. Separateness, she feels, is an illusion.

All matter, both living and inert, is part of the natural world and has equal status in Kaster's ontology. This view leads to well-known perplexities. It implies that the HIV virus and the human body have equal standing in nature. How, then, can therapy designed to eradicate the virus from its human host be justified? Kaster, like many healers, sees the human person as an organism with the power to reach an optimal state of equilibrium. This balance may be expressed as an internal and external harmony (or balance within the self, and between the self and nature). A human being in a state of harmony will have an immune system that can defend the body against the HIV virus. The ideal state for humans is one free of illness, and it is this state that can be achieved through successful meditation. (Presumably the HIV virus does not meditate and so is at a comparative disadvantage.) Kaster does not avoid modern medicine, however. If she is coming down with pneumonia, she goes for an antibiotic without a second thought. But meditation is the more basic approach for her. It does not address disease. It is a method for healing the whole person.

There is also no doubt in Kaster's mind that a few individuals have special healing abilities. Some can easily bring others to the proper meditative levels and release the energies needed to heal the person. Others can appropriate and direct bundles of healing energies at appropriate illnesses and to sites on the body. She reports that when she is the recipient of a powerful healing she finds that her lips will curl up automatically in a little smile. The first time it happened she thought, "like the Mona Lisa," which she reminds us is a painting of a model who was being lavished with all the immediate attention of one of the geniuses of the era. That smile—the feeling of well-being—represents for Kaster the glow of a deliberate type of meditative healing.

The thoughtful reader will also recall the languid smile of the model in Goya's *Naked Maja*. Or the compassion and grief of the Virgin Mary in Michelangelo's *Pietà*. Or, at a more melancholy level, the sad smile of Thomas Canterbury's mother as she died with the comfort of a beneficent and swift passage from life.

LeShan

Lawrence LeShan entered the field of the paranormal because, at one point in his life, he was "very, very tired." He has a doctorate in psychology. His graduate training included the usual empirical methods required of all psychology students, including statistics and research designs. To this day he can run a rat through a maze, though he no longer remembers why anyone bothered to run rats through mazes. He even claims to have invented the ideal maze back in the early 1940s, twenty years too late for most research agendas.

The United States Army summoned LeShan for a tour of duty during World War II. There he received what he still considers superb training in clinical psychology, a field he maintains the Army invented to meet its own medical needs. He spent three years in a psychiatric hospital, working, learning, trying not to do any harm to the patients while attempting to master the main approaches in psychotherapy of the time. He still regarded himself as an experimental psychologist, however, and to this day defines his work in research terms. Put simply, LeShan sees a problem he wants to solve, finds someone (a foundation, a business, an individual) to pay for the research, and does the work.

After leaving the Army, LeShan began working exclusively with dying people, primarily terminally ill cancer patients. His research project was aimed at developing different and more effective psychotherapy for the medically hopeless. The work was exceptionally demanding and conducted with little knowledge of what might work. LeShan did forge a number of effective techniques and supporting theories in the fifteen years he devoted to this effort. But in the end he burned out, even before the phrase was invented. He had always believed that objectivity in psychotherapy is absurd and best deciphered as the therapist's ability to support the mental growth of the patient. This commitment to the patient turned out to be both affirmation and destruction. His patients responded well until they died. LeShan ended up exhausted. He walked away and began looking for something else.

The field of parapsychology intrigued him for perverse reasons. He had always regarded claims for psychical experiences with the usual skepticism of those in conventional forms of psychology. But he was also intrigued by the number of outstanding intellects who took parapsychology seriously. Some of the leading thinkers of the past and current century have accepted the paranormal—individuals like William James, Gardner Murphy—and LeShan wanted to know why. He even whimsically considered discovering and naming the disease afflicting all these famous people, perhaps calling it the LeShan syndrome. It would describe a complicated intellectual failing that at once led scholars into a pseudoacademic discipline while allowing them to do very good work in their own fields.

So LeShan began his studies. In solid Aristotelian fashion he reviewed the literature, sure that he would be able to discover the academically fatal attraction and dismantle it. But many of the research designs, statistics, and data he encountered were impressively tight. He could not find the flaws he had been sure were there. He read further. It began to seem to him that parapsychology was legitimately describing a different way for humans to relate to one another, to communicate and be with one another, and that this set of relations might be the most important task that he could possibly be involved with at this time in his life and in human history. He decided to enlist.

LeShan's first working assignment was with Eileen Garrett, a psychic with a wide reputation for unusual powers. Garrett had invited him to monitor the experiments that psychic investigators conducted with her. LeShan's job was to ensure that the research was methodologically sound. He did this for five years. He came away from this working relationship with two conclusions. One was that Garrett was an ethical and highly principled woman. The other was that she had extraordinary gifts that suggested the validity of paranormal experiences.

LeShan observed Garrett doing things that could not be explained with the standard scientific frameworks he had absorbed for his research in psychology. Very often these feats would be accomplished under LeShan's own experimental conditions. Some of the more impressive exercises were carried out in assisting the police. LeShan says that a man would be on the national missing persons list, someone Garrett had never met and knew nothing about. LeShan would bring her a piece of the shirt the man wore the day before. She would then, according to LeShan, make very specific statements about where the man was or what he was doing: that he was going to Mexico on a bus, or sitting on a porch with some people dressed in outlandish clothes, or that he had lost all the hair on his body. That kind of statement would emerge and turn out to be very accurate. LeShan came to believe that sometimes people had information they couldn't possibly have had, very specific information, and the only way to explain this phenomenon was with psychic frameworks.

Once, in the late 1960s, LeShan was conducting an experiment with Garrett in veridical dreaming. Each morning at 2:00 A.M. a man in Brooklyn would pick out a picture using a random number selector and look at it, concentrating as hard as he could. Then he would call Garrett, waking her up, and ask her to recall her dreams. He would write down the description she provided. Sometimes Garrett would write the report. Then, later, experimenters would try to identify common features of the picture and written report. It is a widely used experiment, and variations on it seem endless.

One morning Garrett came into LeShan's office and related a strange dream. She said that Whately Carington, a well-known psychic researcher who worked with her in the 1920s, had come into her room during the night. This nocturnal presence was especially odd since Carington had died in 1947. Carington told her that she had to do two things for him. One, Garrett was to take care of his wife "because she needs you very badly at this moment." Second, Carington complained that all his papers were being ruined because they were under a bed and a wallaby was sleeping on them. LeShan remembers that he and Garrett giggled a bit, and then the researcher came in and reported an absolute bust for the morning's correlation. The dream had nothing to do with the picture.

The next day Garrett reported having a variation on the same dream. This time Carington had come into her room in an angry state. He said to her that he had asked her to do something for his wife and she had done nothing. He told her it was a very serious situation. He was so mad, Garrett reported, that he had thrown her out of bed. She had awakened on the floor.

Garrett was troubled. "I know myself," she told LeShan. She felt that they should do something about the situation. A group effort began to locate Carington's wife. Someone called Garrett's secretary and instructed her to join the search efforts. Someone else called the Society for Psychic Research in London. No one knew where Mrs. Carington was. Finally Garrett called someone very high in Internal Revenue, someone she both knew and had something on. He reluctantly agreed to assist in the efforts. An hour later he called back and said that Carington's wife lived in a cottage out on the moors in Devon. Garrett made one more demand. "Call the Devon tax office and on any excuse send one of their people out there." The man agreed to make the request.

Six hours later the phone rang. Yes, Mrs. Carington is fine, the Devon tax office reported. She is in the hospital. The tax assessor had gone out to her cottage and found her. She was lying on the floor with a broken hip. She had been in that position for two days, eaten one apple, soiled herself, no one expected for two more days. She would almost certainly have died had not the tax assessor appeared.

Later Garrett arranged a search for the despoiled papers. They were found also, under the designated person's bed, but they were absolute useless nonsense—a collection of tax bills, laundry lists, things that should have been thrown out years ago. The second part of the spiritual request did not match the profundity of the first part. But LeShan had witnessed the report of the dream, taken part in the effort to locate Mrs. Carington, was present in the office when the phone call came through reporting the rescue. He cannot stretch empirical frames of explanation to fit such situations without giving up his sanity.

Still, even after his five years with Garrett, LeShan remained puzzled and uncertain about the paranormal. One problem that persistently bothered him was the theory-deprived state of paranormal inquiry. The study of the paranormal had started as a set of theories in search of data. The acceptance of spiritual causes and mystical explanations, after all, can be traced to the origins of human history. But then the various mechanistic and general empirical approaches to experience celebrated in modern science displaced spiritual theories of being. The anomaly, on LeShan's understanding, was that the data on paranormal events began accumulating more rapidly under scientific controls. The result was a mass of data looking for a theory. LeShan resolved to provide such theory and the techniques for teaching psychic skills, or find a method to explain away what he was observing.

But why turn to psychic healing? LeShan has a pragmatic approach to theory. He insists on subjecting theories to tests of usefulness when deciding on his research priorities. The paranormal is important to him because it demonstrates that people are related to one another in some way beyond the senses, and this knowledge is important in a secular age of isolated individualism. But LeShan also requires that theory be expressed in a language that fits reality and that it be made into a practical tool. Which part of the paranormal can be a useful tool? Telepathy? No, electronic communication will always be better. Clairvoyance? No, because if you want to find out what is in a sealed envelope, get a letter opener. But psychic healing might be useful, for the restoration of health can always be improved, even given the advances in conventional medicine. So LeShan moved into psychic healing.

The first question he raised in his early inquiries is basic enough. Is there a phenomenon? He reviewed the data and concluded that even in the best cases 90 percent of the claims had to be thrown out. The patient forgot to mention that he had received a penicillin injection that morning, or the placebo effect could explain the improvement—that sort of disqualifying consideration discredited most of the best psychic healings. Also, spontaneous remissions fall within medical expectations, and many healings could be explained that way. But he found some cases, maybe 10 percent of the very best, that he couldn't throw out easily. To do so would be to stretch coincidence or spontaneous remissions too far. LeShan looked at these cases with one controlling question: How does psychic healing work when it succeeds?

LeShan pressed this question on healers from the ancient Greeks to the present, scanning written explanations and interviewing serious healers when possible. He catalogued four types of accounts. One, God healed. Two, spirits did it. Three, energy brought healing. Or, four, it was mysterious, inexplicable. None of these met LeShan's intellectual needs. God requires human hands to work, he believes, and so the first explanation devolves to human levels, which leaves the causal powers still unexplained. He refused to do research on spirits, since they seem to appear and disappear at will, leaving the failed healing effect too glibly explained as "the spirits are not here." He viewed energy as a hopeless variable. Healers "didn't know anything more about energy than a cat knows about Christmas." They mixed it literally and metaphorically, sometimes referring to the energy in a Picasso painting, the energy in a group discussion, the energy in an electric light bulb. It made no sense to LeShan.

But he did isolate two categories that appealed to his sense of intellectual economy and decorum. One category was heterogeneous and could be set aside. It consisted of the full range of idiosyncratic things that healers did. They would line up facing in some geographical direction, or they would chant, sing hymns, pray, or they would wash themselves, whatever—all of the different groups of healers would have specific rituals that often distinguished them from each other. But they all did one single thing, a move that was generalizable to all of the healers he studied. It constituted LeShan's second category. At some point in their procedures, all of the healers changed their consciousness. They claimed to have shifted away from the conventional or commonsense reality where the world is a uniform whole. Most of the healers he scrutinized did not regard this shift as important, but to LeShan it looked like the critical variable. And it was a variable he could isolate and study empirically.

LeShan began trying to change his own consciousness. Meditation seemed to be the key. He studied and used every meditative technique he could find. Ever the pragmatist, LeShan saw meditation as an instrument to alter the state of one's mind, much like Nautilus machines are tools to change one's body. He followed a strict regimen, meditated six to eight hours a day, five days a week, for about a year and a half, surpassing some of the most assiduous body builders in dedication to craft. He would try each of the various meditative techniques for about six weeks, carefully evaluating the method for its effectiveness. Then he would retain the methods that worked, discard those that failed. He also paid careful attention to the explanations offered for the steps purporting to lead from ordinary consciousness to the "world of one" consciousness. At the end of his studies and efforts, he felt he had identified and mastered (at a reasonable level) a set of procedures that could take him to the altered state of consciousness found in psychic healings.

At this point he was still skeptical. It was when he started getting results as a healer that "scared the living hell out of me" that he became a believer. His first case was pure drama. A woman came to him with severe arthritis in her hands. She had not been able to close her fingers into a fist for over a year. There was a heavy calcium overlay on the joints. LeShan recalls that at that point in his work he had to have absolute silence to ensure the level of concentration needed to enter the different state of consciousness. (Later he learned how to do it even while at Times Square.) The woman's family tiptoed into the next room, and he was left with a "patient" who asked him, "What do I do?" LeShan had no idea. He asked her what she wanted to do. She said that there was an article in the New York Times that she had been trying to read. LeShan said, "Fine. Read it." Then, while the woman read the Times, LeShan shifted his consciousness several times, clearly holding the altered state for maybe two or three seconds (as much as he can achieve even now, he humbly reports). In this state he and the other person in the focus of his consciousness are one, and he claims to enter a universe of inexorable logic where all things flow into each other. Separateness is revealed as an illusion.

At the end of the meditation, LeShan turned to the woman and asked, "What did you feel?"

She answered, "Nothing."

LeShan persisted. "What happened?"

"Nothing," she replied. Her family came into the room and asked her what had happened.

"Nothing," she said, "except that in Washington, D.C., the politicians are doing . . . ," going on to relate the contents of the article she had read.

"How are your hands?" they asked.

"Just the same," she said, and at that point she raised them up to demonstrate and flapped them back and forth. Somehow complete mobility had been restored. Both LeShan and the woman's family virtually went into shock. The woman did also when she realized what had happened. X rays taken thirty-six hours later revealed a 50 percent reduction in the calcium overlay. LeShan had no idea where that calcium had gone. He did know that if that level of calcium were injected suddenly into the lymphatic system the patient would be lucky to survive. He didn't, and doesn't, know what happened. But that is the kind of result he says he started to get through psychic healing.

LeShan admits that a good healer who is honest will admit to maybe a 20 percent success rate, one in five cases that are genuine cures, *on a good day*. He considers himself a moderately competent healer, a good hack. The theories he studied suggest that healers must be in a state of grace, or possessed of a personality quirk, to work their craft successfully. He has never noticed either of these two features in his own set of characteristics. Nor has he ever had a paranormal experience. He has simply observed them in others. Yet meditative healing worked when he tried it. So he regarded it not as an arcane talent, but as a set of acquirable skills. He resolved to teach these skills to others.

The training sessions he developed with Joyce Goodrich were the result of this resolution. When he first put them together in California, he developed the reputation of conducting the only residential seminars where everybody slept in their own beds. This was not because of LeShan's moral concerns, but because the participants were so exhausted at the end of the day that they looked forward only to sleep. He works novitiates hard. He uses techniques that urge meditation of body, emotions, and mind (or intellect). LeShan believes that the fastest progress is made by jolting individuals back and forth between these three types of meditations, the day consisting of a constant shifting from one to the other. Everyone is also placed in the role of both healer and subject. The sessions are intense. LeShan claims that 80–90 percent of the participants get it at the end of a five- to six-day seminar. Some are more successful than others. But in his experience, success is correlated with practice, not some innate talent (whatever that means). Meditation for LeShan is a very tough discipline, and he is all business in teaching and using it.

The screening methods used in the seminars do not seem very rigorous from an outsider's point of view. Using interviews, the seminar conveners screen out those people on power trips. They also make every candidate promise that they will never (a) take money or gifts for their healing efforts, or (b) treat anyone who is not under a doctor's care. Also, they try to deny admission to those who have rigid personalities. Otherwise, a wide variety of individuals seek and gain admission.

One mark of a developed science is that the researchers know why things do *not* work as well as why they do. LeShan, though, has no idea why healing fails. He claims that we have working knowledge of only one of the three variables that seem to operate in psychic healing. One is what the healer should do. This is where LeShan claims knowledge. A second is what the patient should do. Here LeShan admits to ignorance. The third variable comprises a set of factors that he argues cannot even be identified, much less used as explanatory devices. Here LeShan classifies all of the considerations in mystic philosophies from the beginning of history: Homer's gods, spirits of all types, God in every religion, karma—the concepts, in short, that explain what leads to success or failure in some grand sense beyond the immediate pragmatics of the experience.

LeShan's approach to this third set of factors is at once tentative and ambitious. He reads the esoteric schools (those who advance philosophical or theological explanations for psychic healing) as agreeing on two ways of being in the universe, the way of the one and the way of the many. We are half divine, half empirical self, part mind and part body. All of the philosophies of psychic healing agree that full humanness requires both of these dimensions of reality. LeShan believes (with many others) that we are highly practiced experts in the way of the many, able to negotiate our journey through a sensory reality that we often take as the only level of being. But he maintains that denying the way of the one is to distort existence. It is to cut ourselves off from that spiritual nourishment that provides the needed balance away from the way of the many. For LeShan, the effective healer invites the person into the way of the one for a moment, allowing the person to realize a human potential that is beyond that fixed by the sensory world. In this sense, LeShan asserts, there is technically no psychic healing as such. There is self-healing, made possible by entrance into a different and vital level of being.

LeShan professes ignorance about the extent of such healing possibilities. He claims success in speeding the mending of fractured bones and wounds, alleviating arthritis and bursitis, migraines, and so forth. But he regards psychic healing as an undeveloped field, with knowledge gaps so great that no limits can be set on what might be possible. He concedes that there are probably only six or seven experiments in the paranormal field that really stand up before any bar of science. They are tight and convincing but limited in number and scope. In LeShan's view, paranormal studies have not advanced since the year 1800. He says this cannot be said of any other field, including medicine, dentistry, painting, sculpture, and architecture, though he might be persuaded to concede philosophy as a regressive case.

The puzzle for LeShan is not the status of neurology. He admits that we know what is going on in only a few small areas of the brain. But the deeper conundrum as he sees it is in the connections between the functions of the brain and consciousness, the bridges between the electrochemical changes in the physical brain and the complex functions of the conscious self. He still regards Descartes as having made the first heroic effort to connect body and mind, but with little success. LeShan quotes Arthur Eddington's famous observation approvingly: "The brain function resembles consciousness as a telephone number resembles the subscriber."

In the early 1940s, LeShan was working his way toward a master's degree and was teaching a speech class that addressed the problem of stuttering. Children would come in convinced that they were beginning to stutter because, like the centipede that couldn't walk when asked how he did it, others had pointed out a small speech impediment and had made them self-conscious. They wanted to learn how to take conscious control of their speaking abilities. LeShan's technique was to convince them to lose control and forget their "problems." One day he gave the students an unusual assignment. They were to listen to Lowell Thomas, the master radio commentator at the time, and count the flubs he made. The students said Thomas never made a mistake. LeShan said, "Count them tonight." They concentrated. Lowell Thomas made twelve errors. The students were elated. The point was made that everyone committed errors. But then LeShan was inspired to go further. He asked the class to relate the news Thomas had delivered. They had no idea. They hadn't been listening. They had given up the symphony for the notes.

LeShan uses this story to illustrate levels of reality. One can construe reality as a seamless garment, fixed at a holistic level, or one can see it as a place where discrete items define experience. Either way is valid in LeShan's approach. But psychic healing requires that the individual shift consciousness, move from the notes to the music, and know in the shift that the universe is constructed as a uniform whole where one's own consciousness fuses with the other's consciousness. LeShan believes that this shift can be achieved through a teachable method of meditation, sometimes by the numbers and sometimes tailored for the particular person, but in either case leading to remarkable and only partially explained healings of both body and mind.

LeShan greatly admires Gertrude Schmeidler and loves her metaphor for the paranormal. Imagine being in a forest where we keep hearing the noises of a large animal thrashing about. We see branches waving and broken off, large footprints, bark sheared off trees, stool droppings. We smell the animal. We sense its presence. We know there is something huge in this forest, even though we have not seen it. LeShan believes that we occasionally even have a photograph of it. This usually terrifies people into a kind of irrational denial, because to accept the photograph, to see the animal, to believe in the paranormal, would require abandoning conventional understandings of reality. LeShan is convinced that this is impossible for most people, and so he sees the paranormal chronically being denied, even though its presence is everywhere around us.

Spiritual Discourse

The one truth that both spiritual and secular thinkers might accept without dissent is that humans are located in a universe that exceeds their best efforts at understanding. There is no reason to think that this arrangement is necessary. Evolutionary theory might invite a different conclusion—that cognitive life should evolve toward an intellectual mastery of the environment that nurtured it. But it is not so in human experience. The gap between the realities in which we find ourselves and the explanations of these settings is enormous.

The most important difference between spiritual and secular discourse may be how that acknowledged truth is accommodated. Secular philosophies are developed within the parameters of human categories of knowing. When they are expressed using scientific discourses, these categories are both explicit and elaborated by linear forms of reasoning. Spiritual discourses are not contained by these patterns. Though spiritual believers do use rigorous forms of argument and often rely on scientific principles of inquiry, there is something else going on in the beliefs and justifications offered in spiritual talk. Efforts are made in spiritual practices to accommodate a reality not confined to sensory experience, and these efforts inevitably control the forms of reasoning deployed in spiritual discourse.

Reasoning is notoriously contextual. Almost any feature of both theoretical and practical reasoning is influenced by the type of discourse in which it is found. But it is still helpful to identify, even provisionally, a skeletal frame of reasoning that then can be introduced to particular conversations as a way of demarcating patterns of thinking. Such a frame can assist in recognizing particular types of reasoning that are generalizable to a range of different conversations. It can also demonstrate the decisive effects of spiritual beliefs, especially the acceptance of an external reality, on all forms of practical reasoning.

One helpful type of practical reasoning is deductive. Imagine, in simplest terms, that reasoning is a tiered exercise that begins with universal statements or principles, negotiates an array of bridge rules, and concludes with a directive for action. The immediate advantage of such a deductive model is in its bookkeeping powers. Put bluntly, it allows us to see how relevant considerations might be organized to reach a conclusion about what to do. But the imperative force of a syllogistic form of reasoning is truly in the eye of the beholder (as in observer). A number of discretionary devices allow individuals to control the flow of the syllogism.

The status given to first principles can yield different patterns of reasoning. Some might say that individuals choose or endorse first principles as they wish. For example, the principle of equality may be seen as a useful first choice to govern social distributions, though competing with other useful principles like liberty. Nothing may be compelling or axiomatic about either equality or liberty, or some other distributive principle. Others, however, may regard first principles as items to be discovered in experience rather than chosen or endorsed as a condition for their binding powers. Natural law theories and a number of spiritual perspectives see first principles in this way. The effect of these competing theories is to subordinate the deductive model to arguments over the status of first principles (for no reasoning can occur until some set of principles is in place).

The elasticity of practical reasoning is felt even more powerfully in the determination of evidence or relevant considerations. Suppose that one believes in a God who controls the entire universe. On this belief, events that are unremarkable from a secular point of view are sometimes seen as signs that disclose messages or patterns from a different reality. This evidence of divine intent will be a relevant consideration in spiritual discourse, of no relevance in secular reasoning. Again, the flow of practical reasoning, even in deductive form, is dependent on the beliefs introduced to reasoning.

We can conduct similar exercises on the logic of defeats or exceptions, logical terms like "sameness," and definitions of controlling vocabularies. For example, whether and how to count defeasible conditions in moral reasoning is a function of principles that lie outside the deductive flow of reasoning, and, like auxiliary hypotheses in science, they cannot always govern the discourses they mediate. Or, on the second point, what it means for items to be the same can vary across discourses—even the formal vocabularies of logic cannot govern reasoning. On the third point, the meanings of key terms like "reality" and "human individual" are not settled by practical reasoning but fixed by beliefs brought to reasoning.

These observations suggest that practical reasoning is an expression of beliefs rather than a device to control them. An understanding of spiritual discourse, then, must be charted from the effects of spiritual beliefs on forms of reasoning.

The single most important belief in spiritual discourse is that human experience is one dimension in a larger reality governed by design rather than by chance. This larger reality is also regarded as more important than, and the source of meaning for, human experience. Since this more expansive reality is not knowable in its entirety by humans, the role of the unknown is crucial in interpreting experience. Spiritual healing follows contact with some part of this larger reality.

Two kinds of effects occur when one subscribes to this belief. One bears directly on the framework of practical reasoning. First principles are more likely to be discovered (even revealed) rather than chosen, since the origin of experience is outside human choice and even control. Also, the range of human experience, and thus what counts as evidence, will be expanded. For example, spiritual events (visualization of angels, etc.) are considered real. The reasoning agent also is redefined. Individuals are seen as entries in a cosmic framework, either indivisible and unique (as in Christianity) or part of a uniform (and perhaps indifferent) reality outside of sense experience. A second effect transforms reasoning itself. Instead of the linear forms of reasoning expressed most strongly in deductive models, belief in a larger reality requires a narrative frame of communication in which truth is deciphered rather than presented.

Listen to the stories told here. Each individual who believes in a larger reality attempts to render that more comprehensive world intelligible by telling stories to represent a truth that cannot be expressed explicitly. The members of traditional faiths are typical examples. Faith Jamison and Reverend Penfield say that they are able to talk with God. Jamison sets up tests for God and feels herself enter a new level of awareness when God speaks to her. Penfield senses entries from outside the sequence of his thoughts when God contacts him. Both individuals offer narratives of events that they believe disclose a larger design governing their lives. Fathers Crossland and Brantley see evidence of God's power on the patterns of their own lives and the lives of others. Crossland's "sign" of God's will was first a persistent rhythm of factory machines, later a buzzing in his ears. Brantley witnesses events in his prison ministry that he cannot explain without introducing the will of God to the narrative. Thomas Canterbury, recipient of Crossland's faith healing, tells stories that are filled with unseen designs that can be glimpsed if we believe in God.

Those who follow more recent psychic therapies also use stories to express truth. Practitioners of therapeutic touch explain their methods in part by providing a history based on Estebany's discovery of his powers to heal (unlike some other healers, they may introduce clinical data as well). The therapists and patients who use meditative healing techniques must use narratives to explain healing. The critical experience is a type of mystical event, and one of the defining features of a mystical experience is that it is outside conventional languages. It follows that the oblique references of narratives, rhetorical devices like metaphors and similes, must be used in any intelligible account of meditative healing.

But remember that belief precedes reasoning. The interpretive or narrative form of practical reasoning in spiritual discourse is effective in revealing what experience means, but only to those who are able and inclined to share in those background beliefs in a larger reality upon which the stories are predicated. Interpretive or narrative reasoning (not the linear forms in scientific discourse) is forced upon spiritual thought by the ineffable nature of spiritual knowledge. Once one accepts the truth of a reality outside human experience, narrative modes of expression are inevitable. But the narrative itself cannot establish truth. One first must believe in order for such reasoning to work.

L U K E

The self. *My* self. Myself. These locutions were always puzzling to me. At earlier points in my life I was prepared to say that I was a complex, a congeries of parts that included my body.

How could human identity be otherwise? Even the most rudimentary aesthetic experience seems to stretch to both mind and body. On sunless fall mornings I can see low cloud banks, white vapor of some sort, just beyond the tree line bordering a low field in back of my house. The arrangement of colors—white over shades of green—always holds me in place for long moments of viewing, a vision of the natural world as it might have appeared at the beginnings of human time. Yet this mental connection to the scene has always been accompanied for me by a physical resonance, a feeling of chemical alteration in my body as it, too, responded to the clouds and foliage.

I regarded the biological entity, then, as the unit responding to these surroundings, the individual as the entire complex of items that constitute the living creature. Now I am distant within this complex, my sense of self restricted to the brain in a body that does not feel like it is me. I can think now as a self in a body, detached to a point from the physical. A drifter in the vehicle that conveys me from one geographical point to another.

I have become more aware of the inner self of consciousness, the small and irreducible something that is myself inside the body I occupy. No ghost in the machine, no epiphenomena drifting over the brain like those clouds over the field, but still something that is not the machine. What?

There is thinking going on in the area where I exist. Sometimes the thoughts come so rapidly and forcefully that I scarcely know whether to call them my own, much less use them as proof of my existence. There is also a self here, myself, an active something that restricts, conditions, structures, defines the experiences that I have. The perception of white clouds low over the fields, hovering like white smoke or opaque wraiths.

The problem is in the myth that we know the one true concept of the self, one's own self as each of us experiences the world, when the idea itself may be unintelligible. We all play parts, assume roles. There are life roles, niches in conventional reality designated with terms like "husband," "worker," "friend," and so on. These roles often compete in identifying the self. Sometimes they occur in succession over the course of life, adding to the confusion with the question of whether the youth is the same as the mature metamorphosis of the self. Actors play parts, "become" others temporarily while holding on to the self. Madness is a kind of role, not chosen but compulsively imposed on some individuals by neurology and by others in defining actions and thoughts as unacceptable. Some play at madness, pretending to be other than they are (whatever that means). Then there are fantasies, play-acting at what is not real (whatever that means). Life is a costume party, and selves are multiple, serial, revolving, fusing, partitioning.

Yet there are shields among this multiplicity, interior features of the self. There are things about others that I do not know, cannot know without inhabiting their interior worlds. So it must be that there are things about myself that others cannot know, facts within the phenomenological life of consciousness that only the experiencing subject can know. Layers of experience accessible only to the self. Particular experiences. Secrets also. Falsehoods. I do not pretend to know myself completely, since knowing is embedded in theories—and I do not have most of them. But I know that I am not fully visible to others.

The illness has made me thoughtful, perhaps religious. I believe that I am a single perspective, a point of view, a kind of privileged access to experiences. Sometimes this perspective is lost. The sense of self that consciousness seems to provide dissolved in action. In games, before my illness, I would have moments when I would be at one with the action. A team sport like basketball, when the flow was right and we entered what others have called "the zone," there was no individual, no I separate from experience. There were just the movements, the blur of the court, the whirl of the crowd, the unthinking coordination of the team, the ball, the basket, the crowd sound so loud that we seemed to be playing in silence, the brain so alert that the action was slowed in perception, until finally we were playing in some transparent ether where each individual was only a part of some larger whole not governed by time. Then we would come back down, the spell broken, the breathing painful again, and the sense of separateness restored. The point of view back in place.

During some of these epiphanies in action I would seem to divide, my consciousness split between reflection and engagement. At one level, so immediate and intense that it seemed to control my body from the outside and extinguish myself, I was so much in the action that I *was* the action. At another level, cool as spring rain, I was the inert eye always saying the same thing at some point in the movement, silent and seeming to issue from a reserve deep within myself: "This is magic."

Since my illness I have been consciousness without a sense of body. My powers are exhibited in pure form, modeled as architecture exposed in bright sunlight.

Here is what I do essentially, where my identity as a self is located. I am reflexively conscious. I am able to be conscious of myself as a self, to *self*-reflect, to be aware of and to think about myself as a conscious creature. I am a kind of trap, a closed loop of referential power that links the symbolic with the physical in a continuous interface. I am a location closed and open simultaneously, a recursive function that in addressing itself provides the paradox of conscious existence.

There is more. I am also a four-dimensional collection of simples, an arrangement of parts extending across time from past to future. This arrangement of basic elements is my particular identity as a person. I am the six-year-old boy who contracted leukemia and was cured. I am also the adult who was divided and subdivided by my body's destructive reaction to a penicillin compound.

I am not the other, not the persons who occupy places in my conscious landscape, and these individuals are not me. Yet I have, with others, a kind of power to extend my identity, to see the world with another perspective in place.

Once, before the reactive illness, I was unfaithful to my wife. I took a young woman I worked with to a hotel room near the airport where we enjoyed one another for several hours. At that time I thought there was no high like sex, and no feeling of certainty and sanity like that following physical love. Guilt was not my normal companion. But the woman tracked regret over the next year like a predator after prey. That I was married weighed on her mind with an emphasis I could only label as disproportionate. In the first month of summer following our tryst, she wrote to my wife confessing her error and describing our couplings.

I was out of the country traveling when my wife received the letter. But the young woman had called earlier in the day from New York to tell me what she had done. I began to see, feel, "know" my wife's experience.

Ann is standing on the sand at night just in back of our house on Cape Canaveral. She is holding the letter. Her nightdress is white, and she is trying to imagine herself as a kind of spirit in the moonlight, a figure who might suddenly stop the conversations of those who come upon her.

The letter is light, almost weightless in her hand. The paper is a thin bond that permits erasures without blemishes. Ann had once remarked that God has a strong sense of symmetry. She is thinking of that right now, wondering if the cosmic order includes revenge. She runs her fingers over the chain of her St. Christopher medallion, moving the clasp directly behind her neck. Small specks of sand graze her skin, giving her the sensation of sunburn after a day of tennis or swimming. But on this day she has stayed in, locked in a self-imposed retreat in our bedroom.

I am on a plane, somewhere over the Atlantic. The stewardess comes by with earphones for the movie, a killing story of some sort that stars Charles Bronson. I wave her away. I know about the letter. I am imagining my wife's reaction.

I see her standing on the beach, looking out at the dark horizon. I can see the scene, feel the detached anger and puzzlement, the uncertainty about what to do in the center of a vast calm inside her. White light plays in bursts on the lower part of the sky like heat lightning, though the flashes extend deep into the ocean. I share Ann's curiosity that no sound correlates with the light, no thunder or noise of any kind.

Am I inventing this? No, I see the scene, share the pain my actions have caused. It could be me, will be me, standing on that beach with a letter in hand relating my spouse's indiscretions.

Later, when we face one another, it is like looking in two mirrors that reflect images in an infinite series. Then, later still, when we have reconciled in our own couplings, we can each feel the other's clean relief and love.

Are we one person? Once I told about my encounter with an unusual animal in our garden that I could not identify. I noticed Ann smiling at me while the others in the room listened. Then I knew. It was her experience I was telling.

Are we one person? We put on the frame the other uses, we enter and share each other's pains and elations. But we are two persons, always at every moment, and only our shared lives allow us access to the experiences that the other has.

I cannot be myself without anomaly. But even the shift in my sense of self caused by the illness and resulting detachment, even the rearrangement of my chemical elements, has not extinguished my identity as a distinct self. I still have a location. How can I be another?

8

POLITICAL DISCOURSES

Truths and Realities

One of the strongest human instincts may be the desire to resolve conflict with truth. Let the true story dominate, and justice will be served. Unfortunately for the cultivation of this instinct, realities compete with one another in human experience. Followers of allopathic and holistic medicine do not simply see the world differently; they see different worlds. Truth seems to follow these differences, multiplying with ease across beliefs in healing possibilities and the meaning of health itself. This kind of deep pluralism has produced the institutional arrangements of procedural democracies, which respect both the private truths of individuals and their rights to introduce these visions to public space as political truths.

All of the claims for unorthodox healing examined here rely in some way on beliefs in alternative realities. Both religious and psychic approaches to spiritual healing assume that the structure of the ordinary world, governed by those familiar assumptions of cause and effect, separate and distinct individuals, spatial arrangements of objects, and time's arrow, does not exhaust reality. There is a reality, or realities, fixed somewhere outside of the domains of ordinary human experience and, the claims continue, contact with these alternative realities is the source for eliminating or curing illnesses.

Unorthodox healing practices amend ordinary reality in various ways. The framework of the ordinary world may be maintained with different entries in the set of beliefs. Causality, for example, is sometimes endorsed as an adequate account of how events are related to each other, but then what is accepted as a cause of illness or healing differs radically from conventional to unorthodox practices. An antibiotic and the power of God are different ante-

213

cedent variables, however common the causal framework is in these two competing explanations of medical recovery. At other times, the entry undermines the framework, an effect illustrated by mental telepathy. Holistic therapists who diagnose and prescribe therapy by "entering" the mind of the patient amend the separation between individuals that is part of the structure of ordinary reality. Sometimes therapy requires a loss of the self. This abandonment radically changes and can even override the framework of a reality that depends on separate individuals.

The structure of that ordinary reality found in both secular and spiritual communities is obviously influenced by contemporary science, and thus is biased toward the secular. But the acceptance of such a reality does not limit beliefs about the real. A minimal structure of reality simply identifies provisional benchmarks with which to measure or at least mark the range of deviation from the conventional. In a sense the use of any benchmark biases the case by accepting conventions that may themselves be arbitrary and perhaps even false in some important way. But the data suggest that distinctions between ordinary and unconventional realities are found within all spiritual communities. The starting assertion of nondual philosophies, for example, is not that conventional reality is just an imaginary construct, but that it is an illusion mapped into the very center of human beliefs. The business of real thinking then is to expose and eradicate this false sense of reality. The use of a provisional structure for ordinary reality proceeds along similar lines. The logic of unorthodox healing may require that this structure be dismissed, but setting up the structure tells us exactly what is being dismissed as well as provides a rough measure of how radical the claims are for alternative understandings of the real.

It is also important to understand that there is little independent evidence that can settle the truth or falsity of alternative realities. For example, suppose that the shift in consciousness that produces those experiences said to be of another reality are occasioned by drugs. A skeptic will immediately (and reasonably) conclude that the experiences are hallucinations brought on by drugs with no correlates in any empirical reality. But the believer (and again reasonably, though on different criteria) can maintain that drugs are the devices that provide access to a different reality and so may label the experiences visions. The observer standing outside these two assertions must conclude that if hallucinations cannot be segregated from visions, or veridical perceptions in general, not much remains at a more fundamental level to determine the truth or falsity of the competing claims.

Implications

The implications of competing claims about the scope of reality are not trivial. Sometimes they are even astounding. If a standard question in philosophical inquiry is raised, "What would the world be like if psychic or spiritual experiences were real?" the answer would differ for different experiences. All such experiences, however, require some modification, and sometimes a radical restructuring, of ordinary reality.

Accommodations of psychic experiences are common. Many demonstrations of what seems to be ESP can be explained by expanding standard causal frameworks. Pets can sometimes sense the intentions of their owners through a keen awareness of bodily movements, hormone excretions, tone of voice. Some people may simply have such a heightened sensitivity in being able to "read" others. But this skill is not mysterious; it amounts only to a mastery, perhaps at a subconscious level, of those indicators and inference rules that lead us to deeper understandings of situations and other individuals. Calling such understandings intuitive only designates them as extraordinary exercises of powers that all of us may have in one degree or another. Much of parapsychology aims to document these and similar abilities.

But some psychic claims do exceed conventional realities in dramatic ways. For example, predictions of the future are claims that have strong amending powers. Precognition is an entry that accepts time's arrow yet changes the framework of ordinary reality, even when such change is not intended by those who claim powers of precognition. For some reason disasters are the focal points of many premonitions, though the predictions are typically vague and are usually made public only after the tragic event has occurred (thus allowing for retrospective, and usually erroneous, "preseeing"). A number of individuals had strong and inexplicable premonitions of the sinking of a large ship before the *Titanic* disaster. In Wales, on October 22, 1966, a massive slide of coal and mud destroyed a schoolhouse and killed 144 persons. Dozens of individuals later claimed to have had some precognition of the tragic event, including a ten-year-old girl, killed in the avalanche, who reportedly had a dream the day before the disaster that the schoolhouse had vanished because something black had come down all over it.

Set aside the problems and opportunities in settling on the truth of such predictions. The point is that for precognition to be a genuine power requires a world radically different from the one accepted now on conventional beliefs and theories. The dominant metaphor for time in Western societies is a moving point on a line. The past falls on one side of this point. It is an area populated by events that have occurred. We store them as memories and in historical records that include both physical and social data. On the other side of the point is the future. It consists of the set of events that have not yet occurred. These events obviously do not have the same status in human experience. The present is represented by the point itself, where immediate experience is located. The point moves toward the future in the metaphor.

This metaphor of time is more than just a literary device. It represents basic understandings of reality, from explanations of the origin of the universe in a primal explosion in the past, to the use of causal variables in physical and social theory that precede the events to be explained, to general understandings of empirical evidence as accruing or diminishing over time, to the specific accumulation of geological evidence, to theories of evolution and probability, the concept of change itself, the acceptance of memory, history, a sense of outcomes, expectations, and much more. One might argue that all of conventional reality is constructed on the acceptance of time's arrow.

Premonitions based on knowledge of the future tell us that the future is real, that it exists in some form that can be known. This thought will not fit time's arrow. What is required instead of a line is a tableau. Everything—past, present, and future—is real, has in some sense happened. And we can know parts of this tableau, though not (presumably) all of it at once. To accept this notion—that all of temporal reality is arranged without regard to time—is to give up the main understandings of reality that inform ordinary conventions.

Many beliefs in the healing powers of alternative realities seem to fall somewhere between the modest changes in ordinary experience ESP requires and the more radical amendments precognition demands. To many health care professionals, medical practice seems to reside in an undefined area between spiritual or psychic experiences and traditional science. Observations of symptoms, diagnosis as inference from evidence on the patient's condition, applications of known remedies—though the imaginative use of data in diagnosing and treating illness is always respected in medical practice, the physician's approach to illness can be a textbook case of traditional science (especially now with increasingly precise sources of data on a patient's condition). But it is also true that therapeutic skills vary substantially among physicians, and healing practices contain inexplicable cases of recovery. Few practitioners in the health professions are comfortable in classifying medicine anywhere on a continuum between paranormal and "normal" science.

The methods of pure spiritual healing, however, stand outside conventional medicine, since the practice of medicine is conducted by joining insight and healing gifts to clinical theory and empirical knowledge of the biological world. Spiritual and scientific discourses have their own rules and vocabularies within which the possible is defined. For the spiritual healer, the hand of God, or an external reality in itself, provides the clairvoyant insight and the action across distance that seals the wound. The medical practitioner, insulated from the full ontology of spiritual discourse, holds on to different realities and, as a consequence, different possibilities. Separate truths about diagnosis and therapy ordinarily follow. The result is a set of differences that can lead to the sharpest of disagreements and then disputes over proper medical care. The absence of a common reality, moreover, means that there may be no shared criteria to resolve or even manage the conflict that can result from these differences.

Moral Discourses

At the Family Court hearing that determined Caleb Loverro's treatment for leukemia, the feelings in Tioga County were high and almost totally sympathetic to the Loverros. Stephen Dubansky remembers being worried about his physical well-being and even for his life. The pretrial stories in the newspapers and attendant editorials usually portrayed Dubansky as the heavy, the outsider who was imposing his authoritarian will on a pleasant and loving family in the local area. Some stories had Dubansky forcibly experimenting on Caleb, compelling his mother to hold him while the boy screamed and fought to get away from spinal taps and injections. At one point Dubansky was sitting in the courtroom listening to one of his colleagues testify when a man directly behind him said, "That Dr. Dubansky who caused all this, if I see him I am going to kill him." The person sitting next to this citizen killer was a social worker, who promptly had the man removed from the courtroom. He turned out to be the editor of the local newspaper. Dubansky would not go anywhere in Owego after that without an armed guard.

Each side in the trial felt morally betrayed by the other. The Loverros thought that they had a contract permitting them to withdraw Caleb from the protocol "without prejudice." But when they did so they were arrested for child abuse and neglect. Joseph Loverro was particularly incensed that he was charged with medical neglect. In chiropractic college he took many of the same courses that medical students did, and in fact his college shared faculty with the local medical school. His curriculum included microbiology, histology, pathology, biochemistry and physiology as well as courses in neurobiology, kinesiology, and nutrition. He also took clinical courses in geriatrics, pediatrics, obstetrics, gynecology, emergency care, and the full array of courses in chiropractic. He is unable to understand why his reflective choice of an alternative method of therapy, to be supervised (he hoped) by another physician, was irresponsible. He also believes that Dubansky intimidated potential witnesses from the medical profession who might have testified on the efficacy of diet in cancer therapy.

Dubansky felt that the Loverros turned away from the only treatment that could save Caleb, and simply could not or would not provide any compelling reasons for doing so. He was also shocked by what he considers a personal betrayal. When he was trying to reassure Gillian Loverro that he would not allow Caleb to be removed from their home, he told her, in confidence, of the pain he had suffered in 1970 when he was divorced and lost custody of his son (common at a time before father's rights were prominent). He told Mrs. Loverro that he knew how painful it was to live without one's child and so he would never consider inflicting such a burden on her, as long as Caleb continued treatment. Then, while he was testifying in the trial, the Loverros' lawyer asked him, "Isn't it possible that your zeal in prosecuting these people is based on the fact that you have had a problem with a child taken away from you?" Dubansky had no idea at first what the lawyer was talking about. Then, when the lawyer said, "Think clearly, Doctor," and went over to the table to confer with the Loverros, it struck him. She had told the lawyer the story of his son.

Much later, after Caleb's therapy was resumed with a different physician at University Hospital, Gillian Loverro called Dubansky and asked for a meeting. She had a request that Dubansky found puzzling. "Would it be possible for you to take care of Caleb again?" (The Loverros had insisted as part of the initial court settlement that Caleb be removed from Dubansky's care.)

"Wait," Dubansky said. "You said I was so abusive and evil. Why?"

"Well, we think that you really care about him and he likes you."

Dubansky never hesitated. He told her, "Absolutely. As far as I am concerned, I have never taken our disagreements seriously." This statement he now admits was a lie. He uttered it for Caleb's sake.

Gillian Loverro asked, "Can we hug and make up?" So they did hug, there in the conference room at University Hospital.

Dubansky lied again. "As far as I am concerned, it is all long gone and forgotten." He says he will not forget what was said about him. He cannot forget that. But he wanted to guide Caleb through therapy and prepare him physically for a long and healthy life.

It is impossible to read about these people and their disputes without a moral perspective in place, even one that is the servant of some understanding of reality. The problem is identifying a logic of moral reasoning, since morality is not an abstract calculus that can be pulled clear of its context and inspected part by formal part. The principals supply the cues. The demands for a dialogue between the two adversaries, pressed by Stephen Dubansky at every interval, and the need for reasons to support claims, are clearly a part of moral discourse. Dubansky's most consistent disappointment was the absence of any supporting arguments for the Loverros' position that he could understand. To the moral and legal question, "Who knows best the child's interests?" he answers it depends. In the case of Caleb Loverro, he thought that he knew best because the Loverros, from his point of view, had a morally indefensible position on therapy.

The Loverros stressed the moral authority of parents over their children and their discretionary liberty to select therapy for their son. It is interesting to note that had a physician licensed in New York been willing to supervise the macrobiotic plan, then the court in all likelihood would have allowed the Loverros to implement a diet therapy in place of chemotherapy. The moral weight of parental authority is considerable in the law. The Loverros simply wanted to be shielded from state authority in making decisions in their child's interests, a demand that is normally granted. But because the effectiveness of nutritional therapy for Caleb's illness could not be proved legally, the court intervened in the conflict to ensure Caleb's health by ordering more conventional therapy.

But the moral considerations cut deeper than a (by now almost standard) dilemma caused by conflicting moral principles and disagreements over the efficacy of therapy. The conflict also raises questions about the nature of the self, the agent in human experience who is both the subject and focus of these dilemmas. Both sets of adversaries had reasons for their actions that they were prepared to generalize well beyond the particular case, but neither could communicate with the other because of the distance between their understandings of reality. Their moral discourses, typically a way of thinking that is not confined to any single set of conventions, were effective only within the theories of reality they had embraced. But everyone understood that the principals were deliberative creatures who could use evidence in reasonable ways, who could enter (and abandon) contracts and personal commitments, and therefore were responsible for their actions.

The exception was Caleb. Precisely because he was too young to make decisions in his own interests, the case went to court to settle on who should decide for him. He was not competent, but he was a person in inchoate form—not a thing or an animal but someone with rational expectations. The issue in the dispute was the life of a human being who in normal circumstances would acquire the capacity to deliberate and make autonomous decisions on his own definitions of self interest. It is precisely these primary goods—life, health—that introduce political imperatives to conflicts that admit no private or moral resolution.

Stanford

The competition among discourse communities in health and healing, and the moral problems that follow such competition, can sometimes find expression in individual physicians. David Stanford is an internist who had wanted to practice family medicine from the time he decided to be a doctor. Family practice was the only kind of medicine he ever knew growing up in a small town in Massachusetts. He was a healthy child and never had to see a medical specialist. Even now, over twenty-five years after completing medical school, he gives donations to his alma mater only if the money is targeted to students interested in family practice. He is enough of a realist to suspect that the set of recipients is probably quite small.

Stanford was an English major at Dartmouth. He had a difficult time in medical school. At times he felt that his brain, the seat of his consciousness, was disassociated from his body. He had taken all the pre-med courses as an undergraduate, including the usual retinue in chemistry, physics, and biology. But he had problems with the technical languages in medical school and with some of the doctors who were supposed to be role models. He didn't like many of the ways that patients were approached. He also thought the doctors treated the students very badly. The competition among the medical students was intense. At Dartmouth the classes were small and the students were on intimate terms with many of the professors. In medical school, lecture courses of seventy-five students were not uncommon. When students started flunking out, none of the faculty seemed to care or even know about it. There was also a fair amount of cheating among the students. Stanford realizes that his lack of ability in science may have distorted his judgments, but he remembers medical school as a dehumanizing experience.

At one point Stanford dropped out. He had been taking graduate courses during the summers to get an advanced degree in English. His ideal role model was William Carlos Williams, whom Stanford hoped to emulate with some combination of literary writing and medical practice. But when he failed his second course in medical school during his second year, he applied for and received a fellowship to do full-time graduate work in English literature. His family and friends prevailed, however, and he returned to medical school in the fall. He thinks it was the right decision. He finds taking care of people a very rewarding experience.

From the beginning of his medical practice, however, he has been intrigued by some of the claims and techniques in holistic medicine. He chose to settle in a small village in upstate New York where he has been part of the community for over a quarter of a century. He hears about everything and everyone. People stop him in the street to tell him that their child is better, or his own children report that so-and-so is well. Among the bits of information that came his way in the 1960s were reports of alternative healing techniques. Self-help and self-actualization movements seemed to be everywhere. Stanford began listening to stories of unconventional healings. He started going to conferences, trying to learn about alternative medicine.

The ideas and methods he picked up piecemeal from meetings, conversations, and reading turned out to be useful in his practice. At the very least he discovered theories to justify the pragmatic techniques he had developed over the years. For example, he had unknowingly used role-reversal therapy for some time. He would assume the role of father, husband, wife in interviews with patients to get at the whole history of their health problems. Or he would ask a wife to pretend that she was her husband and try to think like he was thinking as a way of understanding her complaints about her spouse. Then at conferences he realized that these techniques were developed in any number of theories with supporting data.

Stanford had also tried to instill in his patients a positive state of mind. One of his patients was a woman who had moved to his village. She had experienced three terrible births with an eminent obstetrician in the large city where she had previously resided. In this, her fourth pregnancy, the labor was a breeze, one of the easiest births Stanford had attended. He wondered why aloud to her afterwards. "Well," she replied, "each time I came in you said you thought this pregnancy was going so well that the labor will be easy." Stanford realized that he had left a hypnotic suggestion with the woman, and it had worked. So he took a hypnosis workshop to learn how to modulate his voice, calm people down by talking to them a certain way, influence their responses to therapy.

In all of these efforts he was groping toward a better understanding of the doctor-patient relationship. In the 1970s, he participated in group discussions of holistic medicine. The group consisted of doctors, psychiatrists, physical therapists, and exercise instructors. The aim was to identify the whole patient instead of just a medical part of the body and get the diverse professionals to think holistically about their patients. One of the participants went down to New York City and attended a Lawrence LeShan work-shop. When she carried the word back to the group, Stanford decided to attend a session. There he learned about psychic healing. He also attended institutes stressing yoga techniques and studied some of the work demon-strating interaction between stress and blood pressure.

He does not profess an understanding of all that he has tried to absorb. That there is a separation between mind and body is fairly clear to him from his own practice. But he does not always follow the ideas on spirituality or alternative realities. In the LeShan workshops, the participants are tested for latent healing powers. Stanford was poor at spiritual healing but quite good at (Type II) diagnosis and healing of particular areas of the body through touch. Individuals would be brought in fully clothed. Stanford would ex-plore their bodies and be able to tell when a knee, for example, was hot, and have arthritis confirmed in the joint. This kind of thing often happened to him. He realizes he cannot set up shop for spiritual healing because people come into his office with strep throats and the like. They want and need therapy for specific physical ailments, which he provides in his practice. But he finds the general psychic approach helpful. Patients are to him whole and complex persons, not entries in a lecture on biology.

Stanford wants medical practitioners to be more willing to work out spe-cific protocols for particular individuals. He points out that for thousands of years there were no medicines and most people still survived. People with rheumatic fever got better. Others had heart attacks and lived. He concedes the obvious: modern medicine has made it easier to overcome diseases. But he cannot dismiss people just because they do not completely buy into the Western medical system. He cannot tolerate some types of resistance to medicine. For example, he will not treat people who refuse to immunize their children. He knows the risks involved in immunization, and he recog-nizes that the probabilities of a severe neurological reaction and possibly death from the pertussis vaccine make it rational for parents to question this particular immunization and perhaps resist it. But he also believes in public health measures. Parents who oppose immunization receive a lecture from Stanford on responsibilities to others. If they still refuse, he sends them to another doctor.

But Stanford does accept a wide range of patients who dissent from con-ventional medical practice. He regards a request to have a baby at home as perfectly rational, for example. He observes that pregnancy is not a medical disease. It was not invented by doctors nor is it curable by doctors. In point of fact, Stanford believes that for most births the woman and baby are better off with a skilled caretaker who does not intervene than with one who does. But still the medical profession tends to regard women who want to have a home birth as noncompliant and a little crazy for putting their life and their baby's life in danger. Some studies have shown that home birth is actually safer than hospital birth as it is currently practiced, though obviously in some circumstances it is safer to deliver in a hospital. A woman who has had two Caesarean sections is probably better off in a hospital, though even here the evidence is mixed. The point Stanford stresses is that it is not convenient for the doctor to deliver a baby at the woman's home. But this does not make the request any less rational.

Stanford frequently tells a story he heard in Washington, D.C., about a young Hmong man who was diagnosed as having severe liver disease. He checked into a hospital where they stopped feeding him, put him on intravenous feeding, and told him that he needed a liver transplant. All of this is standard procedure. But in Hmong culture, the liver is the seat of the soul, the repository of the human personality (much like the heart is viewed in traditional Western culture, in which individuals can have a cold, hard, or big heart according to their personalities). In effect, the attending physicians were asking the young man to give up his soul and accept someone else's soul. This was impossible for him. Also, by denying him his staple diet of rice they were creating conditions in which he believed he would die from inadequate nourishment.

The man was rational. He signed out of the hospital and sought help from elders in the Hmong community in the area. Fortunately it was a well-organized community with multiple connections to the Anglo world. The elders approached another physician in another hospital who was also very skilled but willing to negotiate a medical protocol with the young man that took into account his cultural beliefs. The first change was in the diet. If all the man could take while being treated for liver disease was fluids, why couldn't he take rice water? So the staff made rice water for him. Then the doctor presented options instead of mandates. He explained to the man that his liver was very bad and that his chances of dying were very great. But he gave him alternative choices on treatment with his best-guess prognostications on survival in each option. Also, the doctor respected his refusal to submit to a liver biopsy since that would amount to a loss (however small) of a piece of his soul. The man began treatment as an outpatient along one of the therapy lines offered to him.

One day the man came to the hospital for treatment when his doctor was on vacation. Another doctor was covering and the man refused everything the substitute doctor recommended. Again the man was labeled a bad apple. The problem was background beliefs again. The man's culture held that loyalty to a healer must be absolute, that one should not take treatment from someone else without getting approval from the healer. Since the man did not believe that the other doctors were healers, and since he could not check with his healer, he rationally turned down all the proposed medical advice. As soon as his doctor (the healer) returned, he followed all the recommendations on therapy. The man got better. He is still living and doing well. He did not die, as the best reasoned projections of the time said he would.

Stanford reports that unexplainable cures do occur, which is what one would expect given the resilience of the human body. He once had a patient with cancer of the cervix, proven with multiple biopsies, who went to her spiritual guru and received a proper order, "Thou shalt drink grape juice," (or whatever). She rejected surgery to follow the guru's orders. But she agreed to follow-up examinations with Stanford. He monitored her and observed her slowly converting from carcinogenic to normal Pap smears. Years later, there still is not a trace of the cancer. Stanford has also seen people with inoperable brain tumors who were radiated to give them three more months to live. Twenty years later they are still alive. Stanford believes in medical miracles because he has seen them.

He admits that such miracles are not suspensions of natural laws but their fulfillment. It is possible that brain tumors could be diagnosed as malignant when they are benign, and that radiation to buy three months of life could knock out a benign tumor, allowing for a long life and only residual problems following therapy. He also is sensitive to both negative and positive placebo effects. He thinks it is uncanny that many people come down with cancer within eighteen months of the death of someone else in the family. Immunity can apparently be conferred or reduced by emotional states. But for Stanford it is precisely that mental influence over the physical that seems to require that doctors respect the beliefs of their patients, even when these beliefs run counter to the imperatives of modern medicine.

Stanford views the world as exceedingly complex with many factors that no one understands. He is not sure that anyone knows why treatment succeeds or fails. Perhaps prayer is an independent variable, with some people subverting therapy by praying against it, others accelerating healing by praying for it. To Stanford, nothing in medicine can rule out these possibilities. He occasionally introduces psychic healing in his practice. Very few people even want it explained to them. He has heard that spiritual healing is good for babies with colic. When a mother calls to complain that her child is up all the time crying, and they've tried changing the formula, calming the baby down, and so on, Stanford might say to her that spiritual healing could be the answer. Then he will describe what it is like and suggest that if she is interested he can meet with her either in person or talk to her on the phone when she can set aside some time for him to explain meditative techniques. (He will not schedule such discussions during office hours because he does not believe that anyone should charge money for spiritual healing.) Usually by the time he has explained the procedures the mother will say something like, "Oh my God. I probably ought to get another doctor." No one has accepted Stanford's advice on meditation. As a consequence, he claims no skills in the area.

Yet he does practice Type II healing sub rosa. If during a physical exam a patient complains about pain in his shoulder, Stanford will try to heal the joint through touch and meditation carried out silently. He reports that when he has asked his patients how a birth, illness, surgery, or treatment was in general, they will often answer it was x, y, or z, but "when you put your hands on my abdomen [or shoulder, or whatever], I do not know how to explain it but something felt real good." Sometimes Stanford feels that he should have been a chiropractor.

Stanford is an orthodox Jew. Yet he believes that the logic of medicine is Christian and the model healer is Christ. To Stanford a central feature of Christ's mission was accepting everyone, no matter how sinful or ugly the person might be. That is why Stanford is appalled to find doctors making judgments about the acceptability of patients. Some patients are regarded as good guys, others as bad guys. The bad guys are alcoholics, those lacking in hygiene, and most of all those who will not listen to their doctors. Stanford says that doctors label these patients as noncompliant, meaning that they do not bend to the doctors. Stanford believes it is the doctors who should be able to bend.

He recognizes limits. He does not want his cancer patients to go down to Mexico to buy apricot pits (laetrile) because he believes they will get "ripped off" in doing so. He does not think the placebo effect should cost in the neighborhood of eight thousand dollars. But he would take care of his patients again when they return from such follies. Nor is he sanguine about dangerous or unproven therapy. Some patients tell him that coffee enemas can cure cancer. Stanford's reaction is direct. First, he will tell the patient that there is not a shred of evidence that cancer can be cured in that way. Second, he will relate to them the background of the theory that purgatives can cure cancer. It will consist of a brief summary of that time in Western history when people believed that they had to take a purgative every day to cleanse their bodies of toxic substances. He will show how the theory still has no supporting evidence today. Third, he will warn of the dangers in this practice. He will point out that individuals who administer such "cures" often do not sterilize their equipment and end up transmitting enteric infections among their patients. People die from such infections. Stanford still believes it is the patient's prerogative to go get an enema if that is what he believes will work for him—so long as he is an adult and competent. But Stanford tries to put such therapy in the proper perspective for the patient.

Stanford understandably attracts a number of "noncompliant" patients, perhaps 20 percent of his practice. They are the types who read books on their illnesses and sometimes, he admits, know more about the diseases afflicting them than he does. He addresses their needs with his technical expertise and his efforts to identify with their experiences. He tries to give meaning to their experiences, help his patients through the medical therapy, be there for them when they are in the depths of pain or depression or anxiety, and be there when they come out at the end of therapy. He uses his practical knowledge gained from treating patients for over twenty-five years to communicate with the people he treats. Stanford reminds us that the medicine man used to come into the house and stay for eight days or longer if necessary. He believes doctors today also have to stay with their patients.

Stanford also directs a hospice. He feels that he should be in better touch with his own mortality. His body is reliable in all manner of stressful conditions. He does not have the vaguest idea what patients mean when they tell him, "I know that I am going to die and I know what it is like." But he still feels that he is effective at taking care of dying people. He does not claim to be some spiritual wonder. He tries to bring things together, to transmit the experiences of his patients back and forth among them. In this way the individual experience of illness and mortality is illuminated by universalizing it.

Of all the experiences of death that Stanford relates, the most vivid is that of the death foretold by the patient. He has gone into a patient's hospital room to prepare him for surgery and heard the patient say, "Doc, I am not going to make it. I'm going to die." Then, in surgery, Stanford has watched this same patient die as he predicted he would. Stanford believes that there is probably not one surgeon who has not had that experience. The usual judgment at the time is that the patient is just depressed or scared. After the surgery the physician will inevitably regret not listening to his patient and cancelling or at least delaying the operation. Here is the conundrum of medicine, however. Stanford believes that doctors have to listen to someone who shares a perception that something is going to happen. But he also knows that for most patients who have that perception, nothing happens and the surgery succeeds.

In Stanford's view, the physician must be both scientist and spiritualist, although he recognizes the incompatibilities between the two. He believes in modern medicine. It is his chosen profession. But he also believes in a healing force and feels that doctors must find ways to bring it to bear on their patients. He knows, however, that the methods employed by the scientist disregard the spiritual side of human experience, and spiritual techniques often require ignoring the demanding test of scientific reasoning.

When Stanford last visited his family home, his father told him that he is proud that his son reads so many books, reminding Stanford that he, the father, has read one book all of his life, over and over (the Bible, of course). Then he asked Stanford if he goes fishing anymore. "No," Stanford replied, "I don't have time." As he left, Stanford immediately stepped on a fishing lure in the street.

This kind of coincidence seems to Stanford to be a recurring experience in his life. He entertains the possibility that his unconscious directed his foot to the lure. But these correlations happen so frequently that even this type of explanation seems inadequate to him. He reports driving to a convention in some city and suddenly thinking of someone he has not seen in years. Then he will meet this person randomly on the street the next day.

Stanford is a physician who practices the very latest and best techniques in contemporary medicine, yet he believes in an energy field and that healers can tap into its powers. He does not know how the field works. He is only sure that it is somehow at work in human experience.

Allopathic and Holistic Medicine

Conflicts between conventional and holistic medicine occur in a variety of forms. One of the sharpest cutting edges may be the one waged within the self. Physicians like David Stanford, who believe in spiritual healing, are sometimes like the divided selves identified in early Christianity. The domain of the psyche is a terrain on which opposing forces do battle. The battle is not always a doctrinaire, zero-sum conflict in which no concessions are possible. Much common ground often can be identified and used successfully, as when Stanford endorses home births, meditative healing for psychosomatic disorders, extended identification between doctors and patients, and other techniques that seem to combine dimensions of holistic and allopathic medicine. But in other areas, such as interpreting and using precognition about death, Stanford is a divided self with no ready instrument to coordinate the two parts of his psyche.

A second conflict arises between the individual and others—family, loved ones, friends, colleagues. An endorsement of psychic healing of whatever variety can be expected to produce astonishment in direct relationship to the orientation of the social context. To declare in a secular academic context, for example, that God can enter the temporal world and heal injuries is to risk social as well as intellectual censure. Pastors Penfield and Jamison broke at the margin with friends and families due to the emotive base of their (Pentecostal) conversion. But the religious background of their lives made the change less radical. When Stanford introduces the possibility of meditative healing in a hospital, he admits that he waits until the other doctors have left the room before advising a patient that there might be other sources of healing. Sometimes the spiritual contract can require a complete break with all friends and the acceptance of an entirely different social network.

The narrowest and in many ways the most stressful conflict occurs between the patient and physician. Stanford draws the noncompliant, the patients who break with their personal physicians because no accord can be reached on therapy that is satisfactory to both parties. Again, a break over holistic versus allopathic techniques need not follow differences in belief. Mrs. Canterbury not only urges both faith healing and conventional medical therapy on her husband but prays for her doctors. In one reported session, a physician despairing over ever helping his depressed patient finally suggested that they pray together (they are both Catholics). The impromptu prayer session helped restore some buoyancy to the patient and more standard medical therapy could resume. That Stanford could himself treat recalcitrant patients is one indication of holistic-allopathic congenialities. On the other hand, the fact that patients leave their regular physicians in search of unorthodox therapies also suggests the inherent conflict between unconventional and regular medical care.

Another conflict arises between and among discourse communities. It is a mistake to think that holistic and even psychic healing are part of some homogeneous set of beliefs. Deep incompatibilities disrupt the harmony that many seek in holistic therapy. LeShan's distinction between Type I and II healing reflect not only theoretical and practical distinctions but also schools of thought that do not always agree with each other. Religious differences are real and sometimes profound even within the same denominations. There is little doubt, for example, that the styles and religious orientations of Fathers Crossland and Brantley are not compatible. Father

Vecchio cannot accept some of the most central techniques used by his principal mentor, Father DiOrio. To accept one type of spiritual or psychic healing is often to find oneself in an adversarial relationship with rival approaches, though again broad compatibilities mark off the field of holistic therapies from allopathic medicine.

The most difficult conflict to adjudicate is the one that arises between the individual and the state. In liberal societies individuals are free to pursue idiosyncratic medicine so long as they do no harm to others and are legally competent. That is the guiding principle. We know, in fact, that the state will protect citizens from exploitation by disallowing many dubious medical practices. Laetrile is a prime example. Also, it is not always easy, and perhaps not even possible, to define competence in ways that satisfy both religious and secular expectation. The result is often a complex range of disputes between individual and state. Sometimes the dispute can be avoided when individuals flee to a different society to seek therapy denied in the resident's society (U.S. citizens going to Mexico for laetrile). At other times the dispute becomes an acrimonious encounter over the criteria for both medical care and competence in making decisions about such care. The most demanding conflict, however, is over the authority of the state to mandate treatment for children against their parents' wishes and beliefs.

In March 1984, a four-year-old girl died in California of acute bacterial meningitis. She had been ill for over two weeks. Her mother, Laurie Walker, is a Christian Scientist. She had chosen prayer over conventional medicine to heal her daughter. The California Supreme Court ruled that Ms. Walker could be prosecuted in the death of her daughter. In 1986, Robyn Twitchell, a two-year-old boy, died in Massachusetts of a bowel obstruction. The parents, also Christian Scientists, had summoned Christian Science practitioners to pray for their son's recovery. While a practitioner prayed over the boy, he grew progressively worse, went into convulsions, lost consciousness, and died. The parents were charged with manslaughter and arraigned in Suffolk County Superior Court. A jury later convicted them of involuntary manslaughter.

These two cases are disputes between the rights of parents to practice their religious beliefs and bring up their children in accordance with those beliefs, and the state's responsibility to protect life. Most states do exempt parents from seeking conventional medical care for their children when the parents believe in spiritual healing. But these laws do not endorse the efficacy of spiritual healing and (as in the California ruling) may not always extend to life-threatening illnesses. When the life of a child is involved, like that of Caleb Loverro in the dispute over treatment for leukemia, courts of law may favor compulsory medical treatment for the minor. In the California case, the court ruled that a jury would have to decide if the mother was responsible for her child's death.

Another part of this dispute concerns which form of healing is most effective, meaning which view of reality is to prevail when the patient is unable to exercise that liberty granted to competent individuals. Christian Scientists say that (a) there are numerous cases of healing that demonstrate the effectiveness of their approaches, and (b) conventional medicine also fails on occasion, and no one considers prosecuting a parent whose child dies under the care of a licensed physician. Medical authorities, on the other hand, typically do not acknowledge any evidence of healing caused by prayer, and accept spontaneous remissions of disease as anomalies to be expected of organisms as complex as a human being. Diagnoses are missed, and the body can heal itself even in cases of severe illness. But these phenomena are not accepted in medical practice as proof of the efficacy of prayer, and certainly not as reason to forgo medical care in serious illnesses. In this kind of dispute, the state may have to arbitrate among competing realities and may be forced to choose which one is the correct account of health, disease, and healing.

Public Conflict

Resolving disputes within the self is different, and less complicated, than resolving disputes among individuals. The individual can manage internal disputes in the most direct way by partitioning the self. Patients who see both the priest and the conventional physician are examples of partitioned selves. This method suggests deception at some level. Certainly from the perspective of an integrated and internally consistent individual, the self arranged as a package of mutually inconsistent beliefs is not very desirable. But another interpretation fits the data better. Those who use both spiritual and conventional therapy are simply using resources from two incompatible realities. Dividing the self to enter each of these worlds can be seen as a pragmatic effort to use whatever works without worrying about settling the complicated truths of each approach. These partitions in belief can be sustained by sequential arrangement of the experiences as well. Individuals who use rival methods of treatment typically see their respective healers alternately, never simultaneously. Dr. Stanford pursues conventional medical care for his patients, then raises the possibility of alternative therapies at some appropriate later moment.

The opposite of a partitioned self is the whole or integrated self. Here the conflict among alternative beliefs must be resolved in favor of one of the sets of beliefs. The conversion experience is arguably the most dramatic transformation of the self. In conversion, the partitioned self, a concept of the individual that flourishes in the pluralism of a liberal society, is abandoned and a new (or an old) self forged from some critical experience. Joanne Park was healed through a spiritual change that, she reports, made her whole. The hard choice between allopathic and holistic medicine has not been forced on her by circumstances. She is still a doctor. But her views on healing have been modified substantially, to the point that she routinely accepts intuitive or mystical influences in therapy.

Neither of these resolution patterns can be imported into public life without difficulties, since problems arise precisely on the distinctions between individual and collective experiences. The partitioned self is reflected in social pluralism. But social partitions can be tolerated only where vital issues are not at stake, or where the partitioned arrangement is not worth establishing. Imagine a society partitioned along the lines of slavery versus liberated practices. As in the disputes between orthodox and unorthodox medical practitioners when life is at stake for dependent humans, partitions could not be tolerated. Some judgment is usually required on the truth or acceptability of one (or more) of the opposed beliefs. Unlike individual life, collective life is a body of practices affecting other individuals, not just parts of the psyche.

More appropriate for social practices is the concept of an integrated self, especially where integration is secured by endorsing a set of beliefs or by discovering consistencies among competing beliefs. But even here the differences between self and collective are important. One can allow a dimension of the self to dominate other parts of the psyche, much like Plato argued for the authority of reason over spirit and desire. The results may be pleasing to the self as whole. But for society to be integrated, some individuals (not just beliefs) must dominate others, a process more complex morally than getting the psyche in order. In granting authority to the claims of allopathic medicine over holistic diets in the Caleb Loverro case, the state decided that the beliefs and practices of Dr. Dubansky took precedence over the beliefs and practices of the Loverros. One practical result was that Dr. Dubansky dominated the Loverros in determining therapy for Caleb. People, not just beliefs, are overridden in forging an integrated and thus consistent society.

The adversaries in the disputes over health and healing described here are opposed on what to do in the here and now, in effect over prescriptions that guide or compel forms of treatment for illness. They are not so commonly at odds with one another over evaluation, since all of the disputants accept the goodness of health and the badness of illness and death. Even here, however, the disputing parties differ over the meanings of these terms, which introduces additional complexity to all efforts to resolve the disputes.

The two broadest types of dispute follow from reasoning itself. In one, two or more sets of adversaries can use the same model of reasoning but oppose one another on different interpretations and/or extensions of basic terms. Abortion is an example of this type of dispute. Both pro-life and pro-choice advocates argue from acknowledged premises according to acceptable rules of inference and evidence. But the term "person" is given a radically different extension from one side to the other. Pro-life extends the term to the fertilized ovum; pro-choice withholds the extension until (usually) viability or birth. Polar moral, legal, and political views follow this conceptual disagreement. This model also helps to explain the dispute between allopathic and Christian Science beliefs, in which each community gives different interpretations to health and illness.

The disputes between allopathic and the various forms of holistic medicine are depicted more successfully in a different model, however. Even though each set of adversaries claims scientific status (demonstrated in the Family Court hearing over Caleb Loverro's therapy), each finally employs a different kind of reasoning to justify what is being asserted. Conventional medicine, descendant of modern science, relies on linear forms of reasoning where rules, evidence, and conclusions are explicit and open (in principle) to public inspection. Holistic traditions use science but also include different forms of reasoning. By its nature, meaning its reliance on beliefs in alternative realities not within conventional human experience, holistic medicine to some extent must employ narrative forms of reasoning. Intuitive or mystical experiences, or healing secured from a reality that cannot be described within the bounds of language, must be referred to obliquely by a variety of other linguistic devices that typically introduce evidence indirectly. This difference in forms of reasoning also characterizes disputes over therapy. When one observes that the Loverros and Stephen Dubansky were talking past one another, it helps to remember that they do not always share the same model of reasoning.

Disputes become political conflicts when the adversaries stop talking and begin acting. It is one of the marks of moral and political dispute that disagreement is not only a debate over principle and concepts but over directives for action. When the disputes and conflicts within the self extend to the ordering of society, then a political problem occurs. The acrimony of the social conflict can be fixed (in theory) by the relationship of both principles and action.

Conflict can occur when adversaries share the same principle of action. Again, the dispute over abortion illustrates the point. Both pro-life and pro-choice advocates share the same deep concern that urges respect for human life with a no-killing principle. But then each extends the principle in different ways to yield mutually contrary actions (no abortion, abortion by choice). The two opposed groups are in moral agreement at a deep level, but are in political conflict over the translation of a respect-for-life principle into social practice.

A moral conflict also can occur when adversaries disagree on principles yet agree on action. For example, two groups might both take a pacifist position on (a) the overriding and even absolute value of human life, or (b) a utilitarian concern to increase the population for industrial purposes. Two such groups are in a moral disagreement but present no political conflict. Their antagonistic principles lead to a singular action.

Moral and political agreement would require an accord on both principle and action. This possibility is more frequent than might be thought. A number of laws, those prohibiting homicide among them, follow deep and surface agreements on moral principles and the actions logically drawn from them. But an accord at both the principle and action levels of discourse also suggests the polar extreme of disagreement at both levels. Conflict can take the form of competing principles and actions, where no agreement is found either on what to do or how to justify actions. If we track the differences between allopathic and holistic medicine down one gradation away from principles respecting human life and health, then a thorough conflict does seem to occur. The medical principles held in each approach are often diametrically opposed to one another and the therapies that follow from these principles are not usually compatible. This pattern seems to characterize disputes over the efficacy of Christian Science, since prayer and meditation in this religion oppose and exclude medical principles of care. Such conflicts typically cannot be resolved by the disputants when the stakes are high (Caleb Loverro's life, for example) except by introducing the state to the dispute, which then brings in another form of rational discourse. The result is an additional level of conflict among principles, in the Loverro case (and others) the principles of parental authority versus the state's obligation to preserve life.

In some ways the conflict between allopaths and holists is an extreme variation on credentialing patterns. The problems occur on reasonable and well-known conditions. Liberal pluralism typically contains communities that endorse a variety of practices. When individuals in one or more of these practices begin to form a profession or discipline, they must rule out their rivals in order both to have professional standards and to establish those curricula in universities that will train individuals for the profession. (Astronomers ruled out astrologers as allopaths expelled homeopaths.) The problem is that the procedures used to adjudicate disputes may not be neutral among the rival communities. Also, the use of literary devices like stories and myths may only intensify the dispute; for when one of the sides relies in crucial ways on narratives to represent spiritual truths, no obvious algorithm exists to reach common conclusions. One consequence this pattern has for medicine is that the autonomy of dependent patients comes under pressure from the authoritative beneficence of physicians. Physicians, as professionals, must "know best" when unauthorized medical therapy is suggested or demanded. Otherwise professional credentials make no sense.

Resolution Patterns

Dispute resolution is a field of research with a variety of methods to manage or resolve conflict. The dispute, and resulting conflict, between allopathic and holistic medicine may be expressed as (a) differences in forms of reasoning, and (b) a disagreement on both principles and actions. It is an unusually difficult social conflict because it concerns methods of reasoning and occurs at two conceptual levels. Are there types of conflict management or resolution that can address these differences?

One common way to resolve conflict is through conflict itself: one or another of the partners to a dispute wins the battle. By the beginning of the twentieth century, allopathic medicine had achieved dominance over rival forms of treatment. Dominance, "winning," can be accomplished in any number of ways. Rival groups can be destroyed either literally or figuratively. Allopathic physicians discredited promoters of alternative medicines through the various state legislatures, successfully controlling those crucial accreditations that separate the professional from the bogus practitioner. Where licensing was not affected, as with homeopaths and chiropractors, access to hospitals and sometimes state and private funding (including, more recently, insurance coverage for some forms of alternative medicine) was denied. Each of these measures are common features of a conflict in which rivals try to undermine the credentials of the opposition, eliminating the alternative point of view by discrediting its intellectual and professional base.

More benign forms of winning are available. At an earlier stage of the abortion dispute, the conflict was regarded as one of attrition. Demographic data suggested that the pro-life position would slowly disappear because the movement consisted largely of middle-aged people who would naturally age, become less active, and finally die. But we know now, of course, that pro-life ideas have been taken up by new generations of activists. Another early prediction about abortion disputes was that the drug RU486 would be widely disseminated, with the result that first-term abortions would be largely private acts beyond the regulatory power of the state. Abortion would then fade as a public issue as the law became increasingly irrelevant as a controlling device. But the abortion dispute in the United States has extended to the marketing of RU486, with pro-life supporters threatening an economic boycott of pharmaceutical companies distributing the drug. The result has been an absence of RU486 in pharmacies and a continuation of the abortion dispute as a political conflict.

Still, these two methods of dispute management (hardly resolutions) are more civilized, and arguably more common, than undermining rival points of view. In the first case, the players change and the game is altered as a consequence; the conflict dissolves as one set of adversaries ceases to exist through attrition. In the second case, the conditions in terms of which the dispute occurs are changed and the dispute is extinguished as a consequence. In neither case, however, do moral and political discourses find a natural location. "Winning" simply eliminates rivals without respect for the opponent's values. Attrition and changes in the conditions of disputes are historical shifts that redefine disputes out of existence. Moral and political discourses typically seek settlements that in some way continue to recognize the adversaries.

The stronger methods of moral resolution are drawn from conversion theories. One convinces, educates, or persuades the opponent to adopt the morally correct view. A step down from conversion are the less satisfactory methods of mediation, conciliation, and negotiation, in which a resolution is sought that represents some acceptable fusion or combination of moral views. Sometimes bargaining and compromise are necessary parts of the resolving methods. On occasion the disputing parties will turn to arbitration, either binding or nonbinding, to reach a settlement. Normally one moves away from the ideal—successfully convincing the opponent of the rightness of one's course—with these alternative methods. Some methods, like bargaining or compromise, may be hostile to the main features of moral discourse (trading away a moral position seeming to most partisans to be immoral on the face of it). Binding arbitration may put the entirety of one's moral values at risk, since the outcome determined by the arbitrator must be accepted (often in law). But each of these methods attempts to incorporate the moral point of view in the collective outcome, something that cannot be said of simply "winning" the battle.

Therapy disputes of the sort that separated Caleb Loverro's parents and the child's physician, Stephen Dubansky, are not likely candidates for either a simple "winning" formula or moral settlements. First, neither side is likely to go out of existence. Allopathic medicine will likely continue to dominate health care in the West, but alternative medicine seems to be quite vigorous and may even be expanding. Moral settlements are also unlikely. The Loverros and Dubansky did engage each other in protracted discussions during the summer of 1987. Nothing came out of the discussions, and there is no reason to think that a third-party mediator would have been successful in resolving the disagreement. One reason for this failure is that the dispute concerned the primary goods of health and life. Not much can give way when an individual's continued existence is at the center of the dispute.

But the dialogues over cases like that of Caleb Loverro also fail because the rock-bottom assumptions about human experience are so different. One of the editorials in the local paper attacked Dubansky for claiming more certainty for his views than science allows, pointing out that yesterday's heresies are today's orthodoxies. Dr. Nicholas Gonzales, testifying as an expert witness for the Loverros, reminded those in the courtroom that the world was recognized as flat by the great astronomers of the fourteenth century and that this "expert" opinion did not mean that the earth is indeed flat. The conclusions of both the local editor and the expert witness was that conventional medicine cannot be authoritative because all of science is provisional, which then rules out the authoritative dismissal of alternative therapies in medicine.

It is true that in 1978 the American Cancer Society announced that there was no relationship between diet and cancer, and then, four years later, was recommending a high-fiber, low-fat diet to reduce the chances of getting cancer. But Dubansky's supporters could have pointed out that scientific change occurs with the introduction of new evidence and theories. The earth was not declared round by intuitionists but by those scientists who accumulated data to support a different theory of the solar system and its orbiting members. Precisely what Dubansky finds missing in the macrobiotic approach is evidence that diet *cures* cancer. Such evidence, if it could be found, would lead to different therapies for treating cancer. But even Joseph Loverro admitted that the claims for diet therapy are not based on firm studies. The terms of difference between the two adversaries include how evidence is to be used and what counts as evidence, not the provisional status of scientific statements.

Conventional medicine is an unusual species of social practice. It is a type of expert authority in conditions of risk and even uncertainty. Physicians are authorities on medical practice and subfields within medicine (they study general and specialized subjects for years in preparation for their practice). Yet the practice of medicine, especially pronounced in some specialties, is at times exceedingly uncertain. The relationship between aggressive therapy and outcomes cannot be known with reasonable certainty in intensive-care medicine, for example, especially when administered to the very young. At best probabilities can be fixed; at worst prognosis is based on intuition and educated guesses. The result in some areas of medicine is the spectacle of an expert authority proceeding in small, serial steps to an uncertain outcome.

Yet the steps taken in medicine are not pure guesswork. Physicians combine intuitions sharpened by clinical and experimental data, theoretical principles of disease, health, and the human body, and actual medical experience. Medical judgments are the result of a constant reciprocity between facts and theories. Practical results modify theories and practices, and theories reframe and reexplain facts. Nothing could be more pragmatic. But like all scientific effort, the practice of medicine is monitored by professionals who have absorbed the theoretical and practical knowledge of the various fields of medicine. The logic of this collective effort must be conservative (as in conserving) and resistant to alternative approaches that do not yield to the rules of evidence and inference accepted within the practice.

Alternative medicine uses different rules of reasoning. Its most obvious contrast with allopathic medicine is the way it defines the patient. In holistic medicine the whole person must be treated—body and mind or spirit. Therapy for the mind is not a conservative form of psychotherapy that mends and adjusts emotive or even cognitive disorders. The goal of therapy is a transformation of the spirit, of the individual's *identity*. This transformation is secured through contact with an alternative reality that exceeds the senses and in which conventional dualisms, especially between selves, are denied. The most helpful correlate of secular reasoning in these efforts is an intuition not constrained by empirical data but sensitive to the possibilities of alternative realities. Meditation, not scientific studies, is the preparation for these healing efforts.

It is unthinkable that moral discourses will be able to find a common ground between these two approaches to therapy *where they are in conflict*. Holistic and psychic healers often, perhaps typically, find compatible points with conventional medicine. But in the cases involving Christian Scientists' children, and in the case of Caleb Loverro, the lives of individuals are not reasonable terrain for adjustment among perspectives that have accepted competing, and sometimes mutually exclusive, realities.

It is also inconceivable on the logic of each type of discourse that privacy can be a regulatory principle. At the center of the notion of privacy is "competence" and the absence of "harm to another." When communities dispute over the nature of reality and its constituent parts, including the definitions of those who experience reality, and when these disputes extend to health and life, then privacy has no role to play in adjudicating the dispute. Again, these observations are not stipulations formed from the outside of such disputes but a logical implication of the fact that "competence" is not generalizable across the competing communities, and the stakes are high enough that they cannot be left to the discretion of individuals not in agreement over basic terms. To grant discretionary authority to individuals to decide on issues of health and life requires that these individuals be competent. No such assignment can be made except within the discourse communities disputing over medical care.

Nor will the distance between these two approaches to health care be closed with the methods common to current political and moral theory. One cannot *add* the different views produced from allopathic and holistic principles to reach some agreeable collective outcome. Social utility can serve as a universal product of competing values only when the values share some common scale, which allopathic and holistic values do not when they are opposed to one another. Nor will various formulations of consent, even those developed on hypothetical grounds, succeed in reconciling these principles. The basic languages used in each view are sufficiently unlike one another that agreement is unimaginable. Rudimentary maximization formulae are unusable as well, since neither a common scale nor criteria for maximizing a mix of these principles are available. More may not be better from the point of view of those opposed to the values to be maximized or distributed.

The strategy of regulation that seems to be most promising consists of the following steps. First, since allopathic and holistic principles are incompatible along a certain range of values, any regulatory effort must introduce some understanding of costs. In this instance costs do not refer to economic disadvantages but to the realization that some part of the value programs of one or all positions will have to be given up in a social practice that includes both sets of principles. Second, the collective arrangement that includes these principles must be defined even without benefit of the standard devices used to produce social distributions—moral discourse, privacy shields, utilitarian composition rules, social choice or consent, and maximization formulae. Yet the collective arrangement is vital to an understanding of all sets of competing principles, since values that are disparate in independent domains may be compatible as entries in a coherent whole. This whole may even reduce values to more basic items while rearranging them in a heterogeneous social pattern where even primary goods may be partitioned along different dimensions of a single collective practice.

Third, and most offensive to liberal temperaments, force may be a natural concomitant of regulation directed toward principles that compete at fundamental levels. Coercion may even be the welcome alternative to neutrality, a prospect that itself compels an examination of the competing dimensions of political power.

LIBERAL POWER

Liberal Governance

Connections between power and truth are typically complex and uneasy, though they are sometimes seen as simple and direct. Classical philosophers viewed power and truth as intimately connected. Plato's *Republic* made mastery of the higher forms the condition for political authority. For Plato, the state is an expression of basic moral principles. But the critic views power and truth as adversaries competing with each other on the common ground of political space. The critical approach to this relationship informs the modern liberal temperament. A liberal state is grounded not on truth but on the recognition that multiple claims to truth exist in human communities. The ideal relationship of the state to these claims is one of tolerance, a perspective best defined as neutrality toward the convictions of competing groups trying to mold power to their own versions of truth.

The story of liberal governance is benign enough so long as it is maintained as an ideal. It goes like this: Factions compete in public space for allocations of scarce resources and control of the accounts of reality used to define both allocation and resources. The state uses empty procedures that manage and perhaps resolve conflict in an unbiased manner. Politics is a kind of sustained conflict maintained in a shifting equilibrium by a state that avoids endorsing the substantive values of the competing factions. Leavening this pure tolerance is typically a respect for primary goods. The state will often protect and promote goods thought to have strong generalizing powers across communities. Life, for example, is usually viewed as such a good and is protected even by minimal states that do almost nothing else. Even here, however, competent individuals are usually given discretionary authority to act on such goods according to their own convictions so long as these actions do not affect others adversely. The composite picture is of a state managing conflict and protecting those primary goods deemed valuable independent of community beliefs while respecting the privacy of competent individuals to endorse, select, and reject those goods if the negative consequences of their actions are isolated, affecting only themselves.

So many points in the liberal story invite qualifications and critiques that interpretations of liberalism have no natural starting point. Even basic distinctions—between formal and substantive values, for example—plead for more examination. But critical understandings of liberalism can be drawn from two areas. One is obvious: the factions competing in that public space marked off by liberal tolerance do not always subscribe to those liberal doctrines that guide the state in managing conflict. Spiritual convictions about health and healing, for example, require holistic arrangements that are hostile to the dualisms of liberal practices. In spiritual communities truth is singular, not pluralistic, and human experience in general is regarded as holistic, not partitioned. Spiritual communities often dismiss the liberal separation of church and state by endorsing a concept of social harmony and even unity that brings all human events together in a single framework. The practical result of such beliefs is that the liberal state must govern communities on the basis of ideas not necessarily accepted by all those who are governed. The separation of state and church must occur at least de facto on the requirement that the state distance itself from the holism found in so many spiritual communities.

The second understanding of liberalism is introduced with the existence of communities that compete at the most basic levels—over primary goods, rights and liberties, and views of reality. Competition at fundamental levels of human experience is an expectation of liberalism, since tolerance of multiple truths encourages pluralism at all levels. In a standard theoretical phrase, the right dominates the good in liberal practices, meaning that the formal procedures of justice and effectiveness, rather than the particular visions of the good life embraced by citizens in the political society, are the instruments of authority used by the state. In one way, the fact of pluralism helps to maintain the distance of formal procedures from substantive goods, for a state that tries to represent a variety of interests cannot be bound too tightly to any one version of human life underlying any of the competing interests. Nor can such a state fix limits on the range of ontological beliefs. The liberal state, on its own logic, must be prepared to govern competing visions of reality.

A problem occurs, however, when ontologies as different from each other as spiritual and secular enter rival claims in public space that are based on incommensurate understandings of reality. The problem can be stated briefly: no common languages may be available to adjudicate disputes among the entries.

A wide variety of literatures addresses the problem of competing and at least partially incommensurate discourses. Anthropologists and philosophers have long pondered the task of extending explanation and understanding across radically different cultures or systems of belief. The resulting discussions have produced insights and sustained disagreements on translation from one vocabulary to another. One of the more intriguing issues in these discussions is the role of rules, reasons, and causes in social theory. Historians of science must also negotiate this problem when they characterize transitions from one scientific paradigm or discourse community to another.

The political problem is normative. It centers on those circumstances that occasion state decisions to regulate disputes among discourses and to tolerate or override community beliefs regarded as unorthodox on conventional values. The existence of competing discourse communities is not just a compelling theoretical topic in liberal practices but a set of issues that the state must address in one way or another. Incommensurate discourses can and do occupy a single area when competing in public space. And the state, in spite of all liberal needs for neutrality, may have to decide at particular points whose way of life is superior when fundamental beliefs collide.

Translations and Neutralities

Complete incommensurability among human communities may be only an intellectual's thought experiment. One can imagine what incommensurate experiences might be like, even when translation between them fails. In the movie *Altered States*, the main character is transmuted from human to ape for a period of several hours. In recounting the experience after resuming human form he cannot adequately describe what it was like, saying only that he was in a continual state of *now*, with no past or future, and that he seemed to *be* desire (not a reflective self driven by desire). Even the imaginative exercise falls short of complete translation, though it is intriguing as an effort to depict a nonhuman consciousness.

It is more difficult to imagine or find human communities that are wholly incommensurate. What would such communities look like? Perhaps none of the primary goods routinely assigned to human life would be found, or those goods would be inverted in inexplicable ways. Imagine a society that consumed rocks for nourishment, routinely slaughtered its members without any show of resistance by the victims, and did not know or experience affection. The imaginative possibilities seem endless, but would in each case include the feature of unintelligibility. Two incommensurate societies could not find common ground for understanding since nothing could be translated into a language generalizable to both societies' members.

Individuals viewing a strongly incommensurate social life from the outside would not regard it as a human community, because they would have no grounds for identifying it as such, nothing to say that humans rather than, say, androids or alien life forms are populating the community. Even designating what is observed as an action, or a community, or even an experience, might be wrong. Strong incommensurability makes translation impossible. Yet even here the judgment is misleading in suggesting that there is something present that cannot be translated. If one is entirely outside of another form of life, without access to any of its internal meanings, one cannot even be sure that there *are* meanings to be translated. The subject of one's puzzlement might be an insect colony, or some analogous social form without members capable of using language in any conceivable way.

The thought that human communities can be incommensurate may be based on a failure to identify beliefs that are universal in human experience. Beliefs can range over spectrums that seem to have no limits. The dominant characteristic of human communities and individuals may be their capacity to define and redefine experiences in multiple and conflicting ways.

But does the range of possible beliefs extend so far as to escape commensurability? Imagine two societies, A and B. In A the individual members believe in witches and electrons; in B they do not. Suppose also that differences in rules of evidence and inference are so considerable that no common language permits a generalizable answer to the question, do witches and electrons exist? Yet to say that A and B are incommensurate requires a metalanguage that must include both societies. This syntactic language establishes a kind of third community of discourse that describes and may even explain the reasoning typifying A and B. The truth of statements about witches and electrons cannot be addressed in the metalanguage, since to say whether these things exist would require entering and endorsing one of the two sets of community beliefs (A or B). But the metalanguage has thin explanatory powers that at least permit the statements supporting the judgment that A and B are incommensurate. Strong incommensurability seems to be impossible, since it depends on a language that denies its own claim.

It is more likely that communities are partially incommensurate, obscure on some dimensions of social life while accessible on others. Also, we often say that beliefs are incommensurate when they address common terms but give radically different interpretations of them. All human communities must address certain "constants" in experience, for example birth and death. But it is not uncommon for understandings of these terms to differ radically. Even to say that different understandings exist is already to rely on languages that comprehend and express these differences. Differences can be exaggerated by the apparent variability of all terms. Even definitions of what is real vary with ways of life and are often the most decisive variables in human communities. But even these differences can be monitored and understood to some extent.

The crucial point is that competing and often mutually exclusive accounts of human experience occur but are usually accessible. Their accessibility is precisely what raises the problems of understanding and translation across systems of belief. If ways of life were strongly incommensurate, these problems would not occur (and we could not even characterize the disparate patterns of "ways of life").

The issue that helps fix the normative role of the state in societies with rival ways of life is whether access requires endorsement. Belief and understanding each vary in different ways depending on a number of conditions. Education, for example, can and typically does affect understandings of religious experience. The question is whether belief and understanding are variables of one another. There is much to suggest that they are. As one understands a system of belief more fully, a religion for example, one's beliefs as a member of the system can change. Similarly, a believing member of a religious order obviously understands the religion in a different way than someone who does not believe and as a consequence stands outside the system. These connections between belief and understanding can be found in a wide variety of practices and are generally expressed in the thought that endorsing or accepting a belief alters the understanding of the experience in which the belief occurs.

The more interesting issue, however, is whether explanation is influenced by belief. Strong traditions in modern philosophy maintain that explanation and belief can be two independent discourses, at least in the sense that one can explain a system of belief without subscribing to the beliefs themselves. A different version of this independence claim, one prominently displayed in the social sciences, is that explanation must be shielded from endorsement in order to be adequate or successful. In both versions of independence, explanation is said to be adequately conducted without endorsing the beliefs that are being explained. Also, explanation seems immune from those changes in beliefs that can affect understanding. Explanation can stand clear of the mental state of the agent in ways that under-standing does not, especially when it is based on objective standards with general appeal.

But it is equally clear that the criteria for completing an explanation can depend on the acceptance or rejection of beliefs. Think, for example, of an observer studying a religious practice. Say that one of the core beliefs of this practice is that human experience is part of a larger design accessible in part by means of meditation and prayer. A secular observer, one who rejects the truth of this belief, will explain the religious practice in causal terms set within the variables of empirical reality. This observer's explanation of the religion will be considered complete when all observable events have been accounted for with a theory confined to the material or temporal world. A religious observer, one who subscribes to the core belief, will frame a differ-ent explanation. A complete explanation then must include the design re-vealed in part to humans by God.

This linkage of beliefs to both understanding and explanation affects the possibility of neutrality. If one understands and explains things differently according to the acceptance or denial of the truth of beliefs, then there can be no discourse independent of the values informing beliefs. Even the way that social practices are defined would seem to require that the individual take some position on the truth of beliefs in the practice. Religion may be the most difficult practice on which to establish neutrality, since the realities on which religious beliefs are founded would compel the individual to view hu-man experience in spiritual terms. These terms are precisely what are con-tested in those secular societies that value neutrality so highly.

Governing Languages

Imagine moving across the conceptual space between secular and spiritual communities, entering each system of beliefs and *seeing* the rival senses of completeness in both understanding and explanation. The linguistic cur-rency of such a traveler would be metalanguages, those that provide access without resolution. This thin language of access could survey beliefs, ren-dering them intelligible, or commensurate. But the truth of the beliefs would be settled in a thicker language that community members use in en-gaging proper interpretation, evidence, and inference. This thick language is the currency of the community. Visitors would not be able to extend it across domains that have rival understandings of reality.

Any inspection of terms in secular and spiritual languages will demon-strate this point. Elaborating the imaginative exercise can help. Think again of the two domains, spiritual and secular, as separated in conceptual space. Now visualize the languages found in each domain as moving across the empty area separating the regions. The task is to monitor the changes that occur as terms enter and leave each field. The goal is to identify which terms are reasonably constant across fields and which are variable. This will allow us to construct two additional domains, one consisting of terms that are general to both spiritual and secular domains, another consisting of those that vary as they enter and leave the rival areas. State efforts to protect life are based on something like this exercise. These efforts are typically justified on the grounds that life is a primary good, at least of starting value in any discourse.

Unfortunately for liberal expectations, all terms can vary between spiritual and secular domains. Social vocabularies obviously vary. What we can know, and how human individuals are defined, can be extremely sensitive to shifts in domain. Spiritual knowledge relies on the unknown for interpretations of human experience. The unknown may support faith against falsifying events. Secular knowledge claims, by contrast, are more easily falsifiable (and alterable) by experience. Different understandings of the individual follow from these differences in knowing. Spiritual communities, as we have seen in our journeys through various forms of healing, view individuals as dual arrangements of spirit and body. A holistic arrangement dominated by spiritual concerns can even unify these two dimensions by absorbing body into spirit. Secular views of individuals can be complete with an account of body, including brain but not spirit.

Even the biosocial terms often taken to be reasonably constant in human experience—birth, life, health, healing, death—are also influenced by differences between spiritual and secular domains. "Birth" is a contested concept in a variety of community disputes, including those over abortion. "Life" is defined in competing ways in current disputes over life-support maintenance in intensive-care medicine. "Death" can be defined in secular medicine, but new technologies seem to force amendments to each definition. To the spiritual practitioner, death may be only a passage to a different reality. The meanings of "health" and "healing" can differ so widely that they contribute to basic distinctions separating spiritual and secular domains.

Sometimes languages are explicitly contextual. Some spiritual discourses use terms, representing concepts like God, sin, and salvation (in Christianity), that are meaningful primarily within spiritual domains. Other terms, those representing concepts of authority, freedom, legitimacy, and the like, seem to extend across communities, including the community of governance, which might be their natural home. It is precisely the generalizing features of political discourses that suggest a neutral form of governing from outside systems of belief. But when beliefs differ on what to count as real, which is the basis for demarcating secular and spiritual communities, even the languages of governance become subject to contextual influences. This is particularly difficult for liberal philosophies to manage.

Liberalism entertains both minimal and aggressive versions of state power. The libertarian origins of liberal political theory outline power restricted to the protection of citizens from physical assault. Liberal theory also justifies an interventionist state, one that redistributes goods and resources to meet the needs of social justice. The range of state functions extends these minimal protections of life and property to more aggressive interventions that promote the public good, ensure that social distributions are just, and assist the weak and powerless.

Whether one selects a libertarian or interventionist point on this range, the task is the same: how to establish the boundaries between individual autonomy and state power. The principles that liberal political thought commonly uses to set these boundaries are assemblages of negative rights that ensure autonomy by shielding individuals from regulation by the state. Liberal governance then proceeds in those areas outside the spheres of liberty marked off by rights vocabularies.

One of the most important negative rights is *privacy*. As many jurists have noted, it expresses a common theme in negative rights that insulate persons and property from incursions by others and by the state. The rights of free speech, assembly, freedom from illegal searches and seizures, and other protections are shields that give individuals discretionary authority to act autonomously. Privacy describes that zone of moral space established by such protections. Another interpretation of privacy is also vital. It is a principle that allows individuals to control information about themselves. The power to order relationships follows from this control. One discloses more information to intimates, less to acquaintances and strangers. The dispersal of information authorized by the individual establishes the ordering.

The two conditions that establish privacy in liberalism and ensure those shields that permit negative liberty are competence and the absence of harm to others. Individuals who are mentally sound and have sufficient amounts of correct information, and whose actions do not harm others, are free to make choices even when these choices are not in their best interests.

It is easy to see how this model world of liberal choice works ideally. If the individual is the origin of meaning and value in society, and society itself is a convenient fiction to describe arrangements that are reducible to individual properties, then the idea of competent and informed individuals making choices free from interference follows naturally. But the principle fails whenever different understandings of reality compete in a liberal political society.

The failure of privacy to set boundary conditions begins with the contradictions that can occur between negative liberty and information. It is obvious that institutions must provide access to, and amounts of, information if individuals are to be knowledgeable. The power of various institutions to influence, factor, interpret, and in general control information even in liberal societies is widely acknowledged and discussed. Dispute arises over what constitutes correct information. Competing understandings of reality can lead to differences over "facts" and the relationships among events (proper therapy in medicine, for example). When introduced to the naturally coercive powers of information to maintain and change behavior, and to the way facts can lead and even compel choices, negative freedom can be entirely subordinate to different beliefs about reality.

Multiple realities also produce different understandings of competence. Mental soundness can be fixed in universalizable ways. Children are not competent by virtue of age, regardless of their beliefs or acumen. Severe brain damage can incapacitate individuals in any community. But one sign of a cognitive disorder is an idiosyncratic view of reality. A belief that we can talk to God is at least a starting reason to doubt the competence of the believer in secular contexts. But to deny the reality of God's design for the universe may be a sign of cognitive flaws in religious contexts. The problem in liberal contexts is settling on the formal qualities of competence when rival communities have mutually antagonistic understandings of the term competence itself.

The interventionist side of the liberal agenda fares no better in escaping community influence. Suppose that principles of justice indemnify the activities of the state outside established zones of negative liberty. Distributive arrangements can be judged as proper or improper depending on the ways the distribution has occurred (fulfilling liberty, for example) or the fit between the distribution and certain structural principles of equality (or warranted inequality). But principles justifying distributions are elastic terms yielding multiple, and mutually contradictory, meanings. There is no reason to think that any particular interpretation is privileged. Additional values are needed to select from among the various senses of equality and liberty that the liberal menu provides. If these values are drawn from understandings of reality, from spiritual convictions, no objection can be raised on liberal grounds.

The methods used to derive or identify liberal principles of government are also subject to community values. Remember that in liberalism individuals are the sources for social values and principles of governing. Utilitarianism is arguably the most famous sideshow in moral philosophy, producing social values by applying arithmetical composition rules to individual utilities. Social contract theory has used both omniscience and sublime ignorance to identify principles of justice. In both of these traditions, different as they are from one another, the individual is defined as an abstraction, separate from context and not identifiable with any point of view or particular understanding of reality. Rather, the self is an Archimedean point from which the basic values and structures of society may be derived.

The problem with this construction is a familiar one. There is no neutral vantage point, no high ground from which to produce governing principles that is not itself influenced by other social values. The abstract self cannot be the source for social values or the origin of social structures if it is completely empty of social content. A hypothetical self that had no knowledge of causal relations, of human longevity and needs, of family relations and practices, could not possibly choose those states of affairs or guiding principles that liberalism demands. But the introduction of these considerations into utility formulations or the social contract brings community values into liberalism. Who is to say which causal relations are correct? Is human mortality fixed at the death of the body? What are human needs? How do groups define individuals and individuals define groups? The point is always the same: the formal devices used in liberalism to set the conditions for resolving disputes cannot function without first introducing those discourses that occasion the disputes in the first place. The unwelcome point is that community always seems to precede formal constructions of both the social good and justice.

The implications of this point for spiritual communities and the liberal state are both inevitable and distressing for liberal expectations. The boundary conditions between individual autonomy and the state must always be both in flux and subject to the community values dominating a political society at any given time. Privacy is vulnerable to definitions of competence. The social good and justice cannot be identified in the absence of community values that contribute to an understanding of human experience. Put in extreme form, we would say that the formal side of governance is both empty and a fiction. The differences among spiritual communities, and between such communities and conventional medicine, insinuate themselves into the apparatus used by liberal states to govern these differences.

In liberal thought state neutrality requires (1) an objective language of governance, one that is entirely or at least partially outside the languages of those communities being governed; (2) neutral resolutions or management procedures; (3) the existence of core terms that define social practices in generalizable ways; (4) the presence of individuals who are competent according to criteria acceptable to all relevant communities. When we inspect these four requirements, however, we find that they cannot be met in any coherent or comprehensive way. Instead, community values seem to dominate the efforts of the state to remain neutral.

The failure of state neutrality follows the recognition of metalanguages. Since commensurability between radically different communities is too slight to support judgment, impartial governance fails. Both forbearance and intervention are biased, the first implicitly endorsing beliefs and the second rejecting beliefs.

The darker, unacceptable side of this picture is that state power may be arbitrary. An arbitrary choice is one for which alternatives exist, but there are no reasons to favor any one or more alternatives over any others. A version of arbitrariness occurs in the exercise of liberal power. The pluralistic setting of liberal societies, where different and competing discourse communities enter claims in public space, provides a variety of criteria to adjudicate the claims. These criteria, however, can be specific to the communities. When this occurs, the state has competing reasons to favor and dismiss claims but no compelling reasons to do so, since nothing may privilege one community perspective over any other. On these occasions, the state must legislate without reasons that can be generalized between state and community, and on grounds that must be regarded as arbitrary from any point outside the dispute in question.

It is easy, too easy, to conclude that liberal politics is a species of madness, in the direct sense that the state claims neutrality and objective principles when the exercise of power is partisan on any reasonable examination. It is both more accurate and generous to say that the state is simply another player in such disputes, not the umpire outside the action as liberalism has assumed. The state is a community like all others, except that it possesses more substantial amounts of power.

Practical Realities: Christian Science

David Twitchell is a third-generation Christian Scientist. He grew up in a comfortable middle-class home on Long Island in New York. His father had a Ph.D. in business and taught elementary school. His maternal grandmother was a Christian Science practitioner. Both of his paternal grandparents were members of the Church as were his parents. He and his brother were raised in the faith. He went to Sunday school at a local Church of Christ, Scientist, though he attended public schools from elementary through high school. Like most teenagers, he doubted his faith from time to time, especially the doctrine that the only true reality is God's creation and not the physical world accepted in commonsense beliefs. But the influence of his family, the testimonies in the Church, the periodicals and Bible sessions, convinced him that Mary Baker Eddy's writings are true and that the idealistic view of reality that is the foundation of Christian Science is correct.

Twitchell reports that he was not taken to doctors as a child, except for one visit to an otolaryngologist. He remembers that the doctor recommended ear surgery and that his parents decided against it. They opted for prayer. The ear healed naturally, without medicine or surgery. On one occasion he fell off his bicycle while racing a friend downhill during a picnic and cut his hand on a broken bottle. The friend he was racing also fell and cut his hand. Twitchell's mother picked them both up and took his friend home first. The friend's parents took him to the hospital where he received stitches. Twitchell's mother took him home, bandaged his hand, and then prayed for healing. Both sets of injuries healed without incident.

Later, while in college, he fell out of a jeep and "got banged up pretty bad." He was unconscious for a time, and then "mentally totally out of it" for a week or so. A Christian Science nurse and a practitioner prayed for him during this time. His parents decided not to call in a doctor. Twitchell's memories of that week are vague and unreliable. He recalls praying with the practitioner, and even taking part in the decision to forgo medical care, though he remembers that he was "like a child to some extent" because of his head injuries. Again he recovered without medical intervention.

The one exception to this exclusionary practice toward medical care was dentistry. Twitchell's parents regularly took him and his brother to see a dentist. As an adult he has gone to a dentist twice. Both times he tried prayer first, in one case for over six months. Neither problem yielded until a dentist addressed them. One was a broken filling that required root canal surgery because he had waited so long before seeking treatment. He has also had two wisdom teeth extracted. Twitchell follows his parents in taking his own children to dentists. He explains these aberrations in terms of a recognition within Christian Science that bone situations are harder to deal with spiritually than other problems. But he still regards this concession as a deviation from an ideal that others, spiritually stronger than he, may be able to realize.

Twitchell believes that turning to God is the best solution to any problem—emotional, physical, financial, whatever. But the prayer, the appeal to God, does not always succeed. The reasons for failure are always deficiencies in the petitioner. Twitchell likens failures in spiritual healing to medical intervention that fails because of a physician's inadequacy. A surgeon, for example, may not perform an operation successfully because he has limited knowledge or training, or because the case is unexpectedly complicated or different from medical expectations. To succeed in similar cases, he may have to get further education or acquire different skills. Twitchell believes that God's powers are unlimited. But the human practitioner may not have the spiritual knowledge or skills equal to the problem being addressed. Twitchell points out that a child may be able to add 2 plus 2 to get 4 but may be stumped by 240 divided by 4. The rules are still there, however, to be discovered through further study. Twitchell admits that his own failures in spiritual healing can be attributed to his lack of understanding, to not being able to get close enough to God in his thoughts, with the result that he cannot always use God's powers well enough to heal. But he believes that the method of prayer cannot be faulted.

Twitchell views medicine as the best alternative to prayer in addressing health problems. If prayer is not working, Twitchell believes that the next step is medical therapy. The problem is deciding when prayer is not working, and how and when to turn to medicine. He fears the mechanistic logic of medical practice, the inertial tendencies to treat once an individual has entered medical domains. For example, he worries that if he brings his children in for a diagnosis, he will inevitably have to surrender his discretionary power to accept or reject therapy. So he has been cautious in turning to medicine, convinced as he is that partial or provisional treatment is impossible. It is all or nothing in medicine from his point of view, though he would still turn to medical therapy if a serious illness did not yield to prayer. Christian Science strictly interpreted does not permit medical therapy.

Twitchell's views on spiritual healing are orthodox, however. The healing that he sees as following prayer is not mind over matter but God's power over matter. One practical consequence of this view is that the placebo effect can be "real" although finally not important. God heals, according to Twitchell, not the attitude of the patient (or practitioner). This means that all illnesses, not just those intimately linked to mental states, can be cured through God's intervention. Twitchell admits that he has not seen a serious illness like spinal meningitis healed through prayer. But he accepts the written and verbal testimonies of others who have witnessed such healings, much as (he points out) patients who go to doctors have not observed medical successes but are satisfied with testimonies that medicine does indeed work.

Twitchell also accepts the role of diet, exercise, and the like as preventive maintenance, helping the individual avoid illnesses. But he worries that a preoccupation with the body distracts the individual from the spiritual dimensions of life. He is convinced that a preventive prayer system, a "spiritualizing" of thoughts, is more effective than any physical precautions an individual might take. In many states, the children of Christian Scientists are exempted from vaccinations. Twitchell claims that these children are protected from the diseases normally prevented by vaccination through the alternative of prayer. The body must be taken seriously, according to Twitchell, and its integrity maintained, but primarily because its breakdown indicates a spiritual problem ("a smudge on the mirror") that must be addressed. But the proper and most effective method to attend to the body is prayer, not physical modifications and interventions.

David Twitchell attended Principia College, a Christian Science college in Elsah, Illinois, for two and one-half years. Then he transferred to the State University of New York at Stony Brook in Long Island (his native grounds). After graduating in 1978 he worked for Nathan's Famous, a popular and well-known firm on Long Island, and later took an administrative position with Open Door, a retirement home for Christian Scientists. By the mid-1980s he and his wife, Ginger, had two young sons. They had lived in California briefly (and unhappily) and were now residing in the Boston area. Twitchell and his wife are both deeply religious and were practicing the principles of Christian Science in their home. Neither they nor their children were being attended to by medical doctors.

In April of 1986 an event occurred that severely tested the faith of the Twitchells. It evolved into the ultimate nightmare for all parents. On Thursday evening, April 3, the younger of the two children, Robyn, began crying. Mrs. Twitchell heard the two-year-old child and woke up her husband. He went in the children's room and, since Robyn was being toilet trained at that time, he took the child to the bathroom. There was no bowel movement, so when Mrs. Twitchell came in the parents put the child's diaper back on. During the diapering they asked him if he hurt. He put his hand on his abdomen. But he also stopped crying. Then, because the other child, Jeremy (three years old at the time), shared the bedroom with Robyn and was still asleep, the parents took Robyn to the living room. There Mrs. Twitchell stayed with him for the rest of the night while her husband got some sleep. During this time Robyn threw up twice. In the morning Twitchell took the child to the bathroom where he had a bowel movement.

While Twitchell was at work, his wife called a Christian Science practitioner. The practitioner began praying for Robyn, though she did not immediately come over to the Twitchell home. Robyn slept most of the day on Friday and did not eat anything. On Saturday morning he threw up and during the evening hours he spit up, but during the day he was "quite well, he had a good time and played." Saturday was the Twitchells' wedding anniversary and they went out to dinner, though they made it a quick dinner because of their younger son's illness. Both children stayed with friends while they were out. Robyn threw up while the Twitchells were away, but he also ate some rice or mashed potatoes (the family keeping tabs on him was not sure which dish he had).

On Sunday Robyn "still had ups and down." Twitchell took Jeremy to church while his wife stayed with Robyn at home. That afternoon the practitioner came over to see Robyn. The previous day she had advised the Twitchells to call the Christian Science Church to find out whether the law would permit them to continue treatment through prayer in this case. The Twitchells did make this call and were advised by a Church spokesperson that the law allowed them to use prayer as an alternative to medicine. At their later trial this call was used by the prosecution to suggest that they were interested only in protecting themselves legally. But Twitchell is adamant in his view that they believed prayer was best and were only determining if the law permitted them to use this best method for healing. On Sunday the Twitchells also decided to call a Christian Science nurse. She advised them to give Robyn small spoonfuls of liquid or broth at frequent intervals rather than trying to get him to eat at meals. The prayers continued.

Robyn was still not eating on Monday, and still throwing up when he tried. By Monday evening the Twitchells were concerned enough to switch practitioners. These changes are common in Christian Science, for it is generally accepted that practitioners sometimes do not do well with a particular kind of illness. They may have tried before and were not successful, or they may simply feel that something is going on that keeps them from maintaining the spiritual approach needed to heal that kind of problem. When this occurs the practitioner may decide to withdraw, or the family may simply seek another practitioner. But the Twitchells were not able to reach a different practitioner on Monday evening.

On Tuesday morning Robyn seemed much better. In David Twitchell's words, "he made a major turnaround, he was bright, cheery, he was up and about, he was interactive." The parents decided to stay with the original practitioner since they were now convinced that the spiritual intervention had worked, "had beaten the problem, whatever it was." That evening Robyn joined the family at the dinner table and "indicated that he wanted supper." They gave him a few spoonfuls of baby food. Then he drank a large glass of water, after which he "threw up badly." The Twitchells took Robyn to his room and placed him in bed. He was twisting and turning, obviously in pain and unable to get comfortable. David Twitchell's mother was due to arrive by train that evening to help care for Jeremy while Robyn was ill. Just before Twitchell left for the station to meet her, Robyn stopped writhing and seemed to be resting comfortably. Mrs. Twitchell bathed him during this time. In the bath the child vomited again. The smell of this vomit seemed different to the mother, though she did not recognize it as feces. (The doctors for the prosecution testified at the trial that Robyn would have been vomiting his own feces at the end.) She just knew that the vomit looked and smelled different and that things were going badly. She called the practitioner. When she could not reach her she called Nathan Talbot, the Church spokesperson. He tried to calm her down and advised her to call the practitioner again. This time she reached her. The practitioner left immediately for the Twitchell home, arriving just as Twitchell returned with his mother and Jeremy.

The remainder of the evening is a blur of events in David Twitchell's memories. He remembers holding Robyn, his wife holding Robyn, the prayers of the practitioner, then Robyn's eyes closing part-way, and the child slightly shaking or shuddering. Then stillness and Twitchell looking for a pulse and not finding any. Then the words he was thinking spoken by the practitioner, "He must have passed on." The sense of time is lost to Twitchell at this point. He remembers the practitioner praying a bit more, then calling the Church and returning with the suggestion that he call a funeral home. Then the practitioner went downstairs. He called the funeral home and when they found out no doctor was in attendance they told him to call 911, the emergency number. He did, and the personnel there advised him to start CPR immediately. He brought the phone out from the bedroom into the hall so that he could follow the instructions on CPR. His wife was holding Robyn, "falling apart in her own way," and would not let go of the child. Twitchell had to take the child from her, get her to hold the phone to his ear while she was crying so he could perform CPR according to the directions being given on the phone. Then the siren, and the lights flashing on the wall from the arrival of the ambulance, Twitchell running downstairs to let the medical technicians in and seeing the Christian Science practitioner praying in the kitchen, Mrs. Twitchell going to see if Jeremy had been awakened by the noise and lights. Twitchell put on his shoes and followed the ambulance in his car. At the hospital a doctor came into the waiting room and questioned him about the child's illness and what had gone on. The doctor also called Mrs. Twitchell and asked her some questions. Mainly, however, he confirmed the single dominating fact of the evening. Two hours after sitting with his family at the dinner table, Robyn Twitchell was dead. An autopsy the next day revealed that he had died of a bowel obstruction.

One might say that there are two ways to look at the events leading up to and including Robyn Twitchell's death. One is, God's will be done. The other is, if only *a*, *b*, *c* had been done we could have saved the child's life. Twitchell does not believe that any child's death is God's will. He points out that Jesus loved children, healed children. Twitchell says that he would not sacrifice his child. He is not convinced that medical doctors could have diagnosed the disease initially, since the symptoms resembled a mild case of the flu and there is no history of bowel obstructions in his family. At the end they may not have been able to save Robyn since surgery would have been required, and the child already was weakened and dehydrated by four to five days with the obstruction. But on the basic point he is clear. If Robyn could have been saved by medical treatment, Twitchell wishes they would have turned to that and brought the boy to a doctor immediately.

The death of their younger son was obviously a crisis of faith for the Twitchells. David Twitchell believes that if Christ Jesus or one of his disciples, or Mary Baker Eddy, had been ministering to the child that Robyn would have been saved. He believes that his son would have been healed had he, David Twitchell, "done better." But he and his wife have kept their faith and still rely on prayer. He is not sure he would turn to medical care any sooner in the face of serious illness, for he continues to believe that spiritual intervention is more effective than medicine. But if he saw the same symptoms that Robyn exhibited in any of his other children, he would call a doctor immediately.

The death of Robyn Twitchell did not go unnoticed by city and state authorities in Massachusetts. In the early hours of the Wednesday morning after Robyn's death, a police officer arrived at the Twitchell home. Both David and Ginger were still awake, in shock and trying to make sense out of what had happened. The officer asked some general questions and then left. Later that morning the Twitchells received a call from the hospital social service office asking that they bring their other child in for an examination. They objected, but then agreed to do so. A short time later representatives from the state social service office came by their home. The Twitchells ended up meeting with social services four times. They also took Jeremy to the hospital emergency room for an examination, where he was pronounced in good physical and mental health. The Twitchells were concerned to help their remaining son adjust to the tragedy and keep the social service people from getting fearful and taking custody of Jeremy.

Two months after Robyn died, the district attorney's office called. They wanted the Twitchells to come in for an informal meeting just to clear up a few questions. They could bring a lawyer if they wanted. They did not, and spent over two hours in the DA's office essentially presenting again the account that they had given to social services. They explained their beliefs, how they first resort to prayer but are willing to turn to medicine if it is necessary, and reaffirmed their love for their children. At the end of November, they received a summons to appear in court the following week as witnesses in an inquest. They were stunned, and sensed that there was "prosecution in the air." They immediately tried to find a lawyer, finally settling on the law firm of Klieman and Lyons.

In 1971, the state of Massachusetts had amended its child abuse and neglect law to provide an exemption for spiritual healing. Nevertheless, the state charged the Twitchells with involuntary manslaughter in the death of their son. On July 4, 1990, over four years after Robyn's death, a jury of eight men and four women convicted the Twitchells on this charge. It is a measure of the complexity and sensitivity of this case that three of the jurors broke down and sobbed as the verdict was announced by their foreman. The judge in the case later sentenced the Twitchells to a ten-year probationary period that also requires them to obtain regular medical checkups during that time for their three surviving children, Jeremy (eight years old at the sentencing) and two children born since Robyn's death, Brian and Elias.

The Twitchells appealed the conviction, in part because the judge gave instructions to the jury that denied the 1971 amendment as a defense against manslaughter. Some jurors interpreted the judge's instructions as urging a "reasonable person" test for the parents' actions instead of using the 1971 law as a framework to evaluate the sincerity of the Twitchells' religious beliefs. Also, the Twitchells are apprehensive about submitting their children to the imperatives of medical practice before prayer can be tried as a healing instrument.

Joseph and Susan Clark are a married Christian Scientist couple. Susan grew up in the religion. Her mother was a member of the Church and her grandmother was a practitioner. Joseph was converted to Christian Science at the age of seven when his mother underwent what he believes was a miraculous healing. He does not remember the details of the cure, though he does recall his mother sitting up at night for weeks because she could not breathe if she lay down. The doctors had given up on her, and she was ready to die. His father called a Christian Science practitioner even though the family was not associated with the Church in any way, and the practitioner talked to his mother at length on the phone. The next night she lay down in bed and slept, completely recovered. End of problem. Joseph Clark started to go to the Christian Science Sunday school after that and began his long membership in the Church.

Susan Clark absorbed the principles of Christian Science in an experience continuous with three generations of her family. Joseph Clark was a convert at an early age. One difference in these two experiences is that Mr. Clark can recall the changes that the religious conversion brought to his family. He reports that both of his parents "had been about as close to alcoholics as you could get." After joining the Church they immediately stopped drinking. They stopped smoking also. The family had been very poor. They ended up quite comfortable financially. Mr. Clark marks the conversion to Christian Science as "a total turnaround in our lives."

Both of the Clarks believe that Christian Science can effectively address every disease. They reason that God created everything perfect and anything less than that is a lie about creation. Susan Clark testifies to numerous healings in her family. On one occasion, when she was ten years old, her uncle was driving to church on a cold Wednesday evening and hit a patch of ice. The car spun around and threw him from one side to the other, his head striking the windows each time. (This was at a time before seat belts were mandatory items in automobiles.) He was taken to the hospital where doctors advised the family that he would either die during the night or recover to a total vegetative state since his brain had been severely damaged in the accident. Susan's parents and aunt stayed with her uncle through the night, taking turns praying and reading the Bible lesson over and over. After twenty-four hours, her uncle was showing signs of recovery. At the end of his third week in the hospital, he was well enough to go home. After two more months, he was able to return to his job as a CPA. No neurological problems occurred. He received no medical treatment throughout this entire episode.

On the Sunday following Thanksgiving in 1988, the Clarks were sitting at the table with family members after dinner when their daughter Celia, almost four years old at the time, came over to ask a question. Susan noticed that the child had a huge bruise on her chin. She asked her if she had been playing with the magic markers. Celia answered no, and said that she had fallen on her chin. Susan considered this answer a bit odd since Celia was the type of child who would definitely scream and cry if she were to fall with sufficient force to cause such a large bruise. But motherly concern was dismissed with the thought that the bruise would heal. Later in the evening, however, red dots started to form on Celia's arms. Susan Clark went to bed that night praying for her daughter, trying to hold firmly to the notion that "she was a perfect idea of God."

In the morning the Clarks were awakened by the screams of their daughter. They rushed into her room and found her bleeding from the nose and mouth. Blood was all over her face and the pillow. They cleaned Celia up and tried to stop the bleeding in the standard ways, pinching her nose and so on. Nothing worked. So they called Bryan Seth, a Christian Science practitioner, and began praying. In the early afternoon Susan gave her daughter a bath to make her feel better and calm her down. She noticed bruises all along Celia's spine and hips, and sores in her mouth. The bleeding continued. By the time Seth arrived, Susan was alarmed at the amount of blood her daughter had lost. But Seth seemed to bring the condition under control and Celia began to rest more comfortably after the healing session.

At 3:00 A.M. Tuesday, however, Celia awakened spitting blood. The Clarks called Seth and, after he did "some more prayer work," Celia quieted down and went back to sleep. In the morning the child was still bleeding, however, and the Clarks decided to take her to a doctor. They offer three reasons for their decision. One was a caution dictated by the court cases involving Christian Scientists ministering to their children. For protection against laws that might judge them as negligent parents, the Clarks wanted to get their daughter's condition diagnosed. A second was a desire to know what it was that they were dealing with. "Sometimes," Susan Clark says, "if you are dealing with a person you know is a liar, then you are very careful about how you treat that person and what you say to that person." The Clarks wanted to know the nature of their daughter's affliction so that they could tailor their prayers and ministrations accordingly ("identify the error so that it can be destroyed"). Third, they wanted to reassure their neighbors, some of whom had visited their home out of concern for both Celia and their own children, with an identification of the disease and a medical statement on whether it was contagious.

They took Celia to the physician who had delivered her, an individual sympathetic to Christian Science principles. He examined the child and took some blood samples, which were sent to a lab on a rush order. The results came back later that morning while Susan was still at her mother's house in the city. They indicated that Celia either had leukemia or ITP (which the Clarks understood to be acute primary thrombocytopenia). The physician recommended that Celia be taken immediately to the state hospital, and in fact had already set up an appointment for the child given the urgency of the case.

Susan Clark called her husband. He agreed with his wife that Celia should be taken to the hospital and immediately left work to meet his wife and daughter there. At the hospital the physician, a specialist in hematology and oncology, ordered both bone marrow and blood tests. The bone marrow turned out to be normal, which meant no leukemia, but the blood tests showed an extremely low platelet count, so low that the physician told the Clarks, "You are lucky she is alive." (Platelets are cells in the blood that help control the clotting mechanism.) Susan immediately thanked God and knew that it had been God sustaining her daughter through this ordeal. The Clarks called the practitioner to inform him of Celia's condition so that he could continue with his prayers.

The issue that had to be addressed then and there, however, was what to do next. The physician asked the question directly and simply: "What do you plan to do?" When the Clarks said that they would like to return home and continue their prayerful support, the physician told them a story. The previous Thursday, a Jehovah's Witness, seventeen years old, had refused a needed blood transfusion on religious grounds. His parents had taken him home, where he had died that evening. The Clarks, listening closely to the physician and "seeing the concern on his face," talked it over and decided to keep their daughter in the hospital. The physician quickly rushed Celia up to the pediatric hematology unit and started aggressive medical treatment. He also told the Clarks just before taking the child upstairs that "he was very glad that we had made the decision because otherwise he would have felt impelled to get a court order to require us to keep her in the hospital."

Celia did not respond to the treatment. On Thursday, when the medical staff had expected her to be well enough to check out and return home, her platelet count was still dangerously low. The Clarks continued to pray for their daughter and consult with the practitioner. On Sunday, with their daughter still very ill, the Clarks sat outside the hospital in their car reading aloud the Sunday lesson sermon. As they reflected on the sermon they realized that they were addressing the prospect of a lack in God's kingdom. They discussed the first chapter of Genesis, "when God created everything and it was very good." They understood once more that with an infinite God there cannot be any lack. Then they explored their own thoughts and concentrated on certain deficiencies—the concern for funds to finish building their house and buy a second car. They realized that God cannot lack for anything and that humans are made in His image. So there could not be any lack, for them or anyone else. Their concerns over funds had been errors in thought. It was also obvious to them that there could not be a lack of blood platelets. "Celia is the perfect image of God," Joseph Clark recalls saying, "and anything else is a lie." The Clarks concluded that evil had been talking to them and they had accepted it. They decided, in the car on that late Sunday morning, that they were not going to accept evil any longer.

At that moment Susan told her husband that they had to rush back into the hospital to get the report on the last blood count. "Wait a minute," Joseph responded. "We don't need to know what the count is. We know what the truth is." The fear that had controlled them broke, and they went out to have lunch. They returned to the hospital in the middle of the afternoon, long after the blood count had been taken, to encounter some astonished doctors. Celia's platelet count had risen from 100 to over 16,000. The physician told them, "I think you have had a miracle." By Monday morning, their daughter's platelet count was in the normal range and she was considered well enough to leave the hospital.

The miracle continued. The medical instructions from the hospital staff had included prescriptions for medicine and a program for using a special helmet for the next several months to protect Celia's brain from injury that could lead to cerebral hemorrhages. The Clarks had signed all the release forms at the hospital, promising to medicate Celia and keep her from physical activity. But when they returned home they threw the prescriptions out and let their daughter resume normal activities, including the ballet lessons she had started the previous September. No helmet was ever used. They did bring Celia in for the scheduled physical checkups. All of the tests continued to show a normal platelet count. When they finally admitted to their physician that Celia had not taken any medicine since leaving the hospital he was properly amazed. But it was evident that the child had made a complete recovery from an illness that had almost taken her life.

Stephen Dubansky was the physician attending to Celia Clark in the state hospital. He reports that Celia was admitted to the hospital at the end of November 1988 with an acute onset of bleeding from her nose and mouth originating in the back of her throat that was secondary to a low platelet count. The sudden absence of platelets was due to a disease called ITP (the complete name is idiopathic thrombocytopenic purpura). The disease is one in which, for some unexplained reason usually associated with a viral infection, the body begins to make antibodies against its own platelets. The platelet count falls drastically, and this drop may or may not be associated with clinically significant bleeding.

Dubansky recalls that in Celia's case the platelet count, which should be 150,000 to 400,000 per drop of blood, was less than 1,000. She essentially had no platelets in her blood. The day before admission she began to develop nose bleeds and in fact vomited blood. She was also symptomatic: Dubansky remembers the Clarks saying that Celia was slightly dizzy while at home. The hemoglobin count taken at the hospital, a measure of the red blood or anemia status, showed the fluid to be 7.7. This figure, which would be about 11 in a normal individual, meant that the child had lost a lot of blood in a short period of time. The bone marrow examination ruled out a malignancy but was compatible with the diagnosis of ITP.

ITP is usually a transient or self-limiting disorder that resolves itself within six months 90 percent of the time. Most patients, Dubansky says, get better within the first three months, and the majority of those getting better in the first three months get better on their own, without treatment, in the first six weeks. He regards Celia's illness as unusual in that she had more serious clinical manifestations. Most ITP patients do not have bleeding severe enough to cause a hemoglobin reduction and symptoms like dizziness. So Dubansky was concerned. Generally he treats ITP on an outpatient basis, half the time just watching these patients and the other half administering steroids (the treatment most pediatric hematologists choose). But because Celia's disease involved such serious bleeding and Dubansky could not be sure how low the hemoglobin count would fall, he recommended hospitalization and "big-time treatment" consisting of an intravenous form of prednisone called Solumedrol and IV gamma globulin with the aim of increasing the platelet count. Dubansky also tried to respect the parents' wishes to avoid all treatment that was not necessary. But on the second day of Celia's stay in the hospital the continued dizziness and descent of the hemoglobin count did require the transfusion of one unit of blood to ensure that oxygen was being provided to her tissues. The parents agreed to this therapy.

Dubansky reports that out of the twenty or so patients he and his staff see each year with ITP, only two of them on average would have to be hospitalized and only one would have the kind of profuse bleeding Celia had. So she was unusual in the severity of her illness. Also, "she was somewhat sluggish in her response" to the therapy. At one point he and his staff were considering an experimental treatment with a medicine called Rhogam, the same medicine given to Rh-negative women both before and after they have delivered Rh-positive babies. For ITP, the drug is administered intravenously. Dubansky even spoke to the Clarks about this treatment. He found them quite receptive, especially since they are Christian Scientists. He remembers Mrs. Clark being very sensitive to the concerns of the medical staff and appreciative of the serious nature of her daughter's problems. This response surprised him because he thought he would have to do more of a "selling job," spend more time convincing her. But he was grateful that she caught on right away to what needed to be done, even though he knew that she didn't want her child to be in the hospital in the first place.

Dubansky says that Celia's rapid turnaround on the weekend is well within medical parameters. She simply responded slowly, then rapidly, to the therapy. But he is unable to say whether it was a miracle cure. He likes to think that what he and his staff did helped, and he has seen numerous patients in Celia's condition respond beautifully without prayer. The only fact Dubansky accepts without reservations is that Celia was cured. If God played a role in that, he is willing to accept it. He does not regard Celia's continued improvement as miraculous. Normally a patient in Celia's state would have been kept on prednisone for two weeks after being discharged from the hospital. But he says that not all doctors would agree that it is necessary to continue treatment for up to two weeks, and that many patients do not take the medicine when they return home. Normally the platelet count remains high once it has reached normal levels.

Dubansky is "all for miracles." He does not belittle them, and in fact admits to respect for people who believe in them since he himself does not have much faith in their occurrence. He thinks that he has seen two things in his medical practice that he would term miraculous. One was a child in Denver who had a relapse with acute nonlymphocytic leukemia and was sick in the hospital with a severe bacterial infection in his bloodstream. Things had reached the point where the child's parents were not sure if they wanted to have him treated any further. The doctors were willing to go along with them and cease treatment because the child was so hopelessly ill. Long-term survival was out of the question. Finally the medical staff suggested antibiotics. They would not hurt the child and perhaps they would raise the quality of his life for a short time, enough so that his parents could take him home for a period of time before he died. The parents agreed and the antibiotics were administered. The child went home improved. Not only did he get over his infection, a highly unusual recovery given the low number of white blood cells in his blood, but the leukemia—untreated and presumably unaffected by the antibiotics—went into remission. It did not return. The child was cured.

Medical journals have described the association of serious infections with remission of cancer, and some speculation has been offered that an immune system jolted into a response by an infection can sometimes rid the body of cancer as well. But Dubansky still classifies that remission in Denver as a miracle and refuses to be blasé about it.

The other miraculous healing was that of a child who had pulmonary metastases from a kidney tumor. Two lesions in the lung were confirmed through biopsy. In Dubansky's understanding of disease, there is no way that this condition could have healed, or even gotten better. But there was a spontaneous remission of the metastases. Dubansky recalls going to these parents and asking them what they were doing that no one else was doing. The answer was, nothing. They had no impressive or serious beliefs, no wild cards of mental resources or special health tricks. They were simply what Dubansky would call average parents. Yet their child experienced what he labels as a miraculous (inexplicable) recovery.

He also relates yet a third mystery cure. One evening many years ago he was driving back from synagogue during the Jewish New Year and saw a dog lying on the side of the road. He stopped his car and ministered as best he could to the stricken animal. The dog would not move. Dubansky picked it up and laid it in his car. Then he drove over to his girlfriend's house an hour away. The dog was paralyzed during the entire drive. As Dubansky got out of his car and started to carry the dog inside, he remembers thinking, "God, I know this is so stupid, but would you let this dog walk because this is a sweet little dog" (though he admits he might also have said, "If there is really a God, you wouldn't have let this happen to this dog"). In any case, no sooner were the words out of his mind than he reached the front door, put the dog down to ring the bell, and the dog got up and ran away. He was amazed because he was convinced the dog was a case of pure flaccid, and permanent, paralysis. So he admits to three miracles in his experience, though he is embarrassed to include the last one in his enumeration of the miraculous.

Dubansky urges care in evaluating miracle cures. He believes that most are not cures at all. Often the patient never had the disease in the first place. Sometimes, he says, a chest X ray will display a lump or blob indicating the child has a pulmonary metastasis. Then it will go away and one might conclude that the cancer is cured. But the X ray might have picked out only a fold, a little bit of lung collapsing. Or the area might be an infection that could spontaneously heal. The diagnosis of metastasis can be confirmed only with a biopsy. Also, some diseases, like multiple sclerosis, have peaks and valleys. It is a mistake, Dubansky believes, to think that prayer brings about improvement in diseases that from time to time will get better spontaneously.

But whatever the possibilities of miracle cures, Dubansky would not have hesitated to get a court order to treat Celia Clark if her parents had tried to withdraw her from the hospital without treatment. The loss of blood, the weakness and rapid heartbeat, placed Celia in danger of a central nervous system bleed, which could have been fatal. Given a child who is in such a condition, Dubansky again would have called on the legal system to mandate treatment. "I think," he says, "that [such action] is my obligation as a physician."

The Clarks believe that Celia's healing was a miracle because the doctors had not changed the medical treatment when the recovery occurred. Their daughter was not responding to treatment when they had their spiritual revelation. She did not respond either to the steroids or to the blood transfusion. The doctors' expectations were not being met. But at the same moment that the Clarks saw through illusion to the underlying reality of their lives and their daughter's true condition of perfection, Celia was healed. They know prayer and meditation were the effective instruments of her recovery.

Natural Domains

The question raised by spiritual healing practices in a liberal setting is, what type of community is the liberal state? Are there natural commitments of liberalism that can explain and leaven the community bias that seems unavoidable in spiritual and secular disputes?

The role of the state in religious matters in the United States is an instructive case study. The neutrality informing the second of the two religious clauses in the First Amendment—the free exercise of religion—bears two interpretations. One is that the state is neutral if it treats all religions alike *and* treats religions as it treats secular institutions. This essentially non-discriminatory interpretation of the free exercise clause would place members of religious organizations under the laws of the land like all other citizens. On an exemption interpretation, however, the state is constrained to allow members of a religion to act on their beliefs without interference from the state. This can mean granting exemptions from the law when the religious belief compels an individual to act in a way different than the law requires. It is the exemption rather than the nondiscriminatory interpretation that leads to the legal protections granted to Christian Scientists in spiritual healing, and it is the logic of this thinking that assigns privacy to all manner of unorthodox healing methods.

But the state must subscribe to a nondiscriminatory approach in spiritual matters on liberal grounds. The liberal state originates in a kind of dualism. Laws exist to regulate body, not mind. The law compels behavioral, not mental, compliance in that beliefs are to be outside the coercive powers of the state. But the distinction between mind and body cannot always be maintained in spiritual communities. Spiritual healing, for example, claims dominion over the body through powers of the mind. Prayer and spiritual appeals in general are said to work through the soul or mind on the body, and to bring about a healing through that spiritual intervention. The province of the body is empirical in nature, however, and so the tests for genuine healing must come from within the domain of empirical science and thus be governed by the techniques of contemporary medicine. Precisely because the liberal state concentrates on body in order to free up beliefs, it is itself a captive of those scientific traditions that fix the terms of bodily states and movements. In any dispute over the primary good of life set in physical terms, the liberal state inevitably finds itself an ally of conventional medicine. Exemptions can be given for beliefs, but impartiality—what works best on physicalist criteria—must govern any claims on medical treatment. The state is aligned with allopathic medicine against spiritual healing even when trying to be neutral.

It is easy to be misled by terms like "nondiscriminatory" or "impartial." In yet one more form of the fallacy of composition, a state neutral on such narrow grounds will lead to outcomes biased against spiritual claims. Christian Scientists, for example, will not be able to be Christian Scientists in a society where medicine is the arbiter of therapeutic claims, which is one reason these disputes must be regarded as paradoxes of liberalism. But such a society will at least compel the treatment of all individuals who cannot yet decide whether to be treated spiritually or medically, though it will do so at considerable costs to the integrity of the families so targeted and to liberal traditions that celebrate tolerance of spiritual belief.

There is more to this story, or less. A state confined to regulating the domain of body, and historically committed to minimal regulation and individual freedoms, must also rest on a minimalist concept of reality. This concept is successfully elaborated with at least some of the core meaning of everyday reality against which spiritual views are measured: that individuals are in some way distinct from the world they experience and are (or occupy) bodies located in time and space. Also, ordinary experience is organized by time's arrow and objects in space that have mass (or extension). The bulk of secular laws and practices assumes such a view of reality, and departures from it are sometimes regarded as signs of some pathology on a secular understanding of experience.

But, of course, the reality of spiritual healing often exceeds and sometimes rejects this minimalist account. In all cases, it views the account as inadequate and incomplete. Spiritual healers, who see individuals in holistic terms, who often challenge time's arrow with retrocausality and dismiss objects and space as vital dimensions of reality, do not fit within a minimalist ontology. Neutrality may be elusive even on liberal realities.

It is also important to note that unorthodox beliefs on diagnosis and therapy can differ radically on the meaning of relevant experiences. Spiritual claims on health and healing always assert effects over the human body achieved through the intermediary powers of the spiritual world (however conceived). But a difference in temperament and understanding demarcates two species of spiritual claims. One is distinguished by variations in the values assigned to health, illness, and death. Vocabularies of acceptance—deliverance, penance, punishment—can designate as good or tolerable what a secular attitude regards as bad. The believer who, for example, sees illness as a proper assignment for earlier wrongdoing, or death as a desirable outcome, is applying a conceptual framework that questions the worthiness of medicine even when it works. Another understanding, represented by Christian Scientists, shares the values of modern medicine on health and illness but differs on the means to achieve healing.

The first understanding is outside liberal frameworks to a greater degree and so is more difficult to govern on liberal values. Since such views may deny even the primary good of life itself, at least as fixed within secular beliefs, state regulation will naturally be more rather than less adversarial to this position. The second understanding is more congenial with internal governance, for at least in principle it should be possible to test the efficacy of each type of healing by neutral means. Perhaps a common language could be located or crafted to yield a shared authority over proper therapy. But if the competing views of reality control the tests used to establish causal efficacy in healing, then the state is returned to its familiar partisan role in disputes over spiritual and medical treatment.

Power in Conditions of Uncertainty

If multiple senses of reality can accommodate the "same" events, and if the state is unable to occupy a high ground that is free of particular and partisan reality, then liberal political theory is obligated to offer an account of power that accommodates failures of neutrality.

The most satisfying exercise of power must be a coercing to morality on the basis of moral certainty. Imagine forcing someone to accept, or at least to act on, moral principles one knows to be true. Economists use conditions of certainty to elaborate utility-maximizing decision rules. Moral certainty has effects elsewhere, primarily in bringing the errant individual back into the moral fold with due concern over the use of coercion.

Coercive resolutions of disputes over proper medical therapy do not occur in conditions of certainty, moral or otherwise. Regulation must occur in the absence of truth as a basis of coercion, but with strong claims to truth by the competing communities. This raises the question of how power should be exercised in conditions of uncertainty over the truth of *claims* to truth made by rival communities.

The model on which power is typically elaborated assumes that the respondent is unified and discrete. Individuals are thought to be organized internally in ways that make a response to a moral or legal imperative possible. But it is not clear that such selves exist. If persons are comprised of multiple selves that vary with circumstances, or are dual entities with separate spiritual and physical dimensions, then power is complicated in interesting ways. Any account of coercion must be elaborated in terms of both uncertainty and competing understandings of individuals.

1) Power can be either direct or oblique. A direct exercise of power is an unmediated effect exerted by a power figure on a respondent. A mugger who holds a gun to the head of a jogger and demands money is exercising direct power. In general, the police powers of the state are forms of direct power. Oblique power is distinguished by its mediating forms. Here the power figure acts on attendant conditions to control or influence the respondent. Agenda control is a famous type of oblique power. If a power figure reduces or expands alternatives, or alters the conditions in which choices (or preferences) are made (or expressed), power has been exercised in oblique ways.

In each of these forms of power there are moral balances, competing moral features that may be arranged in different ways. Direct power is at once an assault on the freedom of individuals and a confrontation capable of recognizing the moral powers of both power figure and respondent. Oblique power is similarly mixed. To restrict alternatives as a method of control is simultaneously to permit a degree of freedom and to conceal the fact of influence from the respondent. Each form of power has both moral and amoral components.

One consideration favors oblique power in conditions of uncertainty. Direct power aims at closure, meaning that it is an action typically designed to restrict freedom to whatever point may be required to get the respondent to act in the desired ways. Oblique power is more ambiguous by virtue of its form. Acting on conditions is no guarantee that the respondent will do exactly what is desired, since a measure of freedom is often (though not always) found in oblique power. If one is uncertain about the truth of opposing claims, and there is no additional or alternative truth on the basis of which power may be exercised, then the ambiguity of oblique power would seem to be more appropriate to the situation.

2) Power on uncertainty also requires that only compliance in behavior, not belief, be sought. Again a distinction in types of power can guide our thoughts here. One can control to transform or to achieve compliance. A full moral act requires both belief and action, so that coercing to morality has as its standard of full success a respondent who acts in the correct way and believes correctly as well (and perhaps acts because of correct beliefs). This type of coercion is transforming, since one of its aims is a change in the beliefs of the respondent and perhaps in the nature of the respondent as well. But one can also control in an external sense, aiming only to bring the respondent's behavior into compliance with rules or principles. The absence of truth as a criterion in coercion shields beliefs from power, for an absence of principles to adjudicate disputes as true or false halts transforming ambitions. How can individuals be reformed, or beliefs controlled or even modified, when there are no truth criteria to apply to beliefs?

3) The presence of strong claims in a dispute requires that *persons* be recognized as the respondents of coercion. Here the task is less complicated. Individuals are biological members of their species who possess an awareness of the self as conscious and continuing over the span of human life. This self-reflective power, normally labeled "personhood," is usually joined to certain rational powers as well. Given the acceptance of *claims* for health and healing in therapy disputes, one also must accept that individual members of the competing communities are capable of asserting interests, framing arguments, using evidence—in short, are conscious at a reflective level and adept in rational discourse.

The constraints on power following such an admission are qualified by two considerations: (a) the absence of truth criteria limits the rational force of persuasion and prohibits demonstrative argument; and (b) the nature of the dispute is such that the competing parties are rational only in terms of community discourses, and so are impervious to rational appeal on precisely the action being coerced. Still, the acknowledgment that a dispute is occurring between persons inclines the use of power to reach a settlement that is reasonable at least on hypothetical grounds.

But note how different understandings of the primitive term "individual" affect the uses of power. The distinction between compliance in *behavior* and *belief* rests on a dualism corresponding to the physical and mental dimensions within individuals. Also, the reality of split or divided selves may be a pathology that makes any response impossible. If one views the individual in reductionist terms, then even stronger effects occur. Persons who are extensions of circumstances, defined by the conditions in which they achieve identity, must be addressed with oblique power. Only if conditions were modified so that coercion were directed toward the context of action rather than the agent of action could such coercion be successful.

It is helpful to remember that political methods of dispute resolution typically seek an outcome that is not a moral settlement (and thus is not concerned with beliefs). Voting, for example, produces a collective outcome that is justifiable only in the procedural sense. One side gains an arithmetical victory that may not represent any morally best perspective. The distinctive feature of any political settlement is its coercive quality, not its sensitivity to the beliefs of any competing faction. The one method for reaching collective outcomes that combines reflective powers with coercion is a juridical settlement. Juridical methods include reasoned inspections of opposing views followed by resolutions that coerce all parties to compliance. Like binding arbitration, though with the seal of statute law, a judge can provide a reasoned outcome that is also coercive. The recognition of persons as claimants in disputes constrains power to reasoned settlements modeled after juridical forms.

4) The absence both of shared criteria of truth and of any overarching truth means that any reasoned settlement must be strongly reconstructive. Again, some rudimentary distinctions are helpful. Truth (and its cognate vocabularies) can be elaborated in terms of correspondence or coherence. A correspondence theory regards statements as true if they match some state of affairs that has status independent of the statements. A coherence theory accepts statements as true if they fit some assemblage of statements that has as one of its features the power to construct a state of affairs.

The dispute between allopaths and holists cannot be viewed in correspondence terms, for there is no evidence independent of the competing claims for a reality against which true statements can be identified. But a coherence theory of truth is possible. Statements can be regarded as "true," as the basis for a reasoned settlement, if they cohere with some set of statements that can be reasonably constructed from the competing claims. It is one of the defining features of intractable disputes that the contending parties cannot reach a resolution through rational discourse. But a resolution imposed from outside the dispute may be able to reconstruct claims in such a way that the settlement coheres with some reasonable range of community views.

The most effective vehicle of reconstruction is the establishment of a collective arrangement that fixes priorities among healing claims when conflict occurs. Remember that neutrality is impossible. Put in the simplest terms and illustrated with Christian Science, the state fails reasonable tests of neutrality whether or not it intervenes in spiritual doctrines of health and healing. Given the endorsement of life as a primary good, to be protected in the absence of competence or when decisions are made for others, the state encounters one of the common paradoxes of liberal practices: to require standard medical care is to override the religious belief that illness is more effectively addressed by prayer than by medical therapy; to abstain from intervention is implicitly to endorse the belief.

There is one escape route from this dilemma. If all goods were defined by communities, including health and life, then competence and decisions that affect others would not produce issues that lead to state regulation. (Life-threatening illness could then be regarded like other trivial matters, clothing, for example, and idiosyncratic beliefs could remain outside the regulatory powers of the state.) But such a solution is unthinkable on liberal values. The great liberal theories of the seventeenth and eighteenth centuries were developed on the primacy of individual choice, breaking with long classical and medieval traditions that stressed the overriding importance of the political society. *This* life, viewed in an individualistic frame, eventually became the focus of meaning and value in human experience. To deny the value of such life undermines liberalism itself. Given such traditions, it is unlikely that life can escape classification as a primary good without causing additional contradictions in liberalism. The paradox of neutrality seems unavoidable. A collective arrangement of priorities follows naturally from an understanding of the state as an institution compelled to govern community beliefs without the agreeable condition of impartiality.

5) States, at least on occasion, must be empty political vessels in order for doctrinaire positions to be able to enter public space. When doctrines overlap and conflict in this space, states must resolve these conflicts with means that are appropriate to the conditions and assumptions of the dispute. But the state also has other considerations. Communal needs for order and stable change, as well as the maintenance of a range of primary goods that might exceed those found in any particular dispute, must also be the aim of political resolutions.

At this exact point, the two responsibilities of the state become clear. One is to produce a reasoned outcome that is most consistent with community beliefs. The other is to impose coercively a collective ordering of priorities drawn from the liberal recognition of priority goods. If the state assigns higher-order status to life than to other goods, then life must be protected. This reasoning follows liberal philosophies. In liberalism, public space is ideally emptied of political content, but the space must be bent to the needs of secular values on the very logic that keeps the state from making religious commitments and adjudicating religious beliefs. A state crafted on secular grounds that emphasize a celebration of individual life is by definition biased toward the preservation of life. The secular expression of this protection is conventional medicine.

The costs of any political intervention are real and sometimes considerable. Requiring standard medical care for all individuals who are demonstrably incompetent does not undermine neutrality, which vanishes as soon as doctrinaire conflict enters public space. The trade-offs occur primarily in the area of practices that flourish behind privacy shields. The family is the most immediate casualty. There is little doubt that any aggressive state regulation of Christian Scientists that forces standard medical care on children will damage family integrity within the religion. Whether the costs are worth bearing will depend on how important individual life is within frameworks of secular beliefs.

Ontological disputes address the deeper levels of human experience. Machiavelli suggests in *The Prince* that the main imperatives of political power are impossible to carry out effectively if ordinary morality guides the state. Extreme pluralism offers the ground on which these suggestions are true. If several moral principles compete with each other in public life, then power cannot follow a homogeneous and consistent set of these principles. It must select and adjust principles that cannot all be realized at once. The special moral skill of those in power must be the ability to negotiate or impose settlements when the disputing parties have equally powerful and contradictory moral beliefs. When the adversaries compete over understandings of reality, basic social practices, and the purposes of human life, this skill must include the ability to map from one moral discourse to another and to find the proportionate settlements that meet the generalizable needs of communities. Power of this type would be amoral from the different community perspectives competing with each other in public life. But from a location outside of conventional morality, the art of political resolution and management would appear rational and moral on the terms of effective power.

10

NARRATIVE REASONING

Professional Ethics

The practice of medicine has two dominant though not always consistent goals. One is the restoration of health. The other is the maintenance of life. It is not always clear in particular cases how medical ethics are related to these two goals, but in general codes of ethics for medical practitioners have developed as devices to protect and further the interests in these goals shared by both physicians and patients. Since the time that medicine became professionalized, various ethical principles have been recognized, often in law, as governing norms for medical practice.

One of the most important of these principles is beneficence and its classical cautionary incarnation as nonmalfeasance. Physicians are supposed to benefit their patients by helping them secure health, or at least do no harm in treating them. Clinical medicine in America has increasingly stressed informed consent as an ethical principle that can ensure patient autonomy. The most important ethical principle in medicine, however, may be the fiduciary principle. The medical professional must act to ensure that the patient's interests in health and life dominate in the practice of medicine by maintaining a relationship of trust (as in trustee) and responsibility toward those receiving medical treatment.

The means for realizing the goals of medicine are drawn from empirical science. Causal relationships established under controlled conditions, or by controlling for extraneous effects, are the sources of medical knowledge. Research data secured with exacting mathematical or statistical techniques (baseline rather than anecdotal) are used in evaluating medicine interventions. A reality constructed from a secular mapping of the physical body guides medical practice today, even when attitudes are recognized as important variables in recovery from injury or illness.

Religious or spiritual practices have different goals. The two goals of all religions, organized or not, are to render human experience intelligible within some framework that exceeds the conventional boundaries of sensory experience, and to provide an account of human identity within this more comprehensive framework. The means used to secure these goals include various efforts to demonstrate the existence of alternative realities and to compromise conventional realities by placing them in more cosmological frames, on occasion by claiming to reverse their governing laws.

Spiritual healing often follows as a consequence of seeking the goals of religious experience, not (as in medicine) as an end in itself. The most consistent claim in spiritual healing is that access to alternative realities is the source of healing. Following closely on this claim is an understanding that the whole person must be healed, spirit and body. A mapping of the human spirit and those realities that exceed human knowledge is more important in spiritual healing than the concern for physical realities found in contemporary medicine.

Those differences are decisive in settling on ethical principles to govern what healers in both professions do. Ethical principles, like political and moral languages generally, are determined by the particular goals, means, and realities found in medical and spiritual practices. The key to understanding these determinants may be found in the set of concepts on which ethical principles rely. Both beneficence (and nonmalfeasance) and the fiduciary principle rest on interests. What is best for the patient—what benefits, avoids harm, and is ensured by trust—guides healing in both sets of practices. But interests differ greatly from secular to spiritual domains. Material and intellectual goals reasonably dominate secular lives while life after death and a continuing relationship with alternative realities receive priority in spiritual discourses. On occasion religion requires that the spirit dominate the body so completely that the health of the body is not perceived as crucial. In other, more generous accounts, spirit is the instrument used to heal the body. But the body cannot be addressed separately from the spirit nor regarded as dominant over it. Yet the interests of the body are controlling in conventional medical practice.

The concept of autonomy fares no better in escaping the differences between medical and spiritual healing. The autonomous individual is *self-directing*. But the account of the self differs considerably in each form of healing. In recent liberal traditions, the secular self is considered autonomous because it is separate from the influences of others and institutions. A distinct and even atomistic self is the bearer of autonomy. But in spiritual traditions the self is typically joined to other realities and entities. Autonomy is illusory if depicted as a distinct and independent power. An individual surrenders to, or is merged in, some more comprehensive reality as a condition for successful direction. The self forms part of a directive line extending to powers outside the self. One gains mastery over one's life in spiritual perspectives only as a consequence of abandoning liberal notions of autonomy.

Informed consent is a principle that relies on both negative freedom and competence. Absent either of these nexus concepts and consent does not occur. Yet the nexus concepts are deeply intertwined in spiritual and medical languages. Negative freedom is a vital concept in elaborating the secular autonomous self, shielding individuals from external influences that might compromise and even contaminate the choice of alternatives that can include basic moral principles. The individual in spiritual traditions, however, is embedded in social networks and extended realities, free in the positive sense of requiring social and spiritual conditions for genuine choices.

Competence is notoriously jurisdictional. A competent individual in liberal traditions is one who can carry out a task. The semantic sign of competence attaches to the individual as an ability. This ability, in turn, depends on an understanding of situations, the power to comprehend realities. But the exercise of this ability differs exactly as one shifts between spiritual and secular communities. Even what counts as information is a variable. For some religions the palpable presence of a spiritual being is an empirical event, hard data to be studied and interpreted. Secular communities on the whole deny such occurrences. Competence, on any understanding of the term, is a function of spiritual and secular beliefs.

The unavoidable conclusion is that professional ethics and ordinary morality are not the sole governors of healing practices, but the artifacts—the structures of conscience—resulting from sets of beliefs that demarcate the two types of communities. There are obviously general norms that can evaluate both sets of practices. Evangelical healers who hustle their followers out of needed money with no discernible benefit following the transactions are violating their own testimonies of integrity. But the deeper tests of ethics drawn from moral principles seem to be variables of competing senses of reality and the goals of different practices. Even the meaning of the human individual is a variable of membership in communities that differ on spiritual and secular considerations.

True Stories

Each of the individuals in this book tells a story. Many are accounts of strong conversion. A life is led that is not satisfactory. Events occur that shift understandings of reality. The effects are transforming. The individual is remade, "made whole" from ingredients previously scattered across the terrain of the self.

The roll call of strong conversions is diverse and impressive. Joanne Park altered her understanding of reality from sequential to holistic as a result of mirror-image therapy. The other was seen as a kind of reflection of the self, and this recognition of extended identity shifted Park's sense of the real. Faith Jamison and Robert Penfield talked to God. Each was pursuing goals that did not meet their deepest needs. An intervention from what they believe is a higher power enlightened each of them on life's purposes. William Sulzman studied theosophy assiduously and then "saw" the reality of the philosophy in traumatic instances of psychic healing. Philip Edwards and Gloria Kaster witnessed healing that they could not explain in conventional ways. They altered their beliefs about the world and individuals as a consequence. Lawrence LeShan "was very, very tired" and turned to psychic healing from what is generally called a "burned out" stage of life. The healing he was able to generate changed his understanding of human experience.

Two figures of uncertainty are Father Vecchio and David Stanford. Vecchio wants to believe in higher powers that can heal but is sure only of the power of rituals to bring about emotional catharsis. Stanford moves between the worlds of conventional medicine and psychic healing, puzzled at the parameters of each. No conversion experience has graced either of those two lives. Nor has a strong conversion occurred in four other lives where convictions have been formed over a lifetime. The Loverros, the Canterburys, the Twitchells, and the Clarks have maintained their beliefs over time, not acquired them as the result of a conversion (though Joseph Clark assumed the views of Christian Science at the age of seven). But unlike Vecchio and Stanford, these latter individuals are not troubled by uncertainties in their beliefs.

One cannot find the commonplace antagonism between authenticity and reflection or "objectivity" in any of these lives. Each individual constructs a discourse that is designed to show and explain the sequence of events leading to the discovery of a true or genuine self. This discovery arises from an encounter with reality. Discontent about the objective world, instead of being hostile to self-discovery, is the source for realizing the true self.

The plot of each individual's life reexpresses the structures of the real world. Changes in character follow this alignment.

Suppose, however, that we take as true the stories that each individual is telling and we match those stories against the realities of conventional medicine. Two levels of discourse immediately appear. One is the set of internal accounts, the stories as told and interpreted (by the teller, by observers). The other is the overall story produced from these multiple narratives. This overall story is a study in pluralism. If the internal accounts are true, then reality is an arrangement of the separate and contrasting accounts of the real offered in the narratives. The higher truth is that no single narrative can express an overriding truth.

Texts are sequences of information. Stories are imaginative arrangements of these sequences and the information they contain. A story is usually a composition consisting of a plot, characters, description, and an unwritten text constructed or extracted by the readers. A third level of discourse invites us to reconsider the texts deployed in this work. It is the frame provided by the author that combines, presents, and interprets the narratives and the overall story. It is important to note (from the authorial frame) that the overall story displays multiple and conflicting truths.

Stories are important where linear reasoning breaks down. Narratives provide exemplars for action. They lead to conclusions internal to context, like invitations to a party where some truth is disclosed to and for the participants in the course of the evening's entertainment. They also can be instruments of reconstruction, presenting the views of living, particular individuals in imaginative renditions that yet cut closer to social practices than empirical theory can.

Stories provide the frame within which moral discourse occurs, and on occasion can identify those first principles that make a particular moral discourse possible. The most powerful stories can entertain multiple points of view without judgment, avoiding the hard disputes over truth that more linear or explicit forms of reasoning seem to require. Suggestion is enough in a story, an oblique reference to moral truths that the narrative identifies as it unfolds.

But a narrative can also suggest, by using metaphor, symbols, and other literary devices, the contours of alternative realities that we may know only tacitly, without fixing them in explicit modes of thinking. We may find the structures of explicit thinking within stories, though on occasion these structures may serve as instruments to intensify experience without fidelity to truth. Still, characters in stories use evidence and draw conclusions, and the plots and frameworks used to make the story intelligible are at least pragmatic forms of linear reasoning. Stories may even serve the interests of conventional reasoning, as when scientists tell stories to illustrate and expose cognitive truths. In these ways narratives fold back upon conventional reasoning both to extend and to illuminate it. The favors are returned in interpretation. Stories can be the data addressed by precise and even analytic forms of thought. This prospect completes the circle of discourse. But stories can also break through the circle, taking us to realities not circumscribed by conventional (linear, sequential) forms of reasoning.

The story of social theory, and the stories told in social theory, have often sought elevation and distance from the actual world of human experience. The intellectual is sometimes anointed as the bearer of objective truth, occupying a series of Archimedean points that give privileged access to cultural beliefs. The cost of distance is considerable, of course, amounting to the abandonment of the *lived* human experience. It is this tension among levels of discourse that yields the interpretations of the stories told here by the figures in this book.

Luke

The eerie distance I feel from the physical is a kind of detachment, an absence of endorsement, that must be like the impartial gaze of the intellectual. I seem to occupy some space between discourses, a metadiscourse more "enlightened" than the others but missing some parts vital to any engagement of reality.

The problem is that all of our rational powers run short. We cannot master reality. I have floated within my body to the ends of thought, as have others who are more tightly attached to the physical. Thought contradicts itself when that happens.

I know that I believe in God. Yet God has no concept of "God," and so must be outside the sphere of human thought. Should we think of penalties for our beliefs? Not to believe in God and then find He exists. Or to believe and find that the belief has no referent. My mind goes back and forth over the self-reflective paths of truth and falsity set in motion by this thought and others like it.

Perhaps we cannot think of God's rewards except as bright gifts at a great distance, somewhere outside the boundaries of thought. Pure melancholy, reminders of the limits of straight rational thinking.

When I talk to God it is from within myself to myself. Only a story will do.

Neurological Selves

Traditional thinking on the nature of the self seems almost chronically inclined to divide and subdivide the individual. Plato's arrangement of reason, spirit, appetite, Christian dualisms of soul and body, even Freud's classification of superego, ego, and id regard the individual as some composite. The two basic elements in this composite are mind and body. Recent efforts to distinguish human "being" from "person" follow these traditions. The biological marker of forty-six chromosomes determines the physical dimensions of self while criteria like sentience, self-consciousness, even rationality are offered as identifying marks of personhood. The latter is typically advanced as the distinctively "human" part of human individuals and is used to draw up ethical maxims and recognize ethical dilemmas.

Yet holistic or integrated biological selves may be more plausible renditions of humans. These conclusions follow the revelation that the human brain has no fixed categories. Recent work in neurology has dismissed the idea that the brain stores information in local sectors, or has powers that are confined to specific regions. The best theories of the brain depict the organ as a set of maps or collections of neural groups that represent and preserve communication between neural tissues and sensory receptors. This arrangement of neurons is malleable. It adjusts to unexpected experiences by mapping stimuli in a variety of overlapping ways. Information is distributed among many maps found in neurological material, and is sent back and forth among the maps. No event in experience is perceived in a single way. Rather, experience is cut and structured in multiple ways by different mapping functions.

The organization of the brain is explained by the needs of the human organism to cope with its environment. Bats and humans have different neurological procedures for categorizing stimuli because they have different coping requirements. The brain has evolved in response to its environment and according to its biological laws of development. Even within a single human brain, different sectors will employ various coping functions in order to manage stimuli. The environment, especially the presence of physical objects, offers a set of constraints that provide an order for the brain. Dreams, then, may be understood as the release of neuronal maps from the constraints of that sensory order known loosely as the "external world." Reciprocity in ordering functions is strong, however. An awake brain structures experience in terms of the neurological procedures that make experience intelligible on the terms set by the brain.

The individual, on this account, is a shifting arrangement of neurons, stimuli, maps (including maps of maps), and memories structured by neurological procedures. The whole body contributes to the identity of the individual. Emotions, the limbic system, are vital in brain functions. The extended body conditions neurological powers. Brain and body define individuals, but the entire system is physical. The mental is an arrangement of physical variables.

Luke

The problem is that *I* am that arrangement of neurological procedures, the incarnate self that can reflect on and know its own physical environment. Where am I in this arrangement?

Let me ask you something. Every theory of the brain, no matter how reductive, allows for directive powers. Shift the focus, engage a new problem or experience, and the brain issues new maps to address the stimuli. Now what is the driving force that directs the brain, that seems to have a kind of primal influence on its uses and functions?

I say it is the soul that is the a priori energy attending to the neurological arrangement, a self that is an incorporeal force driving the brain from a point somehow outside its own physical endowment.

The brain must cope with its own death and with an environment that exceeds the physical. We think of transcendence, of alternative realities, of God. Is a belief in God a coping mechanism? What is the neural grouping that asserts a Creator? We are more than empirical units defined by a complex array of brain matter.

The limbic system also has a lyrical dimension, a mechanism that issues stories to explain our existence. Does that mechanism help us to survive? Or do we cope with realities that are just beyond our grasp?

My mother used to play bolita in Key West. The drawings were held every Wednesday and Saturday in Cuba. I remember that the radio would be on in my grandmother's home, just off Duval Street, and the winning numbers would be mentioned in the rapid monologue of the Cuban announcer. Dreams were important in bolita, even my dreams as a small child. They stood for numbers. You played the numbers of your dreams in the days leading up to the drawings. Then the numbers would be locked into the world on Wednesday and Saturday evenings as literal, written script. Dreams to stories, and then to the empirical realities of winning and losing lottery numbers.

Let me tell you some stories.

A Christian Scientist was trying to explain destiny to a skeptical listener.

He described how he was an engineer on duty in Vietnam. His work was distant from the more intense fighting going on further north, but occasionally he had to make sorties to bases that came under fire. On one mission he was returning from Danang to Saigon in a small plane. The pilot landed the plane on an airfield at a small base en route so that the man could pick up some structural specifications for fortifications he and his engineering staff were designing. He was inside the office when something told him to return to the plane. He ran outside and saw the plane taxiing to take off. He jumped on board. The pilot had seen something in the jungle that had spooked him. He had decided to leave quickly, without his passenger. They took off just as mortar shells started landing on the runway. That night the base was overrun by Vietcong.

Later, in a session with a Christian Science practitioner, an interviewer is trying to understand complete resistance to modern medicine. He tells a well-worn joke to the practitioner. A flood hits a rural town. A man clings to a rooftop as the waters rush by and continue to rise. A raft with two men on board floats by. The passengers yell for the man to jump on board. He refuses. "God will save me," he tells them. Soon a police motor launch approaches. The policeman urges the man to get on the launch. "No," the man replies. "God will save me." The waters continue to rise. Rain starts falling heavily. A state helicopter arrives and a rope ladder descends to the man. He waves the helicopter away with the words, "God will save me." Soon the waters engulf the house and the man drowns. Approaching God in the afterlife, he cannot avoid expressing his disappointment. "Lord, I served you all my life. Yet in my moment of need, you did not help me." The Lord looks at the man for a moment. "Not help you?" he replies. "I sent you a raft, a motor launch, and a helicopter." The interviewer asks the Christian Science practitioner why modern medicine cannot be considered as part of God's handiwork in helping human beings. Why can't medical practice be God's way for humans to reach health? A long pause follows. "Because," the practitioner finally answers, "we have a better way toward health."

Stories. Do you understand that they can be scripts bent to fit a moral point of view? But sometimes stories are not discretionary. They can be maps to an alternative reality.

A young woman holding a baby walks slowly through a subway car. She stops at each passenger, holding her free hand out, asking without speaking. Each person whispers "no" and looks away. The woman is lovely, extraordinarily so, and dressed poorly but with a fine leather jacket over her blouse. A woman seated at the end of the car reaches in her purse and puts some coins in the woman's hand. A man the woman had passed earlier stands up and drops a coin in her hand. Here is the puzzle as the train starts to slow and stop at the next station. Is the woman running a scam, or is she an angel? The test is to know the difference. If you know she is an angel and give you are saved. But you know the difference only if you are worthy of salvation. Do you know whether to give or not? The woman gets off the train as the doors open. She disappears up the stairs.

Later in the evening a young Puerto Rican moves through the subway station as passengers wait for the train. He is distributing religious pamphlets. A skeptic glances at the literature. "What is salvation?" he asks. The man smiles and replies that salvation is easy, that one only has to. . . . The train comes into the station drowning out the man's voice. His lips are moving, but it is impossible to hear him. As the train stops the man nods, "You see how easy salvation is," and moves away.

A group of men sits in chains in a cave facing a wall. Behind them is a fire. On the wall are the shadows cast by the fire. They gaze at the shadows and take them to be the real world. Now a visitor descends to the cave and breaks their chains. He forces them to ascend the path up toward the sunlight. They resist. They are blinded by the light. They see the natural world of objects illuminated by the sun. They realize that their perceptions in the cave were illusions, that reality was in a dimension of experience outside the world below that they had mistakenly taken for real.

A doctor fresh out of medical school decided to spend two years in the Peace Corps in Madagascar before practicing medicine in the United States. He arrived in Rome en route to Africa just after the P.L.O. attack on the El Al desks at the airport. Everyone was jumpy, with armed guards everywhere. The doctor had to go through security to get to his gate. He was wearing heavy bush boots with considerable metal on them. The alarm system was very loud. He knew that the boots would set off the bells and buzzers, and possibly the automatic weapons of the very young and jumpy carbineers on the other side who were looking around nervously with fingers on the triggers of their weapons. He kept trying to explain to the security check in phonetic English his concern, pointing to his boots, making noises like the alarm, then the mock shooting of a gun. The checker kept smiling and shrugging, saying "Okay, okay." Finally, after the third try at communication, the checker gave him a look of pure mischief and said in perfect English, "Don't worry, Americano. We will not shoot your boots off."

During his first month in Madagascar, the doctor treated a sixteen-year-old with tetanus. He worked on him all day and finally got him to a point of recovery late at night. He left the medicine with the village family with instructions to keep giving the boy the drugs at the prescribed intervals. The doctor returned the next morning to find a corpse, the boy's body already cold and his jaws rigid with lips pulled back from his teeth in a paralyzed grimace. The family had not given him the medicine. They had tried tribal healing rituals instead.

Do you see the point of these stories, what they mean and why they are here? A story can extinguish the self, be developed in dramatic contexts by an omniscient narrator who can shift from one point of view to another. Or a story can generalize a first-person point of view, as I have done in narrating these stories.

I am a story. I integrate the facts of my life in narratives, from dreams to scripts, and provide reflections on experience. I invent myself as you invent yourself. We are all in some sense players in an experience where reality is filtered through thought, and made intelligible by narratives. Change the story and reality is altered.

From a report on out-of-body experiences:

"Rather recently I met someone who talked about out-of-body experiences, soul travel, and healing with sound and light. This piqued my interest. Once again I began to experience the sensation of leaving my body— usually from the dream state, but twice I woke up and had out-of-body experiences from an awake state.

"The most vivid one happened a week ago. It was close to morning and I was beginning to be aware—a kind of semi-sleep state. I felt a hand on my right shoulder and on my abdomen. It was as if I was approached from behind. It was a vivid touch and so real that I woke up, but not quite all the way. At first I thought it was my husband touching me, but then I felt a gentle pull backwards and I left my body. We (whoever was with me and touched me) began to travel very fast. We left my house through walls and were in a place that had many structures. The sound was a swooshing—as though traveling fast through the wind. I felt very free and safe because the person who was with me—I trusted. I looked down and didn't seem to have a body, but yet an essence of myself. It is difficult to explain. I saw what seemed to be chandeliers all around me with large crystals gently moving, as if blown by a breeze. The light was dim.

"While I was 'traveling' I heard my daughter get up and turn on the television. I remember thinking, I hope she doesn't disturb my body as I am not ready to come back yet. I felt so free. I began to turn and move as if floating in air. . . .

"At some point I came back to my room and was in my body. I got up and my daughter was watching TV as I had expected. This time getting back to my body was almost unnoticeable. Sometimes I don't seem to know how to do it, and other times I come back with a jolt to my physical body. . . .

"When I think about all this with my 'rational' mind, it is almost embarrassing to talk about. I don't tell many people about my experiences. I consider myself a well-educated, intelligent, rational person. But I cannot deny that these experiences are real.

"One last comment. My life seems now to be happier and calmer since these OBEs have begun. The inner harmony and peace I feel is a welcome experience. I do, however, want to be careful and not run away from 'reality'. . . ."

Luke

That distance between the physical terrain of the body and the things of the spirit, the lower and higher parts of being. Now negotiate from skin to thought, heat to light and back again. And now imagine cutting that membrane, the coaxial frame mapping that thick space between physical and mental. Can the soul be freed from the body?

From an interview with a psychotherapist:

"Many individuals develop depersonalized attitudes towards their bodies, in whole or in part. There have been a lot of theories on what this is about. For example, [some have] thought schizophrenics sometimes depict an area of the body as dead because they want to get rid of that area, that it is their way of renouncing a part of the body which, because of their socialization experiences, is considered bad or evil. They [believe that they] have no right to possess a part of the body that does those things. The history of Christianity is an attempt to conceive of humans as being without a body, except perhaps for the head. Everything below the neck has been disowned. . . .

"The 'soul' has been the refuge of people who do not want to accept the idea that they have a body. It is a futile attempt. It is bound to fail. Even the idea that there is pure thought—that you have a head with a brain and can focus everything on the functioning of that—as we get more data on how people think we know that body sensations are an integral part of thinking. We may do a significant part of our thinking with the kinesthetic sensations from different parts of the body. Talking is a kinesthetic experience. A lot of our coding of ideas starts here. . . . There are data on people who have spinal cord injuries, who have lost all sensation from the neck down. There are good indications that they do not experience the world the way other people do who are getting sensations from the body. It may be affecting their imagery. It may be affecting the way that they think. . . . For one thing, their emotions seem to be less vivid. There is a kind of blunting of their emotional experience."

Luke

But I can talk to God, spiritual communions without body, without weight or extension. And I still have dreams and memories. Images and events come to me in sleep like fragmented messages from some distant consciousness unlike my own. And thoughts of the past as I saw it filtered through older memories and perceptions. Present circumstances fix my identity. Dreams and memories bind me to myself.

Resurrection Stories (Anonymous)

"I believe we will all be there beyond the shadows, as we want to be, dressed in white. Death will be an awakening into a large room or house where everyone will gather, both the living and the dead; for if there is no death then we are all together in one life. We will dance with each other. The healing must be complete, you see, or it would not be perfect. The sightless will see, the lame will walk, the dumb will speak and even communicate with us. There will be a courtyard and we will dance on the stones. The bark of the trees will be washed in rain, glistening in the light. The sun will be out, no clouds, only a blue sky with no end to it. Everyone will take a deep breath of the air, so clean and fresh, and smile at each other. We will love one another. It will be a dream with no end to it."

NOTES

Introduction

Pages 1–2   The NIMH study is described in Martha Farnsworth Riche, "Behind the Boom in Mental Health Care."

Page 2   The Gallup poll, "Belief in Unusual Phenomena," was released in October 1988. Another study, Anthony Greeley, *The Sociology of the Paranormal: A Reconnaissance*, discovered that those who go to college are more likely to have mystical experiences than are individuals who do not attend college. Yet another study, B. Spilka, R. W. Hood, and R. L. Gorsuch, *The Psychology of Religion: An Empirical Approach*, found that 40–50 percent of the American public claims to have talked to God at some point in their lives.

Page 2   A list of healing miracles in the New Testament is provided by George W. Meck in *Healers and the Healing Process*, ed. Meck, 296–97. See also Joseph Champlin's account of these events in *Healing in the Catholic Church*.

Page 5   One resource I do not use, at least as extensively as I might in a study like this, is the field of professional ethics. The reason for this omission is both simple and complex. I discovered in the research that ethics, and even morality— whether elaborated in terms of rules, principles, even virtues—are not the primary variables in explaining or evaluating conflicts between spiritual and conventional healing. How a situation is defined and interpreted, in particular which account of reality is privileged, controls the moral status of the actions taken. *All* ethical and moral languages are variables of ontology. A work that does use professional ethics and morality in studying religion is Margaret Battin, *Ethics in the Sanctuary: Examining the Practices of Organized Religion*. See especially chapter 2, "High-Risk Religion," where the author deploys ethical terms like autonomy, informed consent, and the fiduciary principle in a context of competing realities.

Page 7   By using the term "fantastic" here, I do not mean to suggest that the beliefs are unusual. The Gallup poll, Greeley, and Spilka et al. studies cited above indicate (along with other inquiries) that such beliefs are widespread and even respectable. Also, my deliberate indifference to the truth of the stories related here follows roughly in the tradition of dream interpretation, which, when legitimate, takes the *report* of the dream as the critical datum providing information about the patient, not the dream as it occurred (or did not occur).

Luke

Pages 9–12   It might be best to allow the Luke sections to stand without extensive comment. But the perspicacious reader might see the influence of Thomas Nagel, *The View From Nowhere*, in certain of Luke's ruminations here.

Other philosophical perspectives also inform this work. If we press an imaginary "reveal codes" key, the anthropic principle would be put on display. This principle states that the universe needs observers in order to exist. It is shaped by observations that a range of constants and initial conditions of the universe both define reality and make conscious life possible, and by the thought that the features of the universe must be a derivative of observation and reflection, in the sense that without consciousness there would be no universe as we know it *by definition*. These arguments, one familiar and the other almost trivially self-evident, support the core statement of the principle: that reality can be what it is only if conscious life is one of its features. One implication of the anthropic principle is that reality must be strongly participatory, a product of an interaction between subject and object that also denies this very distinction as a polar relationship. The anthropic principle is virtually a textual premise here. It moves through all of the arguments and presentations, from Luke's opening reflections, especially in the famous tension proposed between observer and observed and the suggestion that events require an observer in order to occur (page 10), to the coherence account of power in the concluding sections of the book. For a recent contribution to this discussion, see the collection of interviews in Alan Lightman and Roberta Brawer, *Origins: The Lives and Worlds of Modern Cosmologists*.

But, having affirmed a version of the anthropic principle, it is also helpful to distance this book from some extravagant thoughts on the implications of quantum mechanics for the role of consciousness in establishing reality (and from considerable misuse of physics in social philosophy). Theories and experiments in quantum physics, especially Niels Bohr's theories and John Bell's theorem, have complicated and redefined the idea of local realities, with the result that reality at the subatomic level has no attributes until measured. The consequence of this counterintuitive truth is that reality at elementary levels must be a variable of our conceptual systems. The implications of these startling conclusions for macro realities are unclear, though a variety of intriguing paradoxes can be drawn up for ordinary reality from quantum mechanics. No one seriously claims, however, that macro phenomena have the same unsettling characteristics of subatomic particles (though some novel conceptions of nonlocal reality have been proposed on the basis of quantum theory, for example the implicate or enfolded order suggested by David Bohm in *Wholeness and the Implicate Order*). I intend to keep the work here distant from those speculative assertions in spiritual healing that use quantum mechanics to support unorthodox therapies. The connections (if any) between micro and macro realities is simply too complicated. Especially helpful on these points are Nick Herbert, *Quantum Reality*; P. C. W. Davis and J. R. Brown, eds., *The Ghost in the Atom*; and the spirited disclaimers in Douglas Stalker and Clark Glymour, "Quantum Medicine."

Chapter One: Rational Disputes

Pages 13–27 I have used several sources in reconstructing these events. The most important were the interviews with Joseph Loverro on December 29, 1989, and Stephen Dubansky on December 30, 1989 (which provide all quotes from the participants used in the text). The Tioga County (New York) Family Court decision written by Acting Family Court Judge Patrick H. Mathews, *In the Matter of Caleb Loverro* (May 24, 1988), was also very helpful. I also read most of the newspaper accounts written at the time of the dispute and used (though more sparingly) some information found there, including the fine stories by Henry Davis in the *Syracuse Herald Journal* (November 4, 1987, and May 26, 1988).

Pages 27–28 The thought that different discourses have different rules of inference and evidence, and rely on different senses of reality, is found in a variety of works, including William James, *Varieties of Religious Experiences*; Michael Oakeshott, *Experience and Its Modes*; and, more recently, Michel Foucault, *The Order of Things: An Archeology of Human Sciences*.

Pages 28–31 This account of early medicine follows a standard history delineated in numerous texts and encyclopedias. See the references cited in the notes for chapter 3.

Pages 31–32 This account of the liberal state as based on the possibility of neutral procedures is found in Ronald Dworkin, "Liberalism." The ideal of neutrality influences numerous attempts to produce or derive rules and principles of justice in recent liberal theory, including both John Rawls, *A Theory of Justice* and, more recently, "The Priority of Right and Ideas of the Good," and Robert Nozick, *Anarchy, State, and Utopia* (where a kindred term—impartiality—is secured in social distributions from a prior condition of liberty). See also Dworkin, *Taking Rights Seriously*; Michael Walzer, *Spheres of Justice: A Defense of Pluralism and Equality*; Bruce Ackerman, *Social Justice in the Liberal State*. Though "neutrality" is employed in different ways in these works, a core acceptance of the neutral state is found in each account of justice provided by the authors. See Michael Sandel, *Liberalism and the Limits of Justice*, for a communitarian alternative to "empty" liberal neutrality.

Neutrality, even as an ideal, is exceedingly complex. Like many other concepts, its sense varies with changes in its reference, with the consequence that neutrality at macro levels may not be neutrality at micro levels, what is neutral in one practice may not be in another, neutrality toward definitions of the good life may not be consistent with neutrality toward persons, and so on. Also, even as an ideal the concept is flawed in prominent ways and has properly been questioned, and even attacked, lately. The most widely known critiques are in the critical legal studies approach. See Roberto M. Unger, *The Critical Legal Studies Movement*, and Mark Kelman, *A Guide to Critical Legal Studies*. But see also Robert E. Goodin and Andrew Reeve, eds., *Liberal Neutrality*, for critiques within liberal perspectives. I am offering cases like that of Caleb Loverro as empirical evidence that a state cannot be neutral between conflicting ontologies.

Chapter Two: Science and Faith

Pages 36–37   Quote from interview on August 10, 1987.

Pages 42–43   Quote from interview on October 6, 1988.

Pages 43–44   Quote from interview on July 21, 1987.

Chapter Three: Medical Traditions

Page 45   I am grateful to Manfred Stanley for some of the thoughts in these two opening paragraphs.

Pages 46–47   The tendency to ascribe psychological traits to elements and powers survived the passing of Homer's ontology, however. Some might say that various unions of mental and physical languages persisted in strong form until Descartes's famous separation of the two. But however robust the historical extension, the use of mental vocabularies to represent the natural world survives Homer. It is certainly found in Plato, for example, in the *Phaedo*. For a quick and neat historical summary of this Greek period, see William Arthur Heidel, *The Heroic Age of Science: The Conception, Ideals, and Methods of Science among the Ancient Greeks*, part 1; F. M. Cornford, *Before and After Socrates*; and W. K. C. Guthrie, *The Greek Philosophers*. Also, see E. R. Dodds, *The Greeks and the Irrational*, and then Hesiod's *Theogony* for a heroic effort to explain the divine, the physical, and the human cosmos as interrelated parts of a single structure.

Pages 48–52, 65–70   Park's story is drawn from two lengthy interviews on November 14, 1988, and February 13, 1989.

Pages 52–56 This account continues the "enlightenment" history of medicine begun in chapter 1. I offer this well-known story not (obviously) as a contribution
to scholarship, since it is standard fare in medical histories, but as a background
reference against which various healing claims may be measured. Remember
that it is this configuration of discovery and development that informs contemporary medical practice, and relating the story clearly and briefly here, without
substantial critical comment, provides a context for beliefs in material and spiritual healing. Much of this narrative comes from an encyclopedic entry (where
the best "standard" stories are found): "Medicine," *The New Encyclopaedia Britannica*, 23:884–939. But I have also used Thomas Hall, *A History of General
Physiology*; Edwin Clarke, *Modern Methods in the History of Medicine*; Lester
King, *Growth of Medical Thought*; Benjamin Nelson, *On the Road to Modernity*; John Higham, *History*; William G. Rothstein, *American Physicians in the
Nineteenth Century*; and, for an account of more recent changes, Paul Starr,
The Social Transformation of American Medicine. Particular histories of various
healing traditions are abundant. Indian medicine, for example, is ably exam-
ined in Sudhir Kakar, *Shamans, Mystics and Doctors*. I am also grateful to
Robert Brophy for reading and commenting on the way I have retold this core
story of medicine.

Page 52 The antibiotics are listed in John E. Conte and Steve L. Barriere, *Manual
of Antibiotics and Infectious Diseases*.

Pages 54–55 The recent data on surgical devices and typical surgical interventions
are drawn from the medical practices in Crouse-Irving Hospital, a mid-size private hospital in Syracuse, New York. I am grateful to Dr. Edward Swift for providing this information.

Page 55 Janet Carlisle Bogdan, "What Difference Did Doctors Make? Physicians
and Childbirth in Nineteenth-Century New York City."

Pages 57–58 Martin Kaufman, *Homeopathy in America*; Rothstein, *American
Physicians in the Nineteenth Century*; Joseph Kett, *The Formation of the Ameri-
can Medical Profession*; John Davis, *Phrenology: Fad and Science*; John Harvey
Young, *The Toadstool Millionaires*; Eliot Freidson, *Professional Dominance:
The Social Structure of Medical Care*; Charles Rosenberg, *No Other Gods*; and
R. Lawrence Moore, *In Search of White Crows*.

Page 58 Loverro's views here are drawn from the interview on December 29, 1989.

Page 58 One of the classic statements here is Owsei Temkin's "Health and Disease." See also Temkin, "The Scientific Approach to Disease"; Lester King,
Medical Thinking; H. F. Stein, *Content and Dynamics in Clinical Knowledge*;
and Susan Sontag, *Illness as Metaphor*.

Pages 58–59 Joseph Margolis, "The Concept of Disease"; George L. Engel,
"Homeostasis, Behavioral Adjustment and the Concept of Health and Disease";

Norbert Wiener, "The Concept of Homeostasis in Medicine"; Christopher Boorse, "On the Distinction Between Disease and Illness"; Caroline Whitback, "A Theory of Health"; Leon Kass, "Regarding the End of Medicine and the Pursuit of Health"; and numerous conversations with and thefts of ideas from Dr. Robert Daly.

Page 61   Quote from Gabriel García Márquez, *Love in the Time of Cholera*, 110.

Page 61   Oliver Sacks, *The Man Who Mistook His Wife for a Hat*, chapter 24.

Page 63   William May, "The Physician's Covenant," and Morris L. Cogan, "Toward a Definition of a Profession."

Pages 64–65   The thoughts on medical ethics have complicated origins. The dramatic reversal of purpose represented in the phrase, "doctoring to kill" (and the phrase itself) has a distinguished lineage. I recall hearing it originally in Philippa Foot's lectures at Oxford in 1968–69. But the thought that social practices are defined by their purposes is part of a long tradition going back to Plato. The other points on medical ethics in these two paragraphs were provided by Dr. Robert Daly, who discussed these matters in a course he and I taught together, "Ethics and the Health Professions," in spring 1986. See also Benjamin Freedman, "A Meta-Ethics for Professional Morality," and Alan Goldman, *The Moral Foundations of Professional Ethics*.

Pages 69–70   P. Joseph Frawley, "Neurobehavioral Model of Addiction," and Shepard Siegel, Marvin D. Frank, and Riley E. Hinson, "Anticipation of Pharmacological and Nonpharmacological Events: Classical Conditioning and Addictive Behavior."

Page 70   M. T. Notman et al., "Psychotherapy with the Substance-Dependent Physician."

Pages 69–70   The practices controlling access to drugs are very tight in most hospitals. All narcotics and stimulants are usually kept in locked areas and typically can be released only for documented purposes (with an authorized signature). That Park could get drugs with such ease testifies both to the looseness of some hospital security systems and to the skills at deception that Park sharpened over years of illicit drug use.

Chapter Four: Mind and Body

Page 75   Translated by Anthony Kenny and cited on p. 218 in his *Descartes: A Study of His Philosophy*, from *Oeuvres de Descartes*, ed. Charles Adam and Paul Tannery, 6:113.

Pages 75–77   "Psychiatry," *Encyclopedia Americana*, 22:717–19, and "Psychiatry," *Collier's Encyclopedia*, 19:447–50.

Pages 77–83, 84   Interview on November 29, 1988.

Page 79   William Osler, *The Evolution of Modern Medicine*.

Page 83   The quote is from James Baldwin, *The Fire Next Time*, 39. Note also Frantz Fanon's experiences in Algeria, where his therapy practice was divided between torturers and victims. Each suffered from pathologies caused by the hideous conditions of French occupation. Fanon reacted by abandoning psychiatry and becoming a revolutionary. See Fanon, *The Wretched of the Earth* and *Black Skin, White Masks*; Jock McCulloch, *Black Soul, White Artifact: Fanon's Clinical Psychology and Social Theory*; and Emmanuel Hansen, *Frantz Fanon: Social and Political Thought*.

Pages 85–87   Richard Gregory, ed., *The Oxford Companion to the Mind*, 197–98, 740–47. The spectacle of conflicting preferences across conditions begins with Homer's *Odyssey*. (The story is so well known. Can it be told again? Of course.) In his travels Odysseus is warned by Circe of the compelling beauty of the Sirens' singing, which is so attractive that no one can resist moving toward its source. Sailors who hear the singing are drawn to the island on which the Sirens live, there to remain for the rest of their lives, bewitched until they die. Odysseus wants to hear the Sirens' songs *and* escape their spell. In Homer's story, he deafens his crew by putting wax in their ears. Then he has his crew strap him to the deck, bidding them to ignore his pleas when they pass the island. On hearing the Sirens' singing he orders, then begs, the crew to release him so that he can go toward the haunting sounds. But the crew follows his earlier commands, thus saving his life and allowing him to be the single human being to hear the song of the Sirens and escape. Like all of Homer's stories, the tale of the Sirens is enchanting, though it requires almost all of any poet's imagination to see the two contrasting conditions as equally compelling resources for establishing Odysseus's authentic preferences. For more recent variations on this problem see Jon Elster, ed., *The Multiple Self*, and the more elaborate explorations in Derek Parfit, *Reasons and Persons*. Practical expressions of the multiple self are found in those cases of individuals drawn unwittingly into cults and then forcibly removed by deprogrammers. See Richard Delgado, "Cults and Conversion: The Case for Informed Consent," and "When Religious Exercise Is Not Free: Deprogramming and the Constitutional Status of Coercively Induced Belief."

Page 87   Ludwig Wittgenstein, *Philosophical Investigations*, and Saul Kripke, *Wittgenstein on Rules and Private Language*.

Pages 87–88   There are other ways to cut the distinctions between sanity and madness. One is to reserve "sanity" for individuals who can act without compulsions. "Madness" will then refer to individuals who lack control of their actions. Or, more generally, as Robert Daly argues in "A Theory of Madness," madness may be an inability to secure one's prudential interests, sanity the ability to do so. My use of the word "madness" also includes delusions, or flawed understandings of a reality fixed by both conventions and physiology (a condition that clearly can impede the securing of prudential interests). The issue, then, is whether such a reality, any reality, is entirely local or generalizable in some minimal sense across discourse communities.

Page 88   *State Department of Human Services v. Mary C. Northern*, Tenn App, 563 SW2d 197 (1978), and *State Department of Human Services v. Larry T. Hamilton*, Tenn App, 657 SW2d 425 (1983).

Page 88   The Müller-Lyer diagram suggests that the top horizontal line is longer than the bottom line when they are actually the same length.

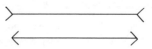

Page 89   Edward M. Hundert tracks the discussion (and debate) over mapping psychoses from flawed understandings of the form or structure of reality; see his *Philosophy, Psychiatry, and Neuroscience*, 165–80. For a brief summary of illusions and hallucinations, see Richard L. Gregory, ed., *The Oxford Companion to the Mind*, 299–300, 337–47. See also K. S. Penrose and R. Penrose, "Impossible Objects: A Special Type of Illusion." An instructive treatment of Escher is found in Douglas Hofstadter, *Gödel, Escher, Bach.* Kenneth Arrow's impossibility theorem is introduced in his *Individual Choice and Social Values.* The paradox developed by Richard Newcomb (then a physicist at the Lawrence Livermore Radiation Laboratory at the University of California) is described by Robert Nozick in "Newcomb's Problem and Two Principles of Choice."

Page 90   The enchanting story of Theseus's ship is another that bewitches the minds of philosophy students encountering identity problems for the first time. In irreverent form, it is the story of a ship, call it the H.M.S. *Enchantment*, that (like all ships) periodically undergoes repairs in port to replace aging sections of the vessel. At one stop a sail is taken down and a new one put in its place. Pieces of the deck are replaced during another stay in the port. At some point a new mast is installed. And so on. Over a long period of time, every piece of the ship is gradually replaced. Question: Is the "new" H.M.S. *Enchantment* the "same" ship? Complications for any answer provided: Unknown to the owners of the ship the owner of the shipyard has retained every old part of the H.M.S. *Enchantment* and used the material over time to build another complete ship. Which ship is the real H.M.S. *Enchantment?* The answer that best fits the arguments of this book: It depends on the discourse. In legal discourses criteria and rules will yield one set of answers, in moral discourses different sets, still others in political discourses, and so on.

Page 91   The extreme position would be the existentialist self as "nothingness," not even the social practices within which selves occur (since to exist as a role in a practice is to be a thing, not a self). See Jean-Paul Sartre's *Being and Nothingness.*

Page 91   From an interview with a psychotherapist on June 21, 1990.

Pages 91–102   Interviews on November 14, 1988, and February 13, 1989 (quotes on page 102 from November 14 interview).

Chapter Five: Spiritual Healing

Pages 103–4   Joseph Kessel, *The Road Back*; Milton Maxwell, *The Alcoholics Anonymous Experience*; Stephanie Brown, *Treating the Alcoholic*; and Ernest Kurtz, *AA: The Story*.

Pages 105–6   The relationships of soul and body are complex even in the New Testament. Hebrew traditions view humans as corporeal creatures in which soul and body are inextricably fused. Resurrection, remember, refers to God raising the *bodies* of the dead on Judgment Day. But St. Paul clearly speaks of an incarnate soul, and much biblical scholarship attributes a measure of dualism to the New Testament and interprets healing as directed to both body and soul. On this and other themes in the section, see Morton Kelsey, *Psychology, Medicine and Christian Healing*, chapters 3–5; Norman Perrin and Dennis Duling, *The New Testament: An Introduction*; and Geza Vermes, *Jesus the Jew*.

Page 106   This is Plato's thesis in the *Theaetetus*, but any reader of the middle dialogues knows that *courage* or *will* also complements knowledge in ensuring good acts. See the *Republic*.

Pages 107–8   Morton Smith, *Jesus the Magician*; Howard Clark Kee, *Medicine, Miracle and Magic in the New Testament* and *Miracle in the Early Christian World*.

Pages 108–10, 112–15   Stanley M. Burgess and Gary McGee, eds., Patrick H. Alexander, assoc. ed., *Dictionary of Pentecostal and Charismatic Movements*; Martin E. Marty, *A Nation of Believers*; Donald W. Dayton, *Theoretical Roots of Pentecostalism*; Margaret Poloma, *The Charismatic Movement*; Rex Davis, *Locusts and Wild Honey*; Richard Quebedeaux, *The New Charismatics*; Walter Hollenweger, *The Pentecostals*; and H. Newton Malony and A. Adams Lovekin, *Glossolalia: Behavioral Science Perspectives on Speaking in Tongues*. The reprint of the old Azusa Street papers collected by Fred T. Corum in *Like As of Fire* provides fine examples of the evangelical energies and loves of early Pentecostalism. The intensities of the movement can also be sensed in books written by those within Pentecostalism, for example, John White's *When the Spirit Comes with Power*.

Pages 110–12   See Watson E. Mills, ed., *Speaking in Tongues*, for collected overviews (and for all of the studies mentioned in the text).

Pages 115–16   The two quotes are excerpts from a service taped in the Reverend Faith Jamison's church on the Sunday afternoon mentioned in the text, May 28, 1989. This section, pages 115–19, is a reconstruction of the interview. Unless otherwise noted, all biographical sections are reconstructions from interview transcripts.

Page 119   Quote from interview on May 28, 1989.

Pages 119–23   This section and all quotes in it are from an interview with Robert Penfield on June 6, 1989.

Pages 123–25   Interview with James Crossland on October 18, 1988.

Pages 125–28   Interview with Charles Brantley on October 27, 1988.

Pages 128–32   Interview with Irene and Thomas Canterbury on January 27, 1988 (including quote on page 130).

Page 133   Kimberly A. Sherrill and David B. Larson, "Adult Burn Patients: The Role of Religion in Recovery."

Pages 133–34   P. Skrabaneh, "Paranormal Health Claims."

Pages 134–35   Quote from interview on March 18, 1989.

Page 136   Interview on June 21, 1990.

Chapter Six: Spiritual Domains

Pages 137–39   St. Augustine, *City of God*; St. Thomas Aquinas, *Summa theologica* and *Summa contra Gentiles*; John of Paris, *Tractatus de potestate regia et papali*; Marsilius of Padua, *Defensor pacis*; and Niccolò Machiavelli, *The Prince*. I am old-fashioned enough to believe that the best history of these philosophical traditions is still Frederick Copleston, *History of Philosophy*, vols. 2 and 3. But see also Dino Bigongiari, *The Political Ideas of St. Thomas Aquinas*.

Pages 140–41   The ideas deployed here on the intentions of the framers are influenced by Michael W. McConnell, "The Origins and Historical Understanding of Free Exercise of Religion." More recent issues in, and interpretations of, the religion clauses are summarized in "Developments in the Law: Religion and State." The reliance of interpretations on understandings of the individual is discussed in "Reinterpreting the Religion Clauses: Constitutional Construction and Conceptions of the Self." Michael Sandel draws important distinctions between conscience and choice in "Religious Liberty—Freedom of Conscience or Freedom of Choice?" See also Robert L. Cord and Howard Ball, "The Separation of Church and State: A Debate"; Carl H. Esbeck, "Five Views of Church-State Relations in Contemporary American Thought"; Bette Novit, "Contradictory Demands on the First Amendment Religion Clauses: Having it Both Ways"; and Barbara Perry, "Justice Hugo Black and the 'Wall of Separation Between Church and State.'"

Pages 143–44   Thomas R. McCoy and Gary A. Kurtz, "A Unifying Theory for the Religion Clauses of the First Amendment." The quote on page 144 is from "Developments in the Law: Religion and State," 1750–51.

Pages 145–46   "Reinterpreting the Religion Clauses."

Pages 147–48   "Developments in the Law—Medical Technology and the Law."

Pages 148–49   Mary Baker Eddy, *Science and Health with Key to the Scriptures*; Lyman Powell, *Christian Science: The Faith and Its Founders*; Robert Peel, *Health and Medicine in the Christian Science Tradition*; and *Christian Science: A Sourcebook of Contemporary Materials*.

Page 149   Quote from Eddy, *Science and Health*, 468.

Pages 150–53   Interview with Bryan Seth on February 21, 1989.

Pages 153–59   Interview with Anthony Vecchio on March 6, 1989; quote on page 159 also from interview.

Page 159   See Michel Foucault, *The Birth of the Clinic*, for a wider discussion of modern medicine.

Page 162   This symbiotic dependence between individual and society is admirably described in Daniel J. Levinson et al., *The Seasons of a Man's Life*, 40–49.

Luke

Page 169   The experience related here is an instance of déjà vu: a perception of a scene accompanied by a compelling sense of familiarity. It is often reported by those suffering from temporal lobe lesions and seems to be one of the experiences of some epileptics. But a majority of "normal" people also have had one or more "already seen" experiences. Many people outside medicine prefer mystical or psychic explanations for the phenomenon, often using it as an indication of a former life. See Gregory, ed., *The Oxford Companion to the Mind*, 182–84.

Page 170   The reality of a disembodied self is described in Oliver Sacks' *The Man Who Mistook His Wife for a Hat*, chapter 3. He describes a woman with extensive damage to the sensory roots throughout the neuraxis. The spinal tap revealed an acute polyneuritis that deprived her of proprioception, a sense of position. The chapter describing this case is titled "The Disembodied Lady."

Chapter Seven: Holistic Medicine

Page 174   The distinction between these two types of healing has been introduced and elaborated by Lawrence LeShan as Type I healing (the meditative alignment with a larger reality) and Type II healing (the traditional action of a healer on a patient). See LeShan, *The Medium, the Mystic, and the Physicist*, esp. chapter 7.

Pages 174–77   The techniques of therapeutic touch are ably outlined in two books: Dolores Krieger, *The Therapeutic Touch*, and Janet Macrae, *Therapeutic Touch: A Practical Guide*.

Pages 177–78   The experiment with mice (and a description of the effects of therapeutic touch on plants as well) is found in B. Grad, "Some Biological Effects of
the Laying-on of Hands: A Review of Experiments with Animals and Plants."
The healing effects on dermal wounds is described in Daniel P. Wirth, "Unorthodox Healing: The Effects of Noncontact Therapeutic Touch on the Healing
Rate of Full Thickness Dermal Wounds." The hemoglobin response has been
found in several studies. See Dolores Krieger, "The Relationship of Touch with
the Intent to Help or to Heal, to Subjects in Vivo Hemoglobin Values: A Study
in Personalized Interaction." Another study has demonstrated an increase in
the activity of the enzyme trypsin as a result of therapeutic touch, in M. J.
Smith, "Paranormal Effects on Enzyme Activity."

Pages 178–79   One of the most accessible pieces on these theoretical categories is
Dora Kunz and Erik Peper, "Fields and Their Clinical Implications." See also
the articles (including this one) collected in Kunz, ed., *Spiritual Aspects of the
Healing Arts*. The Estabany story is everywhere (or so it seems). See, for example, Krieger, *The Therapeutic Touch*.

Pages 179–84   Interview with William Sulzman on October 27, 1989.

Pages 187–89   Interview with Philip Edwards on October 25, 1989.

Pages 190–94   Interview with Gloria Kaster on October 27, 1989.

Pages 194–203   Interview with Lawrence LeShan on December 1, 1989. See also
LeShan, *The Mechanic and the Gardner: How to Use the Holistic Revolution in
Medicine* and *Cancer as a Turning Point*. All quotes in this section are from the
interview.

Pages 203–4   The deductive models of practical reasoning suggested here are found
in both philosophy of science and moral philosophy. See the deductive
nomological explanations developed by, among others, Carl Hempel, *Aspects
of Scientific Explanation* and *Philosophy of Natural Science*, and Hempel and
Paul Oppenheimer, "The Covering Law Analysis of Scientific Explanation."
See also Ernest Nagel, *The Structure of Science*. Then compare with the deductive models of moral reasoning offered by R. M. Hare in *The Language of
Morals* and *Freedom and Reason*. Let us give thanks for the dissenting litera-
tures. See especially Nelson Goodman, *Fact, Fiction, and Forecast*; Karl
Popper, *The Logic of Scientific Discovery* and *Conjectures and Refutations*;
W. V. O. Quine, "Two Dogmas of Empiricism" and *Word and Object*; and the
accounts of practical reasoning based on bounded rationalities crafted by
Herbert Simon, *Models of Bounded Rationality*.

Page 205   For a helpful collection of articles on these ideas, see Martin E. Marty
and Kenneth L. Vaux, eds., *Health/Medicine and the Faith Traditions*.

Pages 207–9   The reader might see the following philosophical views and empirical theories in the Luke reflections here. For discussion of the claim that body is the locus of identity, see Bernard Williams, *Problems of the Self*, and John Perry, *A Dialogue on Personal Identity and Immortality*. The famous attempt to prove self-existence is of course Descartes's exercises in the *Meditations*, since successfully refuted by later philosophers, especially Hume and Kant. The "ghost in the machine" phrase is the familiar depiction of mind used by Gilbert Ryle in *The Concept of Mind*. The use of spontaneous thoughts is a rejoinder to Descartes drawn up by Nietzsche in *Will to Power* and found in various Eastern philosophies, for example, Mahayana Buddhism. No more effective presentation of role playing and madness is likely to be found than in Luigi Pirandello's play *Henry the Fourth*, though the literatures of sociology are filled with discussions of *sane* roles. The experience of entering a "zone" in athletic activity has become a standard mystical event in sports. See Lawrence Shainberg, "Finding 'The Zone.'" The notion of facts existing without our being able to comprehend them (the interior dimension represented by subjectivity) has a distinguished pedigree, but see Thomas Nagel's famous contribution, "What Is It Like to Be a Bat?" for special insights on these issues. (For the record, however, much of philosophy from Wittgenstein's *Philosophical Investigations* to the present has denied both private languages and private selves.) The view of consciousness as "a point of view" is standard in traditional philosophy and has been challenged with variations on split-brain realities, conflicting inner selves, and spectacular thought experiments, none more pleasing than Daniel C. Dennett's ."Where Am I?" And, finally, the understanding of consciousness as an exercise in self-reflection goes back at least to Plato. See, from a large set of interesting recent contributions, Michael Tooley's outline of an aware and continuing self in "Abortion and Infanticide." The use of self-referential paradoxes here is taken from Douglas Hofstadter's *Gödel, Escher, Bach*, and Hofstadter and Dennett, eds., *The Mind's I*, 276–83. The four-dimensional approach is used mainly to explain the existence of objects and their persistence or continuity but also is assigned to human identity. See Mark Heller, "Temporal Parts of Four-Dimensional Objects." The modest exploration of "self" and "other" is elaborated famously (and differently) by Husserl, Sartre, Jacques Derrida, and others. But see also George Herbert Mead, *Mind, Self and Society*.

Chapter Eight: Political Discourses

Page 215   Cited in Robert L. Van de Castle, "Sleep and Dreams." The original study of the *Titanic* premonition is in I. Stevenson, "A Review and Analysis of Paranormal Experiences Connected with the Sinking of the *Titanic*," and that of the coal slide in the Welsh mining village in J. C. Barker, "Premonitions of the Aberfan Disaster."

Pages 217–18   This material is again drawn from the interviews with Joseph Loverro and Stephen Dubansky, the Family Court decision, and the newspaper accounts.

Pages 219–20   One hesitates to suggest a "logic" for moral discourse here or anywhere else. But two traditions must be examined if the disputes related in this work are to be seen in moral terms. One is the quasi-formal or prescriptive view of moral discourse so influential in Britain and America until recently. See the early R. M. Hare in *The Language of Morals*, and Alan Gewirth, *Reason and Morality*. More recent work in this tradition includes the interesting accounts in Bernard Williams, *Ethics and the Limits of Philosophy*, and Stuart Hampshire, *Morality and Conflict*, as well as Hare's midpoint thinking in *Freedom and Reason* and the later thoughts in *Moral Thinking*. The other tradition is represented by a concern for virtue, famously expressed by Alasdair MacIntyre in *After Virtue* and *Whose Justice? Which Rationality?* as an endorsement of theism, and Charles Taylor in *Sources of the Self* as a form of liberalism.

Pages 220–27   Interview with David Stanford on November 7, 1989.

Page 234   See, for example, the heterogeneous collection of work in Louis Kriesberg, Terrell A. Northrup, and Stuart J. Thorson, eds., *Intractable Conflicts and Their Transformation*, and the list of references at the end of the book.

Page 234   A helpful discussion of credentialing can be found in Randall Collins, *The Credentialing Society*.

Pages 234–35   Kristin Luker is the source for the attrition prediction, in *Abortion and the Politics of Motherhood*. I am the unwelcome authority for the thought that RU486 would relocate abortion from public to private domains, in my *Abortion: A Case Study in Law and Morals* (a view accepted at the time by Rep. Henry Hyde).

Pages 236–37   I am using the standard three-place arrangement of these terms. "Certainty" refers to a relationship between alternative and outcome that has a probability of 1. "Risk" describes such a relationship with a probability between 0 and 1. "Uncertainty" refers to alternative-outcome relationships that have no objective probabilities.

Pages 238–39   So much of economic theory depends on shared scales for composition efforts that reminders of the paradoxes multiple dimensions bring are always helpful. Even transitivity, that seemingly empty logical rule, is not spared. Suppose I prefer working two hours as opposed to four hours as a lifeguard, and four hours as opposed to six hours (on the grounds that my leisure time is more valuable to me than the increments of pay that the hourly increase brings *in this sequence*). Now, on transitivity, two hours must be preferred to six. But it may be that in the binary comparison here I prefer six hours to two since the pay difference is now enough to inspire me to work instead of play. This failure of transitivity is probably best explained by a shift in the conditions of the ordering brought on by a concealed threshold effect that makes the increase in hours nonmonotonic. The point for the text is that numerous breakdowns prevent us from aggregating or maximizing principles that occupy different conceptual domains or measurement dimensions. See Michael Stocker, *Plural and Conflicting Values*, for a discussion of some of these problems, especially part 4 for critiques of maximization. Kim DeVogel, one of my graduate students, is the source for the hours-of-work example.

Chapter Nine: Liberal Power

Pages 241–42 The liberal story is still told best by Ronald Dworkin, "Liberalism," and Michael Sandel, *Liberalism and the Limits of Justice*. A more recent book, however, explicitly abandons neutrality by viewing the liberal state as committed to a distinctive conception of the human good, from which follow liberalism's characteristic institutions and practices. See William Galston's *Liberal Purposes: Goods, Virtues, and Diversity in the Liberal State*. This argument, complex and important, is at odds with the conclusions here, though I will mention only briefly where Galston and I differ. I see neutrality failing because even the frameworks for negotiating and managing conflict can be reasonably appropriated by rival factions. Thus, on the views developed here, liberalism fails at some fundamental level. It cannot be rescued by admitting the conditions of "partial agreement and potential mutual advantage" (*Liberal Purposes*), for these terms (and all others) can vary decisively across (for example) secular and spiritual beliefs precisely when coercion *must* be used to resolve disputes. A "liberal" state that requires citizens to act against their own deepest (*and* reasonable) understandings of human experience has abandoned some of its core ideals.

Pages 243–46 Ernest Gellner, *Cause and Meaning in the Social Sciences* and *Relativism and the Social Sciences*; Thomas Kuhn, *The Structure of Scientific Revolutions*; Alasdair MacIntyre, "The Idea of a Social Science" and "Is Understanding Religion Compatible with Believing?"; W. H. Newton-Smith, *The Rationality of Science*; Richard Rorty, *Philosophy and the Mirror of Nature*; Peter Winch, *The Idea of a Social Science*; and Ludwig Wittgenstein, *Remarks on Frazer's "Golden Bough."*

Page 244 This third community of discourse is a perversion of Plato—an abstract world whose formation depends on the absence of truth rather than its attainment. The metacommunity requires that truth remain in the cave, with the systems of belief that the metalanguage describes and compares.

Pages 246–47 One of the more illuminating insights into Rawls's theory of justice, for example, is the (true) observation that the primary goods listed in the work are artifacts of a secular liberal society, and so are deniable on alternative social arrangements. All goods seem local in this sense, thus providing abundant empirical support for the naturalistic fallacy.

Page 247   The observation on languages is from MacIntyre, "Is Understanding Religion Compatible with Believing?"

Pages 246–47   Whether one can enter and provisionally subscribe to hermeneutic styles and methods is one of the great open questions in recent literatures. Is not the traveler forever the outsider, distant from those critical meanings that inform social life? I am trying to say both yes and no with my points on metalanguage and the completeness of explanations.

Page 248   A story that can be tracked (if temporary amnesty can be granted from recent critical dismissals of "traditions") from John Stuart Mill's *On Liberty* through Robert Nozick's *Anarchy, State, and Utopia* (for the libertarian view) and from Jean-Jacques Rousseau's *Social Contract* through John Rawls's *A Theory of Justice* (for the liberating effects of state intervention).

Pages 248–49   Many traditions of Western law are silent on privacy. The principle usually makes its appearance as a summary concept to state the logic and justification of other rights. It achieves Constitutional status in American law as a derivative from a cluster (or "penumbra") of rights, no one of which mentions privacy as such. But taken together they seem to require the principle of privacy as a core statement of what is being protected. The standard justifications for privacy shields in Western societies can be found in Mill's famous brief against state regulation and paternalism in *On Liberty*. See also Hyman Gross, "The Right to Privacy"; Judith Jarvis Thompson, "The Right to Privacy"; James Rachels, "Why Privacy Is Important"; and Gerald Dworkin, "Paternalism."

Page 248   This is, of course, the heart of Mill's libertarian case—that competent individuals can be regulated only when they harm one another, not for paternalistic reasons.

Page 249   See my "Liberal Maps of Consent" for elaborations of these ideas.

Pages 248–50   Again, these are the contrasting views of Nozick and Rawls, both comfortably defined within liberal political philosophy.

   The two principles of justice most characteristic of liberalism are equality and liberty. Each is an elastic term yielding multiple, and mutually contradictory, meanings. Equality can be satisfied by equal access, equal opportunity, strict numerical equality, proportional equality, and other senses of the term. Two individuals can be said to be treated equally, for example, if given the chance to compete for goods (fairly), or if given an equal share of the goods, or if given goods unequally according to just claims (for example, giving more to the one who has greater needs). Liberty is famously divisible into negative and positive, the former interpreted as the provision of conditions needed for action. See Douglas Rae, *Equalities*, for an anticipation of deconstruction with a discussion of various senses of "equality." "Liberty" is demarcated by Isaiah Berlin in *Two Concepts of Liberty*, and compressed again into a single (though more complex) term by Gerald C. MacCallum, "Negative and Positive Freedom."

Page 250   See Dan Brock, "Recent Work in Utilitarianism," for an overview of this political philosophy. See also the collection of papers in Amartya Sen and Bernard Williams, eds., *Utilitarianism and Beyond*. The social contract tradition is more carefully defined by David Hume than other contract theorists in its modern beginnings. See Hume's "Of the Original Contract," in Charles W. Hendel, ed., *David Hume's Political Essays*.

Pages 250–51   See Michael Sandel, *Liberalism and the Limits of Justice*, for the points on what he labels the "unencumbered" self, and Robert Paul Wolff, *Understanding Rawls: A Reconstruction and Critique of "A Theory of Justice,"* for the thought that introducing content to the minimal knowledge of the original position inevitably biases the choices (by historically grounding them, for one thing).

Page 251   It is interesting that a case for the essentially arbitrary nature of politics is also made on entirely different grounds by William Riker in *Liberalism Against Populism*. Riker documents the existence of competing decisions rules to reach collective outcomes, notes that no compelling reasons bid us to support one rule over another, that collective outcomes differ from one rule to another, and so no reasons justify any collective outcome. The fact of political life, from Riker's perspective, is that each rule is used by individuals and groups to manipulate outcomes for partisan reasons.

Page 251   The idea of state as umpire is a reasonable interpretation of the theory of state in Thomas Hobbes's *Leviathan*.

Pages 251–58   Interview with David Twitchell on October 8, 1990, near the Islip Airport, Long Island, New York.

Pages 258–62 and 266   Interview with Joseph and Susan Clark on October 5, 1990, in the Syracuse, New York area.

Pages 262–66   Interview with Stephen Dubansky on October 10, 1990, in Syracuse, New York.

Page 266   The U.S. Supreme Court, in *Jehovah's Witnesses in the State of Washington v. King's County Hospital Unit 1* (1967), has held that the state may justifiably intervene to protect the health and welfare of minors participating in religious practices because "the right to practice religion does not include the liberty to expose the child to ill health or death." The North Carolina Court of Appeals for the Western District, following the *Jehovah's Witnesses* precedent, ruled that the government could enforce the Fair Labor Standards Act against a contractor operating a vocational training program for a church. The program violated the act's provisions for minimum wage, overtime compensation, record-keeping, and employment of minors. One of the implications of the Court's holding is that the right to practice religion does not include the right to jeopardize a child's health. See *Shiloh True Light Church of Christ v. Brock* (1987). Later, in *Forest Hills Early Learning Center v. Jackson* (1989), the U.S. Supreme Court let stand a Court of Appeals decision that the application of state licensing requirements to church-run day-care centers does not interfere with their free exercise of religion and, to the extent that it does, is justified by compelling state interests. One may conclude from the *Shiloh* and *Forest Hills* rulings that if religious practices risk or endanger the health and well-being of individuals, state intervention is permissible in order to avoid adverse health consequences. Also, religious practices are not necessarily exempt from laws of general applicability, especially if courts accept generality as a satisfaction of neutrality. In *Employment Division, Department of Human Resources of Oregon et al., Petitioners v. Alfred E. Smith et al.* (1990), the U.S. Supreme Court held that the free exercise clause does not shield the religious use of peyote in sacramental ceremonies from the state of Oregon's controlled substance law that *generally* prohibits such drugs without specifically targeting religions. (I am grateful to one of my students, Kimberly Sommar, for calling some of these cases to my attention.)

The appellate action in most of the Christian Science cases currently in the legal system focuses on a limited version of due process, in particular (a) whether the parents know before the fact that the state considers spiritual efforts at healing to be a criminal act when a child dies (this issue occasioned by the state laws that shield parents from charges of neglect or abuse when using spiritual healing in good faith), and (b) whether sameness rules are being met, since laws that place spiritual healing on the same legal footing with conventional medical care would seem to require prosecuting parents whose child dies under such care if parents relying on spiritual healing are prosecuted.

The deeper issue in these disputes is whether spiritual healing is effective. Does it work? Since the beliefs of Christian Scientists are based on the empirical claim that prayer is more effective than orthodox medicine, it would seem that some adjudication by means of research should be possible. Unfortunately few neutral studies have been made. One by William Frank Simpson, "Comparative Longevity in a College Cohort of Christian Scientists," indicates problems for spiritual claims. The study compared the longevity of Principia College graduates with those from the University of Kansas and, in spite of the health benefits expected from the Christian Science proscriptions on drugs, alcohol, and tobacco, the study concluded that the "graduates from Principia College had a significantly higher death rate than the control population."

Pages 266–67 Mental states, of course, enter the calculations of the law in both subtle and gross ways. The law, for example, sets degrees of culpability and levels of punishment on states of mind like intentions and motives. Trials of Christian Scientists that fall under the exclusionary provisions of child abuse statutes try to assess the sincerity of religious beliefs, obviously a mental category. But the free exercise clause of the First Amendment frees religious states of mind, meaning beliefs, from state regulation, and the general tenor of liberalism is to shield beliefs from regulation. When laws are broken, however, then the plaintiff's beliefs are natural topics for examination as a way of understanding the offense. The actions, not the beliefs, are on trial.

In a famous case, *Cantwell v. Connecticut* (1940), the U.S. Supreme Court held that freedom of religious beliefs is absolute but freedom to act is not. Religious "conduct remains subject to regulation for the protection of society." The regulation, however, must not unduly infringe on religious freedom. The two-part test that regulation must meet is that it be (1) warranted by a compelling state interest, and (2) the minimal and least restrictive method to advance state interests. These well-known words respect dualisms between thought and action by disallowing an excess of regulation that could crush beliefs through control of actions.

Page 267   To those who might claim that Christian Scientists would only be prevented from being Christian Scientists until they were adults, listen to Joseph Clark's words on children: "In Christian Science we are taught that a child doesn't really know enough about its own existence. The thought of the parents is what governs the child." There is little doubt that Christian Science requires parental dominion over children, and that any denial of this authority would be a denial of one of the central beliefs in Christian Science.

Pages 268–71   The literature on power is predictably complex and uneven. Direct power has been elaborated effectively by a number of scholars, especially Robert Dahl, "The Concept of Power" and "Power"; indirect power, or what I have called oblique power, by Peter Bachrach, *Political Elites in a Democracy*; Steven Lukes, *Power: A Radical View*; and Dahl, *Who Governs?: Democracy and Power in an American City*; and general examinations (and recognition of distinctions between power and exchange) by Brian Barry, ed., *Power and Political Theory: Some European Perspectives*.

Page 269   The distinction between nonreductionist and reductionist selves is from Derek Parfit, *Reasons and Persons*. Nonreductionism views individuals as separate existing entities, distinct from their brains and their bodies as well as from their experiences. Reductionist views define personal identity as no more than certain kinds of relations, like connectedness and continuity. On a reductionist view, individuals are not separate entities.

Pages 271–73   It is not surprising for anyone monitoring the caution of local and state courts that the two most prominent judicial decisions in New York state (where the Caleb Loverro case occurred) addressing compulsory medical treatment for minors focus on the procedural issue of whether a physician licensed in the state has approved the unorthodox therapy being applied. In *Hofbauer* the court allowed laetrile therapy because a physician advocated it, while in *Loverro* the court mandated conventional therapy in the absence of a physician's support for nutritional treatment. Still, in spite of the inclination of both courts to seize on procedure rather than merits, the two opinions illustrate the conjoining of reason and power elaborated in the text.

MATTER OF HOFBAUER [47 NY2d 648]

Statement of Case

Matter of Hofbauer, 65 AD2d 108, Affirmed.
Argued June 5, 1979; decided July 10, 1979

SUMMARY

Appeal, by permission of the Appellate Division of the Supreme Court in the Third Judicial Department, from an order of said court, entered December 20, 1978, which affirmed, on the law and the facts, an order of the Family Court, Saratoga County (Loren N. Brown, J.), after a fact-finding hearing, dismissing a petition under article 10 of the Family Court Act seeking to have Joseph Hofbauer adjudged to be a child neglected by his parents.

In October, 1977, Joseph Hofbauer, then a seven-year-old child, was diagnosed as suffering from Hodgkin's disease, a disease which is almost always fatal if left untreated. The then attending physician, Dr. Cohn, recommended that Joseph be seen by an oncologist or hematologist for further treatment which would have included radiation treatments and possibly chemotherapy, the conventional modes of treatment. Joseph's parents, after making numerous inquiries, rejected Dr. Cohn's advice and elected to take Joseph to a medical clinic in Jamaica where a course of nutritional or metabolic therapy, including injections of laetrile, was initiated. Upon Joseph's return to Saratoga County in November, 1977, the instant neglect proceeding was commenced. The petition alleged that Joseph's parents neglected their son by their failure to follow the advice of Dr. Cohn with respect to treatment and, instead, chose a course of treatment for Joseph in the form of nutritional therapy and laetrile.

The Court of Appeals affirmed the order of the Appellate Division and, in an opinion by Judge Jasen, held that under the circumstances, it cannot be said, as a matter of law, that the parents of a child afflicted with Hodgkin's disease have failed to exercise a minimum degree of care by entrusting the child's physical well-being to a duly licensed physician who advocates a treatment not widely embraced by the medical community.

HEADNOTE

Parent and Child—Abused or Neglected Child

The most significant factor in determining whether a child is being deprived of adequate medical care, and, thus, is a neglected child within the meaning of section 1012 (subd [f], par [i], cl [A]) of the Family Court Act, is whether the parents have provided an acceptable course of medical treatment for their child in light of all the surrounding circumstances and the court's inquiry should be whether the parents, once having sought accredited medical assistance and having been made aware of the seriousness of their child's affliction and the possibility of cure if a certain mode of treatment is undertaken, have provided for their child a treatment which is recommended by their physician and which has not been totally rejected by all responsible medical authority; accordingly, a child suffering from Hodgkin's disease whose parents failed to follow the recommendation of an attending physician to have their child treated by radiation and chemotherapy, but, rather, placed their child under the care of a duly licensed physician advocating nutritional or metabolic therapy, including injections of laetrile, is not a neglected child within the meaning of statute inasmuch as it cannot be said, as a matter of law, that the parents have failed to undertake reasonable efforts to ensure that acceptable medical treatment is being provided their child where there are findings supported by the record that numerous qualified doctors have been consulted by the child's physician and have contributed to the child's care, that the parents have both serious and justifiable concerns about the deleterious effects of radiation treatments and chemotherapy, that there is medical proof that the nutritional treatment being administered the child was controlling his condition and that such treatment is not as toxic as is the conventional treatment, and that conventional treatments will be administered to the child if his condition so warrants.

IN THE MATTER OF CALEB LOVERRO N-774-87

Hon. Patrick H. Mathews

Acting Family Court Judge

Tioga County

Owego, New York

May 24, 1988

On September 3, 1987 Charlotte Keegan of Tioga County Department of Social Services applied, pursuant to 1022 of the Family

Court Act, for a temporary order of removal regarding Caleb Loverro, a 3 year old child. It was alleged that Caleb's parents had failed to provide necessary medical care for his leukemia. Attached to Keegan's petition was the September 2, 1987 letter of Stephen Dubansky of the State University of New York Health Science Center (Upstate Medical), Syracuse, New York. Dr. Dubansky, Caleb's physician, wrote that Caleb's parents had refused to continue chemotherapy and that without chemotherapy the child would likely die. . . .

CONCLUSIONS OF LAW

Article 10 of the Family Court Act is designed to provide due process of the law for determining when the State may intervene on a child's behalf against the wishes of a parent (Family Court Act 1011). Family Court Act 1012, insofar as relevant to the facts of this case, provides that a *neglected child* is a child less than eighteen years of age whose physical condition has been impaired or is in imminent danger of becoming impaired as a result of the failure of his parent to exercise a minimum degree of care in supplying the child with adequate medical care, although financially able to do so [author's note: not an issue in this case].

The standard of neglect against which the facts of this case are to be measured is set forth in *Matter of Hofbauer*, 47 NY2d 648 (1979). Parents, under *Hofbauer*, are required to entrust their children's care to a physician when such course would be undertaken by an ordinary prudent and loving parent. In this regard, the *Hofbauer* Court cited *People v. Pierson*, 172 NY 201 (1903), which long ago established that a parent is obligated to ensure that a child "dangerously ill" be attended by a medical practitioner legally qualified under the laws of New York State. Thus, under New York law, the parents of a child suffering a life threatening illness are minimally required to seek accredited medical assistance and provide treatment for their child recommended by a physician (*Hofbauer, supra*, at 656).

The *Hofbauer* Court recognized the fundamental right of parents to rear their children free of government intervention. *Hofbauer* also noted, however, that this right is not absolute. The State is obligated as *parents patriae* to intervene if necessary to ensure that a child's health is not jeopardized by a parent's fault or omission (*Hofbauer, supra*, at 655).

In balancing the rights of parents against the obligation of the State, *Hofbauer* attempted to defer as much as reasonably possible to the parents. The choice of physician and mode of treatment is for the parent to decide. The State's inquiry, in the case of a life threatening illness, is limited to ensuring that the parents provide treatment which is (1) recommended by a physician of their choice and (2) a treatment which is not totally rejected by all responsible medical authority (*Hofbauer, supra*, at 656).

The first prong of this test is dispositive of this case. The *Hofbauer* Court wrote, "if a physician is licensed by the State, he is recognized by the State as capable of exercising acceptable clinical judgment" (citing *Doe v. Bolton*, 410 US 179, 199) [*Hofbauer, supra* at 655]. *Hofbauer* requires the State to yield to the parents' treatment choice provided that in arriving at that choice the parents relied, " . . . upon the recommendations and competency of the [duly licensed] *attending* physician . . . " (emphasis added) (*Hofbauer, supra*, at 655). The Court finds as a fact that there was no physician licensed to practice in New York State attending Caleb as of September 3, 1987 other than Dr. Dubansky.

. . . On the record of these proceedings, the Court finds that, if there is a legitimate medical controversy regarding discontinuation of chemotherapy in ALL treatment, it applies solely to the maintenance phase of treatment. The Court finds as a fact that no responsible medical authority would recommend discontinuation of chemotherapy shortly after remission.

On the facts as herein determined and the law, a finding that Caleb Loverro is a neglected child is entered. Pending the dispositional hearing all prior orders will remain in full force and effect. This constitutes the decision and order of the Court.

How can one additional fact be entered into these records without undermining the arguments for parental discretion? Joseph Hofbauer died from Hodgkin's disease on July 16, 1980 at the age of ten.

Page 272   I am as aware as anyone that religious beliefs strongly influenced liberal thought from its origins until (perhaps) recently, and that life as we view it today in the West was not regarded so seriously in the past even in liberal practices and philosophies. I am maintaining here only a modest point on the implications of liberal assumptions that "eventually" (over historical time) led to the view that individual life is a primary good. Also, and conceded, the secular state is a recent configuration absent from earlier "liberal" societies. But I still hold to the conceptual point that the barriers between church and state established in the First Amendment, even if inspired by a desire to assist religion, create a secular state charged with an impartiality that is impossible to realize in conflicts over health and healing when reality is at issue and life is at stake.

Chapter Ten: Narrative Reasoning

Page 277   For an impressive attempt at doing what I say cannot be done, however, see Margaret P. Battin, *Ethics in the Sanctuary: Examining the Practices of Organized Religion.*

Page 278   One of the more effective illustrations of the differences between "authentic" and "reflective" discourses is "The Case of W" by Ernst Strouhal, in Ruth Wodak, ed., *Language, Power and Ideology.* W, the young woman being examined by a psychiatrist, tries "to verbalize the inner reality of her experience" while the therapist tries to impose scientific standards on the inquiry. The result is a complete failure of communication.

Pages 279–80   The way that plots function as devices to interpret and summarize texts has been explored in a number of recent works. See Wendy G. Lehnert and Cynthia Loiselle, "Plot Units and Narrative Summarizations," and the exercise using and expanding on this work, Hayward Alker, Lehnert, and D. Schneider, "Two Reinterpretations of Toynbee's Jesus: Explorations in Computational Hermeneutics."

Page 280   Karl Mannheim, for example, trusts the intellectual to find the outside vantage point that will provide an escape from the dilemmas of internal truth, in particular the liar's paradox found in the center of the sociology-of-knowledge thesis.

Page 280   This type of paradox occurs as the statement addresses itself. Pascal's dilemma suggests the difficulties in introducing an overriding value to utility calculations. In such calculations in conditions of risk, probabilities and utilities combine to disclose an ordering of outcomes. For example, in the expression

$$P(O_m)U(O_m) - P(O_n)U(O_n) > 0 \text{ for m} \neq \text{n}$$

the product of the probability (P) and utility (U) of O_m is greater than the product (P)(U) of O_n. Alternative m is then said to have a higher expected value than n (which presumably also leads to an ordering of m > n).

But, as Pascal saw, such calculations work (if they work at all) only when there are reasonable bounds on utility. If an infinite value is introduced to utilities, then even the lowest probability will not affect the peremptory force of the value. (For example, if there is *any* chance that God exists, one must believe it because of the expected benefits of such belief *vs.* the extreme costs of nonbelief.) The difficulty is that possibility then has overridden probability, and one is no longer doing utility calculations in conditions of risk. Probabilities do not calibrate expected values; the values dominate once the alternative is recognized as possible.

Pascal's dilemma can communicate many lessons, most of them obvious or worthless. But suggested in the distorting effects of infinite values on utility calculations is a distinction between complete and limited knowledge. If the range of knowledge is less than infinite, the calculations can work. But a range that moves beyond any limits cannot be expressed successfully in sequential forms of reasoning.

Newcomb's problem introduces these limitations on linear or sequential reasoning in even more enlightening ways. Assume an omniscient God (who is never wrong). Two boxes, X and Y, are presented to a human being, one (X) containing $1,000, the other (Y) containing either $1,000,000 or nothing. The human being may choose either both boxes (X & Y), outcome a, or box Y, outcome b. If God predicts a, then box Y contains nothing (and the reward is the $1,000 in box X). If God predicts b, then X still contains $1,000 but box Y contains $1,000,000 (and the reward is the $1,000,000 in box Y).

Argument 1: Remember, God is never wrong. If a, then the payoff of the choice is $1,000 (for God would have predicted the choice). If b, then the payoff is $1,000,000 (on God's prediction). Since $M > $T, then b > a.

Argument 2: Either the $M is in box Y or it is not. If it is there, then the payoff of a is $M + $T, the payoff of b is $M. If it is not there, then the payoff of a is $T, of b is zero. Since a = [(M + T)v T] and b = (M v O), then a > b.

Embellishment for argument 2: Imagine an observer (human) who is behind both boxes and the boxes are transparent. He sees that the $M is either there or it is not. If he were trying to maximize the interests of the chooser, he would always urge a > b.

Reminder for argument 1: If the outcome is a, then there is no $M under the terms of the paradox. For a > b, God would have to be wrong.

The paradox is often used to demonstrate a logical inconsistency between two decision rules; for the rule of dominance requires a choice of b > a, and a rule maximizing expected value requires a > b (urged by the human observer, since the average payoff of both alternative outcomes in a is greater than the average of alternatives in b). But this conflict is misleading, for both dominance and utility coincide when the human perspective is controlling. It is God's perspective that allows b to dominate a. For example, in the payoff matrix

	a	b
a	1	1 + M
b	0	M

the only outcomes on an acceptance of God' omniscience are a = 1, b = M (or cells {a,a} vs. {b,b}). A dominance criterion requires b > a. But if all four cells are introduced as possible outcomes (on the human observer's perspective, and ignoring God's predictions), then both dominance and expected utility require a > b. On dominance, since 1 > 0 and (1 + M) > M, then a > b. On utility, since a = p(1 + M) + (1 − p) = pM + 1, and b = pM, then a > b. But these calculations do not express Newcomb's problem. They ignore God by opening up the Newcomb-restricted two-place matrix to four outcomes. In Newcomb's problem, $pa(1 + M) \approx 0$ and $pbM \approx 1$. So, again, $b > a$ because $\{a,b\}$ and $\{b,a\}$ are not possible. The tension is between the human perspective and God's predictions, not the decision rules as such.

Newcomb's problem occurs as one shifts between temporal and fixed, partial and holistic, perspectives. God "sees" (not "predicts") the choice as part of a tableau, a scene frozen in time. The experience of the human actor is sequential, a series of actions (deliberations, choices, outcomes) occurring longitudinally across time. God perceives the whole, with knowledge of what from the human perspective is past, present, future. The human actor chooses in uncertainty, a player in a movie (not a snapshot) who does not grasp all of the details. The observer (in the embellishment for argument 2) is a hybrid god, occupying a place between God and human actor.

Viewed in this way, Newcomb's problem is a paradox created by the joining of two different and contrary perspectives on being—omniscience (which collapses time and sees holistically) and that temporal, partial knowledge on which linear reasoning succeeds. The conflict exposed by the paradox is between external and internal realities. The limitations on linear reasoning occur when "human" calculations are extended to the "God" domain in the problem. The alternative reality fixed by God's omniscience requires a holistic seeing of reality rather than a set of sequential calculations. This distinction between domains of the real, and between internal and external reasoning, elaborates spiritual beliefs in realities that can be distinguished from each other.

Newcomb's problem (as noted earlier) was invented by a physicist, Dr. William Newcomb, and exploited (benignly) by Robert Nozick to show a conflict between the two decision rules; see Nozick, "Newcomb's Problem and Two Principles of Choice," in Nicholas Rescher, ed., *Essays in Honor of Carl G. Hempel*. Most of the literature that interprets Newcomb's problem as a game-theoretic problem assimilates it to versions of the prisoners' dilemma, in which the constancy or reliability of God's predictions are introduced to the human player's calculations. See, for example, Steven J. Brams, "Newcomb's Problem and Prisoners' Dilemma," and David Lewis, "Prisoners' Dilemma Is a Newcomb Problem," though Brams is the more sophisticated in his consideration of "decision-theoretic" dimensions of Newcomb's problem that pay proper respect to the deity's omniscience. I am grateful to this literature, and to David Austen-Smith (in a private communication), for whatever clarity this note has, and for suggestions (not always followed) on the game-theoretic matrix and equations to illustrate the problem.

Pages 281–82   This section on the brain is drawn from the overview of research provided by Israel Rosenfield in *The Invention of Memory*. See also Gerald M. Edelman, *Neural Darwinism*.

Pages 285–86   This quote is from a letter sent to the author in March 1990 by a woman who is having spontaneous out-of-body experiences.

Pages 286–87   Quote from interview on June 21, 1990. The complex structure of the brain helps to explain a variety of experiences that are unusual in one way or another, though no account of neurological functions can address the validity of claims for the supernatural.

REFERENCES

The items listed here do not amount to a full bibliography. Except for a few vital additions, they are no more than the full citations for the works entered (and often discussed) in the Notes. Other than the interview material, they are my main resources for this book in the sense that they guide my thinking and provide information used in the text. But I have read considerably more than these materials in my research. So let this list function as a kind of Hemingway short story or Pinter play, one where a minimal linguistic entry can summon from the reader a more complete account. In this way we will avoid a bibliography as long as the Notes.

The risk in referential minimalism is that the author may leave out something that informs what he has written. I believe I have listed here all of the materials directly used in this book. If this belief is false, if I have relied on sources without citation, I apologize to the omitted authors.

Ackerman, Bruce. *Social Justice in the Liberal State*. New Haven, Conn.: Yale University Press, 1980.

Alker, Hayward R., Jr., Wendy G. Lehnert, and Daniel K. Schneider. "Two Reinterpretations of Toynbee's Jesus: Explorations in Computational Hermeneutics." In *Artificial Intelligence and Text Understanding*, ed. Tomfoni Garziella, 49–94. Ricerca Linguistica G. Parma: Ediziora Zara, 1985.

Aquinas, Thomas. *Summa contra Gentiles*. Notre Dame, Ind.: Notre Dame University Press, 1970.

———. *Summa theologica*. New York: Bengign, 1948.

Arrow, Kenneth. *Individual Choice and Social Values*. New York: John Wiley, 1951.

Augustine. *City of God*. Abr. and trans. J. W. C. Wand. London: Oxford University Press, 1963.

Bachrach, Peter. *Political Elites in a Democracy*. New York: Atherton, 1971.

————. *The Theory of Democratic Elitism.* Boston: Little, Brown, 1967.

Baldwin, James. *The Fire Next Time.* New York: Dell, 1963.

Baldwin, Robert. *The Healers.* Huntington, Ind.: Our Sunday Visitor Publishing Division, 1986.

Barker, J. C. "Premonitions of the Aberfan Disaster." *Journal of the Society for Psychical Research* 44 (1967): 169–81.

Barry, Brian, ed. *Power and Political Theory: Some European Perspectives.* New York: John Wiley, 1976.

Battin, Margaret P. *Ethics in the Sanctuary: Examining the Practices of Organized Religion.* New Haven, Conn.: Yale University Press, 1990.

Berlin, Isaiah. *Two Concepts of Liberty.* Oxford: Clarendon Press, 1958.

Bigongiari, Dino. *The Political Ideas of St. Thomas Aquinas.* New York: Hafner, 1953.

Bodgan, Janet Carlisle. "What Difference Did Doctors Make? Physicians and Childbirth in Nineteenth-Century New York City." Paper presented to the Syracuse Consortium for the Cultural Foundations of Medicine Faculty Seminar, 7 March 1988.

Bohm, David. *Wholeness and the Implicate Order.* London: Routledge & Kegan Paul, 1980.

Boorse, Christopher. "On the Distinction Between Disease and Illness." *Philosophy and Public Affairs* 5 (Fall 1975): 49–68.

Brams, Steven J. "Newcomb's Problem and Prisoners' Dilemma." *Journal of Conflict Resolution* 19 (December 1975): 596–612.

Brock, Dan. "Recent Work in Utilitarianism." *American Philosophical Quarterly* 10 (October 1973): 241–76.

Brown, Stephanie. *Treating the Alcoholic.* New York: John Wiley, 1985.

Burgess, Stanley M., and Gary McGee, eds.; Patrick H. Alexander, assoc. ed. *Dictionary of Pentecostal and Charismatic Movements.* Grand Rapids, Mich.: Regency Reference Library, 1988.

Cantwell v. Connecticut 310 U.S. 296 (1940).

Caplan, Arthur A., Tristam H. Engelhardt, Jr., and James J. McCartney, eds. *The Concepts of Health and Disease: Interdisciplinary Perspectives.* Reading, Mass.: Addision-Wesley, 1981.

Champlin, Joseph. *Healing in the Catholic Church.* Huntington, Ind.: Our Sunday Visitor, 1985.

Christian Science: A Sourcebook of Contemporary Materials. Boston: Christian Science Publishing Society, 1990.

Clarke, Edwin, ed. *Modern Methods in the History of Medicine.* London: Athlone, 1971.

Cogan, Morris L. "Toward a Definition of a Profession." *Harvard Educational Review* 23 (Winter 1953): 33–50.

Collins, Randall. *The Credentialing Society.* New York: Academic Press, 1979.

Conte, John, and Steven L. Barriere. *Manual of Antibiotics and Infectious Diseases*. Philadelphia: Lea & Febiger, 1988.

Copleston, Frederick. *History of Philosophy*. Vols. 2 and 3. Westminster, Md.: Newman Press, 1963, 1962.

Cord, Robert L., and Howard Ball. "The Separation of Church and State: A Debate." *Utah Law Review* 1987, no. 4 (1987): 895–925.

Cornford, F. M. *Before and After Socrates*. Cambridge: Cambridge University Press, 1978.

Corum, Fred T. *Like As of Fire*. Wilmington, Mass.: Fred T. Corum, 1981.

Dahl, Robert. "The Concept of Power." *Behavioral Science* 2 (July 1957): 201–15.

———. "Power." In *International Encyclopedia of the Social Sciences* 12, ed. David L. Sills, 405–14. New York: Macmillan, 1968.

———. *Who Governs?: Democracy and Power in an American City*. New Haven, Conn.: Yale University Press, 1961.

Daly, Robert. "A Theory of Madness." *Psychiatry* 54, no. 4 (November 1991), 368–85.

Davis, Henry. "Boy Caught in Medical Tug-of-War." *Syracuse Herald Journal*, 4 November 1987.

———. "Judge Rules Against Parents Who Want to Stop Child's Chemotherapy." *Syracuse Herald Journal*, 26 May 1988.

Davis, John D. *Phrenology: Fad and Science; A Nineteenth-Century American Crusade*. New Haven, Conn.: Yale University Press, 1955.

Davis, P. C. W., and J. R. Brown, eds. *The Ghost in the Atom*. Cambridge: Cambridge University Press, 1986.

Davis, Rex. *Locusts and Wild Honey*. Geneva: World Council of Churches, 1978.

Dayton, Donald W. *Theological Roots of Pentecostalism*. Metuchen, N.J.: Scarecrow Press, 1987.

Delgado, Richard. "Cults and Conversion: The Case for Informed Consent." *Georgia Law Review* 16 (January 1982): 533–74.

———. "When Religious Exercise Is Not Free: Deprogramming and the Constitutional Status of Coercively Induced Belief." *Vanderbilt Law Review* 37 (1984): 107–115.

Dennett, Daniel C. "Where Am I?" In Dennett, *Brainstorms: Philosophical Essays on Mind and Psychology*. Montgomery, Vt.: Bradford Books, 1978.

Descartes, René. *Meditations on First Philosophy*. Cambridge: Cambridge University Press, 1986.

"Developments in the Law—Medical Technology and the Law." *Harvard Law Review* 103 (May 1990): 1520–676.

"Developments in the Law: Religion and State." *Harvard Law Review* 100 (May 1987): 1606–781.

Dodds, E. R. *The Greeks and the Irrational*. Berkeley: University of California Press, 1951.

Dworkin, Gerald. "Paternalism." *The Monist* 56 (January 1972): 64–84.

Dworkin, Ronald. "Liberalism." In *Public and Private Morality*, ed. Stuart Hampshire, 113–43. Cambridge: Cambridge University Press, 1978.

———. *Taking Rights Seriously*. Cambridge, Mass.: Harvard University Press, 1978.

Eddy, Mary Baker. *Science and Health with Key to the Scriptures*. Boston: First Church of Christ, Scientist, 1971.

Edelman, Gerald M. *Neural Darwinism*. New York: Basic Books, 1987.

Elster, Jon, ed. *The Multiple Self*. Cambridge: Cambridge University Press, 1986.

Engel, George L. "Homeostasis, Behavioral Adjustment and the Concept of Health and Disease." *Mid-Century Psychiatry*, ed. R. Grinker, 33–46. Springfield, Ill.: Charles C. Thomas, 1963.

Esbeck, Carl H. "Five Views of Church-State Relations in Contemporary American Thought." *Brigham Young University Law Review* 1986, no. 2 (1986), 371–404.

Fanon, Frantz. *Black Skin, White Masks*. Trans. Charles Lam Markmann. New York: Grove Press, 1968.

———. *The Wretched of the Earth*. trans. Constance Farrington. New York: Grove Press, 1965.

Flathman, Richard. *Toward a Liberalism*. Ithaca, N.Y.: Cornell University Press, 1989.

Forest Hills Early Learning Center, Inc., et al. v. Jackson, Director, Department of Social Services of Virginia, et al. 488 U.S. 1029 (1989).

Foucault, Michel. *The Birth of the Clinic*. Trans. A. M. Sheridan Smith. New York: Vintage Books, 1975.

———. *The Order of Things: An Archeology of the Human Sciences*. Trans. pub. New York: Pantheon, 1971.

Frawley, P. Joseph. "Neurobehavioral Model of Addiction." *Journal of Drug Issues* 17 (Winter/Spring 1987): 28–46.

Freedman, Benjamin. "A Meta-Ethics for Professional Morality." *Ethics* 89 (October 1978): 1–19.

Freidson, Eliot. *Profession of Medicine: A Study of the Sociology of Acquired Knowledge*. New York: Harper & Row, 1970.

———. *Professional Dominance: The Social Structure of Medical Care*. New York: Atherton Press, 1970.

Frohock, Fred M. *Abortion: A Case Study in Law and Morals*. Westport, Conn.: Greenwood Press, 1983.

———. "Liberal Maps of Consent." *Polity* 22 (Winter 1989): 231–52.

Galston, William. *Liberal Purposes: Goods, Virtues, and Diversity in the Liberal State*. Cambridge: Cambridge University Press, 1991.

García Márquez, Gabriel. *Love in the Time of Cholera*. Trans. Edith Grossman. New York: Knopf, 1988.

Gellner, Ernest. *Cause and Meaning in the Social Sciences.* Boston, Mass.: Routledge & Kegan Paul, 1973.

———. *Relativism and the Social Sciences.* Cambridge: Cambridge University Press, 1985.

Gewirth, Alan. *Reason and Morality.* Chicago: University of Chicago Press, 1978.

Goldman, Alan. *The Moral Foundations of Professional Ethics.* Totowa, N.J.: Littlefield, 1980, esp. Introduction.

Goodin, Robert E., and Andrew Reeve, eds. *Liberal Neutrality.* London and New York: Routledge, Chapman & Hall, 1990.

Goodman, Nelson. *Fact, Fiction, and Forecast.* Indianapolis: Bobbs-Merrill, 1965.

Grad, B. "Some Biological Effects of the Laying-on of Hands: A Review of Experiments with Animals and Plants." *Journal of the American Society for Psychical Research* 59 (1965): 95–127.

Gray, John. *Liberalisms: Essays in Political Philosophy.* London: Routledge, Chapman & Hall, 1989.

Greeley, Anthony. *The Sociology of the Paranormal: A Reconnaissance.* Beverly Hills, Calif.: Sage Publications, 1975.

Gregory, Richard L., ed. *The Oxford Companion to the Mind.* New York: Oxford University Press, 1987.

Gross, Hyman. "Privacy and Autonomy." In *Nomos xiii, Privacy,* eds. John Chapman and J. Roland Pennock, 169–82. New York: Lieber-Atherton, 1971.

Guthrie, W. K. C. *The Greek Philosophers.* New York: Harper & Row, 1960.

Hall, Thomas. *A History of General Physiology.* Chicago: University of Chicago Press, 1969.

Hampshire, Stuart. *Morality and Conflict.* Cambridge, Mass.: Harvard University Press, 1983.

Hansen, Emmanuel. *Frantz Fanon: Social and Political Thought.* Columbus: Ohio State University Press, 1976.

Hare, R. M. *Freedom and Reason.* Oxford: Clarendon Press, 1963.

———. *The Language of Morals.* Oxford: Clarendon Press, 1952.

———. *Moral Thinking.* Oxford: Clarendon Press, 1981.

Heidel, William Arthur. *The Heroic Age of Science: The Conception, Ideals, and Methods of Science among the Ancient Greeks.* Baltimore: Williams and Wilkins, 1933.

Hesiod. *Theogony.* Trans. Norman O. Brown. New York: Liberal Arts, 1953.

Heller, Mark. "Temporal Parts of Four Dimensional Objects." *Philosophical Studies* 46 (November 1984): 323–34.

Hempel, Carl. *Aspects of Scientific Explanation.* New York: Free Press, 1965.

———. *Philosophy of Natural Science.* Englewood Cliffs, N.J.: Prentice-Hall, 1966.

Hempel, Carl, and Paul Oppenheimer. "The Covering Law Analysis of Scientific Explanation." *Philosophy of Science* 15 (1948): 135–74.

Herbert, Nick. *Quantum Reality*. Garden City, N.Y.: Anchor Press/Doubleday, 1985.

Higham, John. *History*. Englewood Cliffs, N.J.: Prentice-Hall, 1965.

Hobbes, Thomas. *Leviathan*. Indianapolis: Liberal Arts, 1958.

Hofstadter, Douglas. *Gödel, Escher, Bach*. New York: Basic Books, 1979.

———, and Daniel C. Dennett, eds. *The Mind's I*. New York: Basic Books, 1981.

Hollenweger, Walter. *The Pentecostals*. Minneapolis: Augsburg, 1972.

Homer. *Odyssey*. Trans. Walter Shewing. New York: Oxford University Press, 1980.

Hume, David. "Of the Original Contract." In *David Hume's Political Essays*, ed. Charles Handel, 43–63. New York: Liberal Arts, 1953.

Hundert, Edward M. *Philosophy, Psychiatry, and Neuroscience*. Oxford: Clarendon Press, 1989.

In the Matter of Caleb Loverro N-774 (1987).

In the Matter of Hofbauer 47 NY2d 648 (1979).

James, William. *Varieties of Religious Experience*. New York: Modern Library, 1929.

Jehovah's Witnesses in the State of Washington v. King Country Hospital Unit 1 (Harborview) 390 U.S. 598 (1967).

John of Paris. *Tractatus de potestate regia et papali*. Discussed by George Sabine, *A History of Political Theory*, 280–86. New York: Henry Holt, 1955.

Kakar, Sudhir. *Shamans, Mystics and Doctors*. New York: Knopf, 1982.

Kass, Leon. "Regarding the End of Medicine and the Pursuit of Health." *The Public Interest* 40 (Summer 1975): 11–42.

Kaufman, Martin. *Homeopathy in America*. Baltimore: Johns Hopkins University Press, 1971.

Kee, Howard Clark. *Medicine, Miracle and Magic in the New Testament*. Cambridge: Cambridge University Press, 1986.

———. *Miracle in the Early Christian World*. New Haven, Conn.: Yale University Press, 1983.

Kelman, Mark. *A Guide to Critical Legal Studies*. Cambridge, Mass.: Harvard University Press, 1987.

Kelsey, Morton. *Psychology, Medicine and Christian Healing*. San Francisco: Harper & Row, 1973.

Kenny, Anthony. *Descartes: A Study of His Philosophy*. New York: Random House, 1968.

Kessel, Joseph. *The Road Back*. New York: Knopf, 1962.

Kett, Joseph. *The Formation of the American Medical Profession*. New Haven, Conn.: Yale University Press, 1968.

King, Lester. *Growth of Medical Thought*. Chicago: University of Chicago Press, 1963.

————. *Medical Thinking*. Princeton, N.J.: Princeton University Press, 1982.

Krieger, Dolores. "The Relationship of Touch with the Intent to Help or to Heal, to Subjects in Vivo Hemoglobin Values: A Study in Personalized Interaction." In *Proceedings of the Ninth American Nurses Association Research Conference*, 39–58. New York: American Nurses Association, 1974.

————. *The Therapeutic Touch*. New York: Prentice-Hall, 1986.

————. "Therapeutic Thouch: The Imprimature of Nursing." *American Journal of Nursing* 75 (1975): 784–87.

Kriesberg, Louis, Terrell A. Northrup, and Stuart J. Thompson, eds. *Intractable Conflicts and Their Transformation*. Syracuse, N.Y.: Syracuse University Press, 1989.

Kripke, Saul. *Wittgenstein on Rules and Private Language*. Cambridge, Mass.: Harvard University Press, 1982.

Kuhn, Thomas. *The Structure of Scientific Revolutions*. Chicago: University of Chicago Press, 1962.

Kunz, Dora, and Erik Peper. "Fields and Their Clinical Implications." In *Spiritual Aspects of the Healing Arts*, ed. Kunz, 213–61. Wheaton, Ill.: Theosophy Publishing House, 1985.

Kurtz, Ernest. *AA: The Story*. San Francisco: Harper & Row, 1988.

Lehnert, Wendy G., and Cynthia Loiselle. "Plot Units and Narrative Summarizations." In *Semantic Structures: Advances in Natural Language Processing*, ed. David A. Waltz, 125–65. Hillsdale, N.J.: Erlbaum, 1989.

LeShan, Lawrence. *Cancer as a Turning Point*. New York: Dutton, 1989.

————. *The Mechanic and the Gardner: How to Use the Holistic Revolution in Medicine*. New York: Holt, Rinehart & Winston, 1982.

————. *The Medium, the Mystic, and the Physicist*. New York: Viking, 1975.

Levinson, Daniel J., et al. *The Seasons of a Man's Life*. New York: Ballantine, 1978.

Lewis, David. "Prisoners' Dilemma Is a Newcomb's Problem." *Philosophy and Public Affairs* 8 (Spring 1979): 235–40.

Lightman, Alan, and Roberta Brawer. *Origins: The Lives and Worlds of Modern Cosmologists*. Cambridge, Mass.: Harvard University Press, 1990.

Luker, Kristin. *Abortion and the Politics of Motherhood*. Berkeley: University of California Press, 1984.

Lukes, Steven. *Power: A Radical View*. London: Macmillan, 1974.

MacCallum, Gerald C. "Negative and Positive Freedom." *Philosophical Review* 76 (1967): 312–34.

Machiavelli, Niccolò. *The Prince*. Trans. and ed. Robert M. Adams. New York: Norton, 1977.

MacIntyre, Alasdair. *After Virtue*. Notre Dame, Ind.: Notre Dame University Press, 1981.

————. "The Idea of a Social Science." In *Rationality*, ed. B. R. Wilson, 112–30. Oxford: Basil Blackwell, 1970.

————. "Is Understanding Religion Compatible with Believing?" In *Rationality*, ed. Wilson, 62–77.

————. *Whose Justice? Which Rationality?*. Notre Dame, Ind.: Notre Dame University Press, 1988.

Macrae, Janet. *Therapeutic Touch: A Practical Guide*. New York: Knopf, 1988.

Malony, H. Newton, and A. Adams Lovekin. *Glossolalia: Behavioral Science Perspectives on Speaking in Tongues*. New York: Oxford University Press, 1985.

Mannheim, Karl. *Ideology and Utopia*. New York: Harcourt, Brace, 1936.

Margolis, Joseph. "The Concept of Disease." *Journal of Medicine and Philosophy* 1 (1976): 238–55.

Marsilius of Padua. *Defensor pacis*. Trans. and ed. C. W. Previte-Orton. Cambridge: Cambridge University Press, 1928.

Marty, Martin E. *A Nation of Believers*. Chicago: University of Chicago Press, 1976.

Marty, Martin E., and Kenneth E. Vaux, eds. *Health/Medicine and the Faith Traditions*. Philadelphia: Fortress Press, 1982.

Maxwell, Milton. *The Alcoholics Anonymous Experience*. New York: McGraw-Hill, 1984.

May, William. "The Physician's Covenant." Chapter 4 of May, *The Physician's Covenant*. Philadelphia: Westminster Press, 1983.

McConnell, Michael W. "The Origins and Historical Understanding of Free Exercise of Religion." *Harvard Law Review* 103 (May 1990): 1409–517.

McCoy, Thomas R., and Gary A. Kurtz. "A Unifying Theory for the Religion Clauses of the First Amendment." *Vanderbilt Law Review* 39 (March 1986): 249–74.

McCulloch, Jock. *Black Soul, White Artifact: Fanon's Clinical Psychology and Social Theory*. Cambridge: Cambridge University Press, 1983.

Mead, George Herbert. *Mind, Self and Society*. Chicago: University of Chicago Press, 1934.

Meck, George W., ed. *Healers and the Healing Process*. Wheaton, Ill.: Theosophy Publishing House, 1977.

"Medicine." *The New Encyclopaedia Britannica* 23:884–939.

Mill, John Stuart. *On Liberty*. Ed. David Spitz. New York: Norton, 1975.

Mills, Watson E., ed. *Speaking in Tongues*. Grand Rapids, Mich.: W. B. Erdmans, 1986.

Moore, R. Lawrence. *In Search of White Crows*. London: Oxford University Press, 1977.

Nagel, Ernest. *The Structure of Science*. New York: Harcourt, Brace & World, 1961.

Nagel, Thomas. *The View From Nowhere*. London: Oxford University Press, 1986.

————. "What Is It Like to be a Bat?" *Philosophical Review* 83 (October 1974): 435–50.

Nelson, Benjamin. *On the Roads to Modernity*. Totowa, N.J.: Rowman & Littlefield, 1981.

Newton-Smith, W. H. *The Rationality of Science*. Boston: Routledge & Kegan Paul, 1981.

Nietzsche, Friedrich. *The Will to Power*. London: Weidenfield & Nicolson, 1968.

Notman, M. T., et al. "Psychotherapy with the Substance-Dependent Physician." *American Journal of Psychotherapy* 41 (April 1987): 220–30.

Novit, Bette. "Contradictory Demands on the First Amendment Religion Clauses: Having It Both Ways." *Journal of Church and State* 30 (Autumn 1988): 463–91.

Nozick, Robert. *Anarchy, State, and Utopia*. New York: Basic Books, 1974.

———. "Newcomb's Problem and Two Principles of Choice." In *Essays in Honor of Carl G. Hempel*, ed. Nicholas Rescher, 114–46. Dordrecht: D. Reidel, 1969.

Oakeshott, Michael. *Experiednce and Its Modes*. London: Cambridge University Press, 1933.

Osler, William. *The Evolution of Modern Medicine*. New Haven, Conn.: Yale University Press, 1921.

Parfit, Derek. *Reasons and Persons*. Oxford: Clarendon Press, 1984.

Peel, Robert. *Health and Medicine in the Christian Science Tradition*. New York: Crossroad, 1988.

Penfield, Wilder. *The Mystery of the Mind*. Princeton, N.J.: Princeton University Press, 1975.

Penrose, K. S., and R. Penrose. "Impossible Objects: A Special Type of Illusion." *British Journal of Psychology* 49 (1958): 31.

Perrin, Norman, and Dennis Duling. *The New Testament: An Introduction*. New York: Harcourt, Brace, Jovanovich, 1982.

Perry, Barbara. "Justice Hugo Black and the 'Wall of Separation Between Church and State.'" *Journal of Church and State* 31 (Winter 1989): 55–72.

Perry, John. *A Dialogue on Personal Identity and Immortality*. Indianapolis: Hackett, 1978.

Pirandello, Luigi. *Henry the Fourth*. Trans. Robert David MacDonald. London: Oberon Books, 1990.

Plato. *Phaedo*. Trans. Hugh Tredennick. In *Plato: The Last Days of Socrates*, ed. Tredennick. Baltimore: Penguin Books, 1961.

———. *Republic*. Trans. Allan Bloom. New York: Basic Books, 1968.

———. *Theaetetus*. Trans. F. M. Cornford. In *Plato's Theory of Knowledge*, ed. Cornford. London: Kegan Paul, 1935.

Poloma, Margaret. *The Charismatic Movement*. Boston: Twayne, 1982.

Popper, Karl. *Conjectures and Refutations*. New York: Basic Books, 1965.

———. *The Logic of Scientific Discovery*. London: Hutchinson Publishing Group, 1968.

Powell, Lyman. *Christian Science: The Faith and Its Founders*. New York: G. P. Putnam's, 1917.

"Psychiatry." *Encyclopedia Americana* 22 (1988): 717–19.

"Psychiatry." *Collier's Encyclopedia* 19 (1979): 447–50.

Quebedeaux, Richard. *The New Charismatics*. San Francisco: Harper & Row, 1983.

Quine, W. V. O. "Two Dogmas of Empiricism." In Quine, *From a Logical Point of View*, 20–46. Cambridge, Mass.: Harvard University Press, 1964.

———. *Word and Object*. Cambridge, Mass.: MIT Press, 1960.

Rachels, James. "Why Privacy Is Important." *Philosophy and Public Affairs* 4 (Summer 1975): 323–33.

Rae, Douglas. *Equalities*. Cambridge, Mass.: Harvard University Press, 1981.

Rawls, John. *A Theory of Justice*. Cambridge, Mass.: Harvard University Press, 1971.

———. "The Priority of Right Ideas of the Good." *Philosophy and Public Affairs* 17 (Fall 1988): 251–76.

"Reinterpreting the Religion Clauses: Constitutional Construction and Conceptions of the Self." *Harvard Law Review* 97 (April 1984): 1468–86.

Riche, Martha Farnsworth. "Beyond the Boom in Mental Health Care." *American Demographics* 9 (November 1987): 35–61.

Riker, William. *Liberalism Against Populism*. San Francisco: W. H. Freeman, 1982.

Riker, William, and Peter Ordeshook. *An Introduction to Positive Political Theory*. Englewood Cliffs, N.J.: Prentice-Hall, 1973.

Rorty, Richard. *Philosophy and the Mirror of Nature*. Princeton, N.J.: Princeton University Press, 1980.

Rosenberg, Charles. *No Other Gods*. Baltimore: Johns Hopkins University Press, 1976.

Rosenblum, Nancy, ed. *Liberalism and the Moral Life*. Cambridge, Mass.: Harvard University Press, 1989.

Rosenfield, Israel. *The Invention of Memory*. New York: Basic Books, 1988.

Rothstein, William G. *American Physicians in the Nineteenth Century*. Baltimore: Johns Hopkins University Press, 1972.

Rousseau, Jean-Jacques. *The Social Contract*. Trans. G. O. H. Cole. New York: Dutton, 1950.

Ryle, Gilbert. *The Concept of Mind*. Oxford University Press, 1949.

Sacks, Oliver. *The Man Who Mistook His Wife for a Hat*. New York: Summit Books, 1985.

Sandel, Michael. *Liberalism and the Limits of Justice*. Cambridge: Cambridge University Press, 1982.

———. "Religious Liberty—Freedom of Conscience or Freedom of Choice?" *Utah Law Review* 1989, no. 3 (1989): 597–615.

Sartre, Jean-Paul. *Being and Nothingness*. Trans. Hazel E. Barnes. New York: Philosophical Library, 1956.

Sen, Amartya, and Bernard Williams, eds. *Utilitarianism and Beyond*. Cambridge: Cambridge University Press, 1982.

Shainberg, Lawrence. "Finding the 'Zone.'" *New York Times Magazine*, 9 April 1989, 35–39.

Sherrill, Kimberly A., and David B. Larson. "Adult Burn Patients: The Role of Religion in Recovery." *Southern Medical Journal* 81 (July 1988): 21–25.

Shiloh True Light Church of Christ v. Brock 670 F. Supp. 158 W.D.N.C. (1987).

Siegel, Shepard, Marvin D. Frank, and Riley E. Hinson. "Anticipation of Pharmacological and Nonpharmacological Events: Classical Conditioning and Addictive Behavior." *Journal of Drug Issues* 17 (Winter/Spring 1987): 83–110.

Simon, Herbert. *Models of Bounded Rationality*. Cambridge, Mass.: MIT Press, 1982.

Simpson, William Frank. "Comparative Longevity in a College Cohort of Christian Scientists." *Journal of the American Medical Association* 262 (1989): 1657–58.

Skrabaneh, P. "Paranormal Health Claims." *Experientia* 44 (1988): 303–9.

Smith, M. J. "Paranormal Effects on Enzyme Activity." *Human Dimensions* 1 (1972): 15–19.

Smith, Morton. *Jesus the Magician*. San Francisco: Harper & Row, 1978.

Sontag, Susan. *Illness as Metaphor*. New York: Farrar, Straus & Giroux, 1978.

Spilka, B., R. W. Hood, and R. L. Gorsuch. *The Psychology of Religion: An Empirical Approach*. Englewood Cliffs, N.J.: Prentice-Hall, 1985.

Stalker, Douglas, and Clark Glymour. "Quantum Medicine." In *Examining Holistic Medicine*, ed. Stalker and Glymour, 107–25. Buffalo, N.Y.: Prometheus Books, 1989.

Starr, Paul. *The Social Transformation of American Medicine*, New York: Basic Books, 1982.

State Department of Human Services v. Larry T. Hamilton. Tenn App, 657 SW2d 425 (1983).

State Department of Human Services v. Mary C. Northern. Tenn App, 563 SW2d 197 (1978).

Stein, H. F. *Content and Dynamics in Clinical Knowledge*. Charlottesville: University Press of Virginia, 1988.

Stevenson, I. "A Review and Analysis of Paranormal Experiences Connected with the Sinking of the *Titanic*." *Journal of the American Society for Psychical Research* 54 (1960): 153–71.

Stocker, Michael. *Plural and Conflicting Values*. New York: Oxford University Press, 1990.

Taylor, Charles. "Neutrality in Political Science." In *Philosophy, Politics and So-*

ciety, 3d ser., ed. Peter Laslett and William Runciman, 25–57. Oxford: Basil Blackwell, 1967.

———. *Sources of the Self: The Making of the Modern Identity.* Cambridge, Mass.: Harvard University Press, 1989.

Temkin, Owsei. "Health and Disease." In *Dictionary of the History of Ideas*, vol. 2, ed. Philip Wiener, 395–407. New York: Charles Scribner's Sons, 1973.

———. "The Scientific Approach to Disease." In *Historical Studies in the Intellectual, Social and Technical Conditions for Scientific Discovery and Technical Invention from Antiquity to the Present*, ed. A. C. Crombie, 629–41. New York: Basic Books, 1963.

Thompson, Judith Jarvis. "The Right to Privacy." *Philosophy and Public Affairs* 4 (Summer 1975): 295–314.

Tooley, Michael. "Abortion and Infanticide." *Philosophy and Public Affairs* 1 (Fall 1972): 37–65.

Unger, Roberto M. *The Critical Legal Studies Movement.* Cambridge, Mass.: Harvard, 1986.

Van de Castle, Robert L. "Sleep and Dreams." In *Handbooks of Parapsychology*, ed. Benjamin B. Wolman, 473–99. New York: Van Nostrand Reinhold, 1977.

Vermes, Geza. *Jesus the Jew.* London: Collins, 1976.

Walzer, Michael. *Spheres of Justice: A Defense of Pluralism and Equality.* New York: Basic Books, 1983.

Whitback, Caroline. "A Theory of Health." In *Concepts of Health and Disease: Interdisciplinary Perspectives*, ed. Arthur A. Caplan, Tristam H. Engelhardt, Jr., and James J. McCartney, 611–26. Reading, Mass.: Addison–Wesley, 1981.

White, John. *When the Spirit Comes with Power.* Downers Grove, Ill.: Intervarsity Press, 1988.

Wiener, Norbert. "The Concept of Homeostasis in Medicine." *Transactions and Studies of the College of Physicians of Philadelphia* 20 (February 1953): 87–93.

Williams, Bernard. *Ethics and the Limits of Philosophy.* Cambridge, Mass.: Harvard University Press, 1986.

———. *Problems of the Self.* Cambridge: Cambridge University Press, 1973.

Winch, Peter. *The Idea of a Social Science.* New York: Humanities Press, 1958.

Wirth, Daniel P. "Unorthodox Healing: The Effect of Noncontact Therapeutic Touch on the Healing Rate of Full Thickness Dermal Wounds." *Proceedings of Presented Papers*, Parapsychological Association 32nd Annual Convention, San Diego, California, 18–20 August 1989.

Wittgenstein, Ludwig. *Philosophical Investigations.* Trans. G. E. M. Anscombe. New York: Macmillan, 1967.

———. *Remarks on Frazer's "Golden Bough."* Trans. A. C. Miles. Ed. and rev. Rush Rhees. Atlantic Highlands, N.J.: Brynmill Press, 1979.

Wodak, Ruth, ed. *Language, Power and Ideology.* Amsterdam: S. Benjamins, 1989.

Wolff, Robert Paul. *Understanding Rawls: A Reconstruction and Critique of "A Theory of Justice."* Princeton, N.J.: Princeton University Press, 1977.

Wolman, Benjamin B. *Handbook of Parapsychology.* New York: Van Nostrand Reinhold, 1977.

Young, John Harvey. *The Toadstool Millionaires.* Princeton, N.J.: Princeton University Press, 1961.

INDEX

Basil, Max, 128
Beliefs, 145, 245–46, 268, 270, 277;
    divine intervention and, 134–35;
    and healing, 41, 224; and mental
    disorders, 84–85
Bell, John, 290
Beneficence, 146, 275, 276
Bennett, Dennis, 114
Bethel Bible College, 108–9
Biofeedback, 4, 133
Birth control, 53
Black, Hugo, 143
Blavatsky, Helena Petrovna, 180
Block, Keith, 15, 19, 24, 25
Body, 29, 47, 59, 173, 297; effect on
    the mind, 190; faith healing and,
    132–33. *See also* Mind-body rela-
    tions
Body awareness, 190
Bohr, Niels, 290
Bork, Silas, 33–37
Brantley, Father Charles, 123, 125–
    28, 205, 228

Cancer, 54, 224; diet and, 236; treat-
    ment of, 15–16, 29, 54, 88, 225–
    26. *See also* Chemotherapy; Mac-
    robiotic diet
Canterbury, Irene, 128–30, 228, 278;
    attitude toward faith healing, 131–
    32
Canterbury, Thomas, 128–31, 194,
    205–6, 278; attitude toward faith
    healing, 131–32
Cantwell v. Connecticut, 307
Cardiac surgery, 56
Carington, Whately, 196
Catholicism, 2, 140, 163; healing in,
    123–28, 153–59; and Pentecostal-
    ism, 114
Causality, 213–14; disputes over, 27–
    28

Charismatic movements, 3, 108, 111;
    as extension of Pentecostalism,
    113–15; and faith healing, 114–15
Chemotherapy, 11, 14–15, 27; atti-
    tudes toward, 17–18; effects of, 18–
    19
Chicago Review, 48
Children, state regulation and, 229–
    30, 233, 265–66. *See also* Inter-
    vention: state
Chiropractic medicine, 17, 27, 234
Cholesterol, 60
Christianity, 2–3, 59, 105; faith heal-
    ing in, 114–15. *See also*
    Charismatic movements; Christian
    Science; Pentecostalism
Christian Science, 3, 4, 90, 148–53,
    160, 174, 229, 230, 233, 237,
    253–55, 267, 268, 307; dispute
    with allopathic medicine, 152, 232;
    and exemptions to the First
    Amendment, 266, 306–7; and lib-
    eral governance, 257–58, 273,
    305, 306. *See also* Clark, Joseph;
    Clark, Susan; Twitchell, David;
    Twitchell, Robyn
Church of Christ, Scientist. *See*
    Christian Science
Church of the Foursquare Gospels,
    113
Church of God, 113
Church-State relations. *See* Religious
    freedom
Clark, Celia, 259–66
Clark, Joseph, 258–62, 266, 278
Clark, Susan, 258–64, 266, 278
Cocaine, 69
Coercion. *See* Power
Cognitive disorders, 87, 89; tests of,
    87–88
College of Electors, 138
Commitment, 162

James, William, 195
Jamison, Faith, 115–19, 205, 228, 278; call to the ministry, 116–18
Jefferson, Thomas, 140, 141, 143
Jehovah's Witnesses, 145, 261
Jehovah's Witnesses in the State of Washington v. King's County Hospital Unit 1, 305–6
Jesus of Nazareth, 104–7
Jesus People movement, 120–21
John of Paris, 138
John of Salisbury, 137, 138, 140
Johnson, Duke, 126
Jung, Carl, 111

Karma, 181–82
Kaster, Gloria, 190–94, 278; meditative healing and, 192–94
Keifer, Ralph, 114
Kunz, Dora, 182
Kushi, Michio, 15

Laetrile, 225, 229
Last Temptation of Christ, The (Scorsese), 124
Law of infinitesimals, 57
Law of similia, 57
Laying on of hands, 41, 114–15, 124, 174–75, 191. *See also* Therapeutic touch
LeShan, Lawrence, 187, 191, 194–203, 222, 228, 278; and psychic healing, 197–202; study of parapsychology by, 195–97; training sessions by, 200–201. *See also* Type I healing; Type II healing
Liberal governance, 238–39, 241–42, 268, 302; arbitrariness of, 251, 305; autonomy and, 5, 248–50, 304; Christian Science and, 257–58, 305, 306; community standards and, 249–51, 272; competence and, 219–20; conflict and, 242–43;

neutrality and, 31–32; and parental authority, 219, 229–30, 233, 307–11; and privacy, 238, 248–49, 304; and religious freedom, 145–48; and welfare of children, 229–30, 233, 265–66, 305, 307–11. *See also* Governing languages; Intervention: state; State
Liberalism, 31–32, 84–85, 164, 242; dissent and, 163–64; and the individual, 87–91; neutrality and, 241, 291, 303; and state power, 248, 251
Licensure, 63, 64. *See also* Credentialing
Life support systems, 36–37, 43, 247
Lighthouse Ranch, 121
Lobotomy, 136
Locke, John, 140
Love in the Time of Cholera (Marquez), 61
Loverro, Caleb, 13–16, 19, 21, 22, 217–20, 229–33, 236, 237; state intervention for, 16, 19–21, 25–27, 309–10; treatment of, 23–27
Loverro, Gillian, 13–16, 20, 22–27, 31, 218
Loverro, Joseph, 13–23, 26–27, 31, 58, 217–18, 236; attitude toward medicine, 17–18

Machiavelli, Niccolò, 138–39, 273
Macrobiotic diet, 4, 13, 16, 25, 26, 54. *See also* Diet therapy
Madison, James, 140, 141
Madness, 80, 295. *See also* Mental disorders
Magic, 40, 193; in early medicine, 30; Jesus and, 107–8; and Type II healing, 191–92
Man Who Mistook His Wife for a Hat, The (Sacks), 61
Marquez, Gabriel Garcia, 61
Marsilius of Padua, 138, 139

Odysseus, 86–87, 295
Ohsawa, George, 54
Osler, Sir William, 79
Out-of-body experiences, 285–86

Paranormal experience. *See* Parapsychology
Parapsychology, 195, 197, 215–16. *See also* Psychic healing
Parental authority, state regulation and, 219, 229–30, 233, 307–11
Parham, Charles, 108–9
Park, Joanne, 66–67, 103, 104, 231, 278, 294; alcohol abuse by, 92–94; drug abuse by, 69–70, 91–94, 97–99; relationship with patients, 67–68; spiritual beliefs of, 101, 102; and the study of medicine, 48–52, 65–66; treatment of, 95–97, 98, 99–101
Participant observation, 186
Pascal's dilemma, 312–13
Paul VI, 114
Pediatric Oncology Group, 23
Penfield, Robert, 119–23, 205, 228, 278; views on faith healing, 123
Penicillin, 52
Penrose, Lionel, 89
Penrose, Roger, 89
Pentecostalism, 3, 90, 108–9, 111–13, 122; Catholicism and, 114; and faith healing, 114–15
Pentecostalism Holiness, 113
Pentecostal ministries, 115–19, 119–23
People's Republic of China, 83
People v. Pierson, 310
Perception, reality and, 88–89
Personality, 76, 85. *See also* Divided selves
Physicians, 55, 60, 228; conflict over healing, 227–28; and drug abuse,

70, 294. *See also* Medical professionals
Physiology, 30
Pietà (Michelangelo), 194
Placebo effect, 160, 161, 177–78, 198, 224, 225, 253
Plato, 87, 105, 164, 241, 281
Plessis, David de, 113
Pluralism, 140–42, 164, 231, 242, 273
Politics (Aristotle), 137
Power, 241, 269, 273, 290; individuals and, 270–71, 307; and morality, 268–69, 269–70; and state regulation, 239
Prayer, 4, 228, 230, 233, 253–55
Precognition, 215–16
Prince, The (Machiavelli), 138–39, 273
Privacy: competence and, 250; state governance and, 238, 248–49, 304
Psychiatrist's gaze, 82–83
Psychiatry, 76, 83–85, 87. *See also* Duncan, Paul: attitude toward psychiatry
Psychic healing, 3–4, 187–89, 191, 197–202, 238. *See also* Spiritual healing
Psychic membranes, 61
Psychoanalysis, 30, 76
Public health service, 31

Quimby, Phineas Parkhurst, 148

Ranaghan, Dorothy, 114
Ranaghan, Kevin, 114
Randi, James, 134–35
Rational discourse, 46–47, 113
Rawls, John, 303–4
Reality, 7, 47, 89–90, 145, 213–14, 267–68, 290–91; in Christian Science, 149, 152–53; competence